THE ABBEY OF BURY ST EDMUNDS

The Abbey of Bury St Edmunds
History, Legacy and Discovery

Francis Young

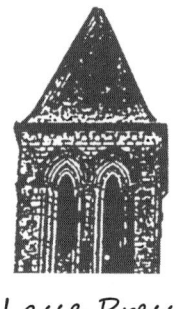

Lasse Press

Text © Francis Young
Design © Curran Publishing Services Ltd

All rights reserved. No reproduction, copy or transmission of this
publication may be made without written permission.

No portion of this publication may be reproduced, copied or transmitted
save with written permission or in accordance with the provisions of the
Copyright, Designs and Patents Act 1988, or under the terms of any licence
permitting limited copying issued by the Copyright Licensing Agency,
Saffron House, 6–10 Kirby Street, London EC1N 8TS.

Any person who does any unauthorized act in relation to this publication may be liable to criminal
prosecution and civil claims for damages.

The author has asserted his right to be identified as the author of this work in accordance with the
Copyright, Designs and Patents Act 1988.

First published 2016
by the Lasse Press
2 St Giles Terrace, Norwich NR2 1NS, UK
www.lassepress.com
lassepress@gmail.com

ISBN-13: 978-0-9933069-4-5

Typeset in Garamond by
Curran Publishing Services Ltd, Norwich, UK

Manufactured in the UK by Imprint Digital, Exeter.

For Naomi

Contents

List of illustrations	ix
Foreword by the Rt Revd Dom Stephen Ortiger OSB, Titular Abbot of Bury St Edmunds	xi
Preface	xiii
A timeline of St Edmunds Abbey	xv

Introduction   1
The site of the Abbey   3
The organisation of the Abbey   5
Town and Abbey   8
Histories of Bury St Edmunds   10

1 Origins, 869–1065   16
St Edmund   16
The community at Beodricsworth   21
The 'foundation' of the Benedictine Abbey   25
The first Abbey buildings   28
Abbot Leofstan. c. 1043–65   30

2 The Golden Age: from Baldwin to Anselm, 1065–1148   35
Abbot Baldwin and the Norman Conquest, 1065–97   35
Baldwin the physician   42
Baldwin the builder   44
Anselm, 1121–48   47
Development of the Abbey Church   50
Master Hugo   51

3 The age of Samson and the age of Magna Carta, 1148–1229   56
Ording and Hugh 1, 1148–80   56
Samson of Tottington, 1182–1211   61
The library and scriptorium   67
Samson the builder   69
Hugh of Northwold, 1215–29, and Magna Carta   70

4 A century of troubles, 1229–1329   75
Richard of the Isle to Edmund of Walpole, 1229–56   75
Simon of Luton, 1257–79   77
John of Northwold, 1279–1301   82
Thomas of Tottington, 1302–12   87

The uprising of 1327–29	87
The aftermath	92

5 Plague, revolt and fire, 1329–1469 — 94
The Abbey and the Black Death, 1348–78	94
Henry of Kirkstead and the monastic library	96
An anti-Abbot: Edmund Bromefield	96
The revolt of 1381	98
William Cratfield, 1389–1415	101
John Lydgate and William Curteys, 1429–46	104
William Babington, 1446–53	107
John Bohun, 1453–69	110

6 The final years, 1469–1539 — 114
Late medieval Abbots	115
The last Abbot: John Reeve, 1513–39	116
Dissolution, 1535–39	123

7 Legacy — 134
The aftermath of dissolution	134
The Liberty of St Edmund and the Liberty of Bury St Edmunds	136
The Archdeaconry of Bury St Edmunds	139
St Edmund's restored, 1615	142

8 Discovery — 151
John Leland and the early antiquaries	151
The seventeenth-century antiquaries: Henry Spelman, John Weever and William Dugdale	155
John Battely	161
Popular antiquarianism	162
Archaeology and imagination	166
Modern investigations	168

Appendix I: Abbots, Priors and Sacrists of the Abbey of Bury St Edmunds	173
Appendix II: A guided tour of the Abbey Church in 1465	177
Bibliography	*189*
Index	*197*

Illustrations

Figure 1	The Norman Tower today	xii
Figure 2	The Abbey Gate, engraved by George Vertue (1745)	xvii
Figure 3	The ruins of the Abbey Church today, looking east from the nave towards the east end	xviii
Figure 4	Ground plan of the Abbey Church by William Yates (1802)	2
Figure 5	Ruins of the Abbey Church, looking east (1804)	4
Figure 6	Seals of the Abbey and of individual Abbots	6
Figure 7	The Abbey precincts viewed from Angel Hill (1818)	9
Figure 8	Title page of John Battely, *Antiquitates Sancti Edmundi* (1745)	11
Figure 9	Fragmentary penny of King Eadmund	16
Figure 10	St Edmund's head	17
Figure 11	Danish memorial penny of St Edmund	19
Figure 12	The site of the Abbey viewed from the River Lark (1804)	23
Figure 13	Ancient stone heads from the Abbey	26
Figure 14	Ground plan of Abbot Baldwin's Abbey Church by Sir James Burrough (1718)	36
Figure 15	The town gates of Bury St Edmunds	43
Figure 16	One of the massive crossing piers of Baldwin's church, looking west (1804)	45
Figure 17	Abbot Anselm's Norman Tower (1804)	49
Figure 18	The west front of the Abbey Church (1804)	57
Figure 19	Penny of Henry II struck at the Bury mint	58
Figure 20	The shrine and feretory of St Edmund	63
Figure 21	Samson's Tower from the south-east (1804)	68
Figure 22	The martyrdom of St Edmund (tomb of Abbot Hugh of Northwold, Ely Cathedral)	73
Figure 23	Plan of the Abbey precincts (1893)	78
Figure 24	The Abbot's Palace, drawn by Sir James Burrough in 1720	85
Figure 25	The fortified Abbot's Bridge (1804), built to defend the Abbey precincts after the rebellion of 1327	89
Figure 26	The west front of the Abbey Gate, rebuilt after the rebellion of 1327 (1804)	93
Figure 27	The Abbey Gate from the east (1804)	97
Figure 28	Decorated era sculpture from the Abbey Gate	100
Figure 29	St Saviour's Hospital on Fornham Road (1804), site of the death of Humphrey, duke of Gloucester in 1447	108
Figure 30	The outcome of dissolution: a view of the Abbey in 1745	114
Figure 31	Gentry imitation of ecclesiastical architecture: the courtyard of Hengrave Hall (1822)	126
Figure 32	The ruins of the north transept of the Abbey Church	133
Figure 33	Samson's Tower in use as a stable (1818)	135

Figure 34	Seal of St Edmund's Abbey, Douai	143
Figure 35	The 'great axis' today: the Norman Tower from the west end of Churchgate Street	152
Figure 36	Opening page of John Battely's *Antiquitates S. Edmundi Burgi* (1745) with annotations in the hand of George Ashby	160
Figure 37	The hand of time: the Abbot's Palace in 1804 and 1720	163
Figure 38	Portrait of Richard Yates	165
Figure 39	The Abbot's Bridge today	172
Figure 40	The ruins of Abbot Baldwin's crypt today	172
Figure 41	The ruins of Abbot Samson's west front of the Abbey Church today	178
Figure 42	The ruins of Abbot Simon's Lady Chapel, looking north towards the site of the Abbot's Palace	184

Foreword

How splendid that Dr Francis Young should have written this book! The curious absence of an Alpha to Omega history of St Edmunds Abbey from its foundation in 1020 to its dissolution 1539 is now rectified, and on behalf of its readers, I offer Dr Young our sincere thanks and warmest congratulations. His labours offer us a splendidly accessible account, a helicopter view, of the 500-year history of what was a very bright star in the medieval monastic firmament, and the appearance of this volume at this juncture is particularly timely because 2020 will be the millennium of the Abbey's foundation by King Cnut in 1020. Dr Young covers the entire history of the Abbey from that date to its dissolution under Henry VIII in 1539, and he also does us the great service of describing the impact of the monastery on subsequent generations; the legacy was a significant one: witness Thomas Carlyle's depiction in 1843 of Abbot Samson of St Edmunds as a role-model of leadership. This comet has a long tail.

I declare a personal interest in Dr Young's work. I have been a Benedictine monk of Worth Abbey in Sussex for more than fifty years and, after serving as Abbot for some years, I was offered a titular abbacy, that is, the honorific title of Abbot of an ancient abbey; my happy choice was Bury St Edmunds. I have visited the Abbey several times, mainly on foot but once rather differently: I was able to fly over the ruins in a small aeroplane; I therefore resonate with 'helicopter view'. A significant difference between a ruling abbot and a titular abbot is that the latter has no trouble with his monks; mine have been quiescent since 1539. I can, and do, also take pleasure in being a successor, however tenuously, of men of the calibre of Abbot Samson: 'there were giants in the earth in those days'. Yes, indeed. I am very grateful to Dr Young for asking me to write a Foreword to this important and welcome book and I wish it every success.

+ Stephen Ortiger OSB
Titular Abbot of Bury St Edmunds

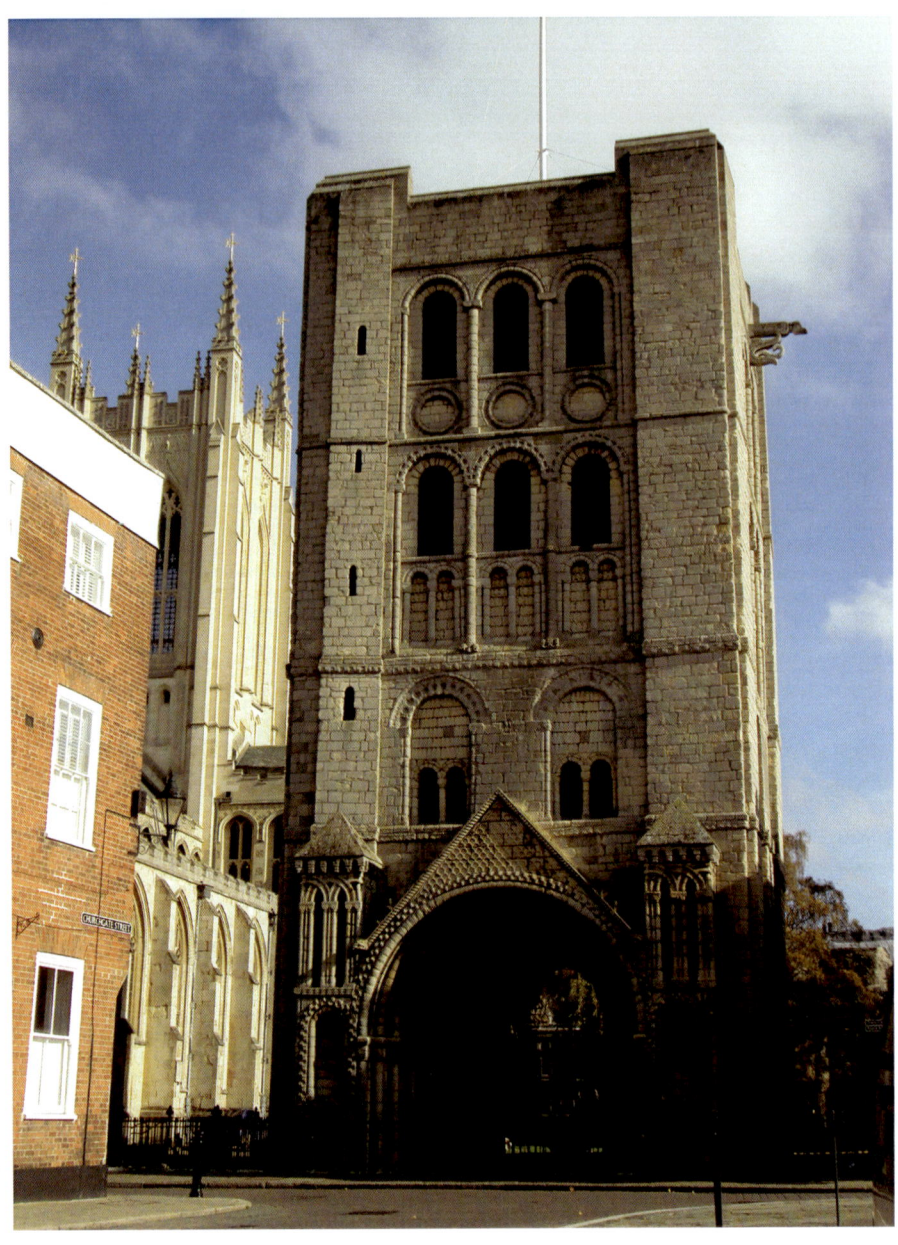

Figure 1 The Norman Tower today. Photograph by the author.

Preface

'Love of the place persuades me that, since it is my native soil, I should gather together in one heap, collected from everywhere, whatever I will be able to find written about it in edited or unedited authors.'[1] So wrote John Battely, the first historian of the Abbey of Bury St Edmunds, in around 1691. His words betray the daunting nature of the task that faced him, as virtually the first person since the dissolution to try to make sense of the scattered but plentiful records of the great medieval abbey. Fortunately, the historian of the twenty-first century is in a much more advantageous position than Battely, and I owe a great debt of gratitude to him and to all of his successors for rebuilding in print, as it were, the lost glories of St Edmunds Abbey. In writing this book I faced a different kind of challenge. Battely never completed his history, finishing in 1272, and no historian has attempted, until now, a narrative history of the Abbey from foundation to dissolution. My task has been one of synthesis, interpretation and exposition rather than discovery.

The Abbey of Bury St Edmunds: History, Legacy and Discovery is the first history of East Anglia's greatest medieval abbey from foundation to dissolution. However, I also felt it necessary to take the history of the Abbey beyond 1539, to demonstrate how the events of the distant past are still shaping the present. This is the first book to tell the story of how historians, antiquaries and archaeologists – as well as enthusiastic amateurs – steadily uncovered the truth about the Abbey's archives and its enigmatic ruins. It is intended as an introduction to the history of the Abbey and, quite deliberately, it depends on secondary sources rather than attempting a new analysis of the original documents. Recent years have seen an explosion of authoritative studies on different aspects of the history of the Abbey and the cult of St Edmund. This book does not compete with those studies, but rather brings together the findings of these scholars and makes them accessible to students of medieval and monastic history and the general reader alike.

I was fortunate to grow up surrounded by relics of Bury's monastic history. The back garden of my parents' home, located just south-east of Heyecross, one of the four crosses marking the ancient *banleuca* of Bury St Edmunds, contained fragments of medieval architectural stone: a threshold and pieces of what was probably an elaborately carved door frame, in pride of place in the rockery. These were probably stones taken from the medieval Hospital of St Peter, founded by Abbot Anselm for 'infirm brethren' in the twelfth century, and used after the dissolution as field-markers. Eventually they became ornamental features in the suburban gardens of Edwardian houses. A short walk away was the base of Heyecross itself, the so-called 'plague stone', where according to legend coins

---

1 John Battely, *Antiquitates S. Edmundi Burgi ad annum MCCLXXII perductae* (Oxford, 1745), p. 2: *Loci tamen, cum mihi sit natale solum, suadet amor, ut quaecunque de eo apud autores sive editos sive ineditos scripta invenire potero, undique collecta in unum acervum congererem.*

were dipped in vinegar before people were allowed to enter the town. My sister and I spent much time clambering over the Abbey ruins. Some of my earliest memories are associated with them, but it was many years before I began to make sense of the Abbey as a building.

As a teenager I spent hours poring over (and saving up to buy) old books about the town in the Bury Bookshop in Hatter Street, and it is fitting that the idea for this book came from a visit to another bookshop, Churchgate Books, in August 2015. A customer was shocked to discover that no history of the Abbey existed in print. Upon investigation, I too was surprised to discover that no history of the Abbey from foundation to dissolution had ever been written. Although my academic background lies in the study of Suffolk in the early modern period (c. 1500–c. 1800), I am convinced that the history of the Abbey is essential to understanding the history of Suffolk, even long after the dissolution. I therefore offer the reader a narrative history of the Abbey of Bury St Edmunds, hitherto unavailable in an accessible form, from its earliest beginnings to the dissolution – and beyond.

Following the usage established by Antonia Gransden, I refer to the Abbey throughout the text as St Edmunds or St Edmunds Abbey (without an apostrophe). St Edmund's (with an apostrophe) refers to the Benedictine monastery founded in Paris in 1615. 'The Abbey' (capitalised) always refers to St Edmunds Abbey, and 'Abbot' is likewise capitalised whenever it refers to the Abbot of St Edmunds. Occasionally I use 'Bury' as shorthand to refer to the Abbey rather than the town, but it should be clear from the context whether the town or the Abbey is being referred to.

In the majority of cases, I have modernised spelling in quotations from Middle English sources. Biblical quotations are from the Authorised Version. Translations from the Latin are my own where the original Latin is given in a footnote; I am grateful to John Trappes-Lomax for his kind advice on the translation of William Hawkins's *Musae Juridicae,* and to the Revd Tapani Simojoki and Dr Korey Maas for their insights on Robert Barnes and Richard Bayfield. I thank Clive Dunn for supplying the splendid colour photographs for the front cover and elsewhere, and Susan Curran for guiding this book so smoothly towards publication.

Dates before 1752 are given according to the Julian Calendar, with the year taken to begin on 1 January. I am very grateful to Colin Currie for reading an initial draft of this book from the perspective of a medieval historian and for his valuable insights. The staff of the Suffolk Record Office, Bury St Edmunds and Cambridge University Library have been, as usual, unfailingly helpful and I acknowledge their assistance with thanks. As always, my greatest debt of gratitude is to my wife Rachel for her unfailing grace and patience.

Francis Young
Ely, Cambridgeshire
February 2016

Abbreviations

Three sources are referred to frequently in the footnotes and bibliography and are therefore abbreviated:

ODNB	*Oxford Dictionary of National Biography*
PSIA(H)	*Proceedings of the Suffolk Institute of Archaeology (and History)*
SRS	Suffolk Records Society

A timeline of St Edmunds Abbey

869	Eadmund, King of the East Angles, killed by the Danes
c. 890	Minting of St Edmund Memorial Coinage in Danish East Anglia
c. 925	St Edmund's body moved to St Mary's Church in Beodricsworth
945	Edmund I of England allegedly grants the *banleuca* to the community at Beodricsworth
951	Bishop Theodred bequeaths lands to St Edmund
985	Abbo of Fleury visits Ramsey Abbey and writes the *Passio Sancti Eadmundi*
1010	Æthelwine the Sacrist takes the body of St Edmund to London
1013	Æthelwine brings St Edmund back to Beodricsworth
1014	Death of Sweyn Forkbeard
1020	Traditional foundation date of St Edmunds as a Benedictine Abbey by King Cnut
1032	Consecration of the Rotunda of St Mary and St Edmund
1034	Translation of St Edmund to the Rotunda
1043	Edward the Confessor grants the eight-and-a-half hundreds of west Suffolk (the Liberty of St Edmund) to the Abbey
c. 1048	St Edmunds granted minting rights
1065	Baldwin elected Abbot
1070	Herfast, Bishop of Elmham, attempts to relocate his see to Bury St Edmunds
1081	William I rules against Herfast and in favour of Baldwin
1093	Consecration of the choir altar of Baldwin's new minster
1095	Translation of St Edmund to the new minster
1097	Death of Abbot Baldwin
1121	Anselm of St Saba elected Abbot
1129	Henry I orders observance of the Feast of the Conception of the Virgin Mary
c. 1130	Master Hugo begins work at St Edmunds
1136	Abbot Anselm elected bishop of London
1138	Abbot Anselm returns to Bury after his confirmation as bishop of London fails
1142	Completion of the nave of the new minster
1150	Infirmary damaged by fire
1173	Roger Bigod and Knights of St Edmund defeat Robert, earl of Leicester at the Battle of Fornham
1181	Jews accused of the murder of 'Little St Robert'
1182	Samson of Tottington elected Abbot
1185	Foundation of St Saviour's Hospital
1190	Massacre of Jews on Palm Sunday; Abbot Samson expels the Jews from Bury St Edmunds
1192	Abbot Samson visits Richard I at Dürrenstein
1193	Abbot Samson leads the Knights of St Edmund at the siege of Windsor Castle
1198	Shrine of St Edmund damaged by fire
1208	King John confiscates the Abbey's possessions
1210	Abbey's central spire collapses
1211	Death of Abbot Samson
1213	Hugh of Northwold elected Abbot
1214	Barons gathered at St Edmunds swear to compel King John to grant Magna Carta
1215	King John confirms the election of Abbot Hugh
1229	Abbot Hugh consecrated bishop of Ely
1233	First challenge by the Franciscan friars against the Abbey's privileges

1257	Simon of Luton elected Abbot; Franciscan friars admitted to Bury
1263	Franciscan friars ejected from the town
1264	Rebellion of the Guild of Youth
1266	Justices search Bury St Edmunds for rebel barons
1275	Building begins on a new Lady Chapel; foundations of Rotunda discovered
1290	Townsfolk attack the cellarer's dam at Tay Fen
1296	Parliament meets at Bury St Edmunds
1300	Foundation of the Chapel of the Charnel
1305	Townsfolk accused of throwing stones at the Abbey Church
1326	Queen Isabella's army passes through Bury St Edmunds
1327	Rebellion by the townsfolk; Abbey ransacked and Abbey Gate destroyed
1329	Townsfolk kidnap Abbot Richard of Draughton and imprison him in Brabant
1338	Burial of Thomas of Brotherton, earl of Norfolk, fifth son of Edward I
1349	The Black Death arrives in Bury St Edmunds
1361	Year of three Abbots; plague breaks out again
1362	Henry of Kirkstead elected prior
1369	Third outbreak of plague
1379	Edmund Bromefield enthroned as anti-Abbot
1381	The Peasants' Revolt; rebels kill the prior and baroner
1389	William Cratfield elected Abbot
1398	Pope Boniface IX rules that Abbots of St Edmunds no longer require Papal confirmation
1423	John Lydgate elected prior of Hatfield Regis
1424	Abbot William Exeter rebuilds St Mary's Church
1427	Burial of Thomas Beaufort, duke of Exeter, third son of John of Gaunt
1429	William Curteys elected Abbot
1430	West tower collapses
1433	Henry VI visits St Edmunds
c. 1435	Abbot Curteys builds a new monastic library
1449	Death of John Lydgate
1447	Parliament meets at Bury St Edmunds; death of Humphrey, duke of Gloucester at St Saviour's Hospital
1450	Richard, duke of York meets the duke of Norfolk at St Edmunds
1465	Abbey Church gutted by fire
1486	Henry VII visits St Edmunds
1503	Abbot William Bunting rebuilds St James's church
1513	John Reeve elected Abbot
1515	Abbot Reeve visits the holy maid of Ipswich
1517	Cardinal Wolsey rules in favour of the Abbot in a dispute with the townsfolk
1526	Reformer Robert Barnes visits St Edmunds
1528	Rising of the Poor Men; Reeve imprisons Richard Bayfield for being in possession of heretical books
1530	Abbot Reeve charged with praemunire for aiding Wolsey
1531	Richard Bayfield, monk of St Edmunds, burnt as a relapsed heretic
1533	Funeral of Mary Rose Tudor, sister of Henry VIII
1534	Act of Supremacy cuts St Edmunds off from the Papacy
1535	Visitation of the Abbey by Sir John Legh and John ap Rice; relics confiscated
1538	Visitation of the Abbey by John ap Rice, John Williams, Richard Pollard, Phillip Parys and John Smyth; shrine of St Edmund despoiled
1539	Abbot Reeve surrenders the Abbey to the commissioners; Abbey Church demolished
1540	Death of Abbot Reeve

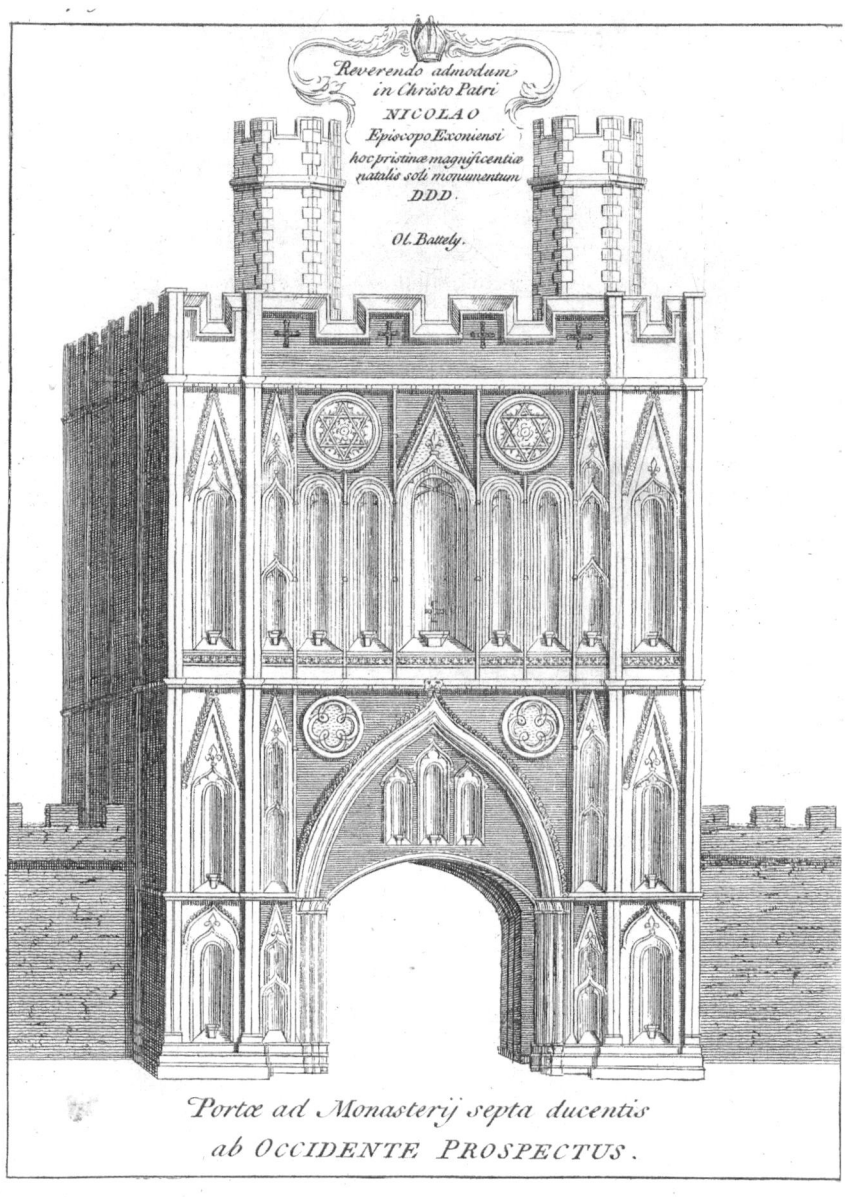

Figure 2 The Abbey Gate. Engraving by George Vertue for John Battely, *Antiquitates Sancti Edmundi* (1745), plate facing p. 1.

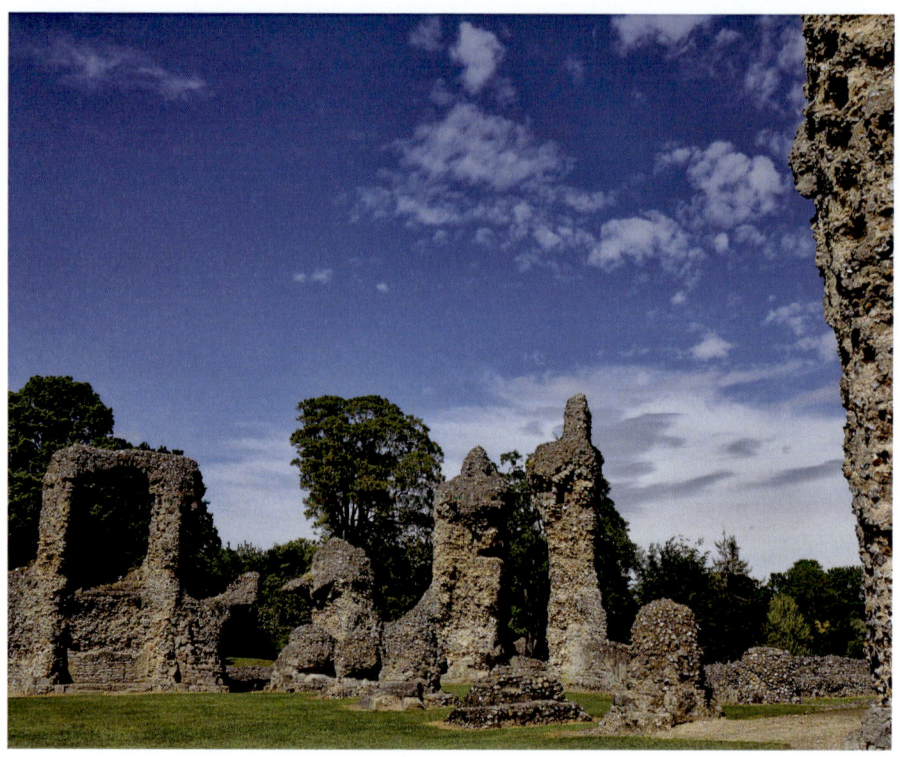

Figure 3 The ruins of the Abbey Church today, looking south-east from the central crossing. Photo by Clive Dunn.

Introduction

One sunlit day between 1535 and 1538 Henry VIII's royal librarian, John Leland (c. 1503–52) rode into Bury St Edmunds. Leland was impressed by what he saw, and was moved to exclaim:

> A man that saw the Abbay would say verily it were a Citie: so many Gates there are in it, and some of brasse, so many Towres, and a most stately Church: Upon which attend three others also standing gloriously in one and the same Churchyard, all of passing fine and curious Workmanship.[1]

Leland was, if anything, understating the magnificence of the scene before him. The Abbey Church of St Edmund was one of the largest churches in the world, with an approximate floor area of 13,648 square metres.[2] If the church were still standing, it would be exceeded in floor area only by the largest church in the world, St Peter's Basilica in Rome (15,160 square metres), which was still in the early stages of construction when St Edmunds was destroyed. The Abbey Church at Bury can be compared in size only with three other Romanesque churches: the cathedrals of Speyer (begin 1033) and Winchester (begun 1079) and the abbey of Cluny (begun 1088).[3] We can never know the true size of the Abbey Church because we do not know its height (and therefore cannot calculate its volume). It is possible that it was the largest completed church in the world when Leland saw it. Yet the Abbey was a building already doomed, and the purpose of Leland's visit was to take an audit of its library with a view to transporting the books, after the dissolution, to London.

It is ironic that the last man to bear witness in writing to the Abbey's physical appearance may also have played a part in ensuring that we now know so much about it. The real legacy of the Abbey of Bury St Edmunds is not its ruins – which are unimpressive in comparison with those of many other English abbeys – but rather its chronicles, books and archives. More cartularies survive from Bury St Edmunds than from any other medieval English abbey, and the textual sources for the study of the Abbey are remarkably

---

1   Quoted in William Camden, *Britain, or A chorographicall description of the most flourishing kingdomes, England, Scotland, and Ireland* (London, 1637), p. 460.
2   Calculated from William Yates's survey of 1802, reproduced in Richard Yates, *An Illustration of the Monastic Antiquities of the Town and Abbey of St Edmund's Bury* (London: J. B. Nichols and Son, 1843), plate facing p. 34. This estimate does not include the floor area of the west front chapels, octagons or apsidal chapels.
3   Eric Fernie, 'The Romanesque Church of Bury St Edmunds Abbey', in Antonia Gransden (ed.), *Bury St Edmunds: Medieval Art, Architecture and Economy* (London: British Archaeological Association, 1998), pp. 1–15, at pp. 4–5.

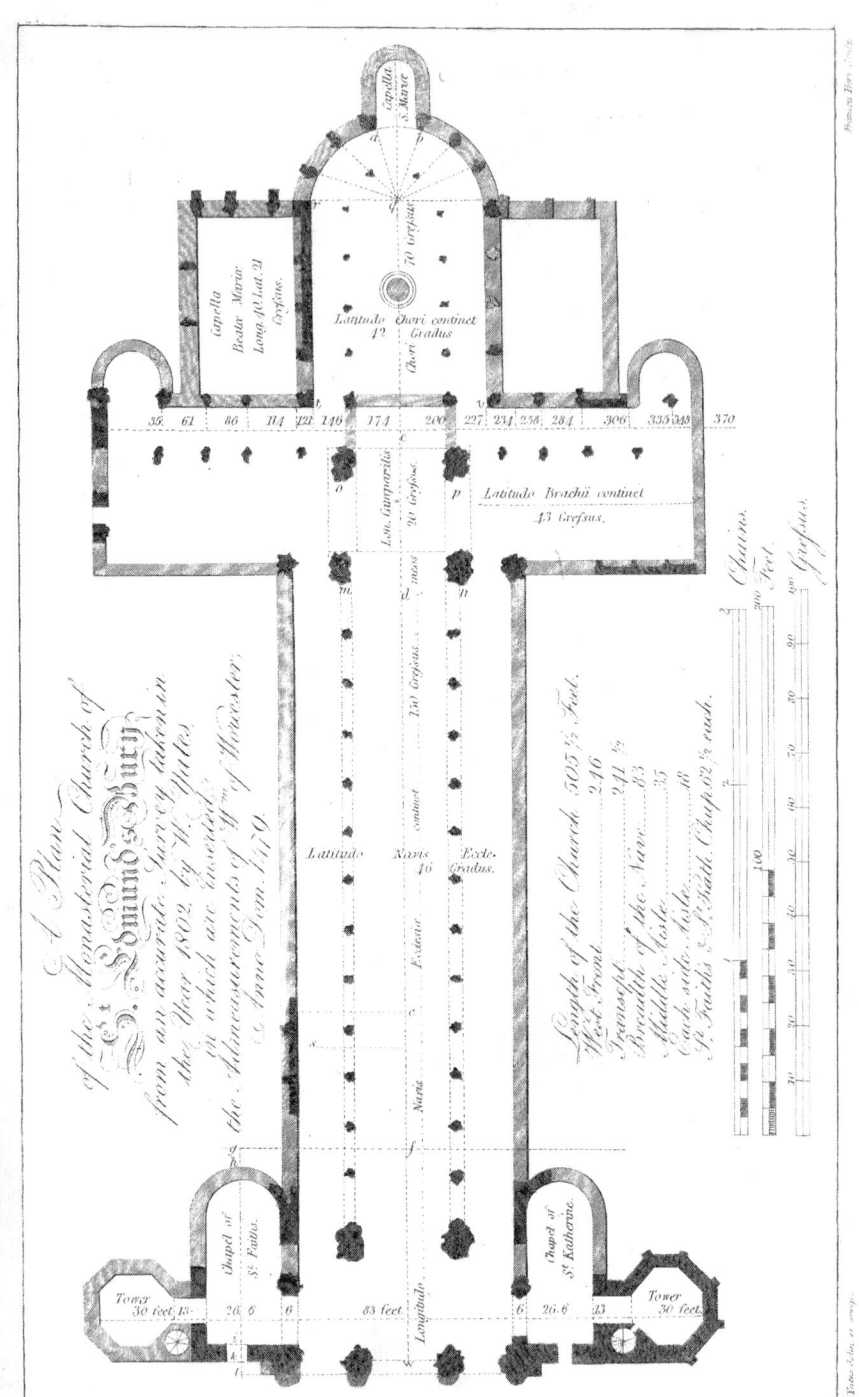

Figure 4 Ground plan of the Abbey Church by William Yates (1802). Engraving from Richard Yates, *An Illustration of the Monastic Antiquities of the Town and Abbey of St Edmund's Bury* (1843), plate facing p. 34.

rich.[4] The most famous of them is undoubtedly the monk Jocelin de Brakelond's colourful *Chronicle* of the reign of Abbot Samson of Tottington (1182–1211), a classic of medieval biography that has even been published as an Oxford Classics paperback. The Abbey of Bury St Edmunds is a treasure trove for historians rather than a feast for archaeologists.

A small number of the Abbey's treasures also survive, giving a tantalising glimpse of the splendour it once contained. They include the eleventh-century Bury St Edmunds Psalter, a beautiful Anglo-Saxon manuscript now in the Vatican Library; the magnificent twelfth-century Bury Bible in the Parker Library at Corpus Christi College, Cambridge; and an exquisite twelfth-century cross of walrus ivory in the Metropolitan Museum of Art in New York. Both Bible and cross have been attributed to Master Hugo, the first named artist working in England. The Abbey also left less tangible legacies: the cult of St Edmund, which was a Europe-wide phenomenon; Abbot Baldwin's introduction of the medical works of Galen into England; and Abbot Samson's idea of providing free education – along with the destructive legacy of antisemitic blood libels.

The magnitude of the Abbey's legacy is even more evident in East Anglia. The County of West Suffolk, which existed until as recently as 1974, was based on the boundaries of the Liberty of St Edmund, given to the Abbey by Edward the Confessor in 1043. Until the middle of the nineteenth century the Liberty remained a distinct judicial and ecclesiastical jurisdiction with its own justices and its own archdeacon. Without the Abbey, the town of Bury St Edmunds would not have its famous 'Norman grid' plan, the result of innovative town planning by Abbots Baldwin and Anselm in the eleventh and twelfth centuries. St Edmund's Fair, in late November and early December, endured until the 1870s. Until the 1930s, the limits of the town were still those established, according to tradition, in a charter of King Edmund I issued in 945.[5] Perhaps most importantly of all, in 1914 the choice of Bury St Edmunds rather than Ipswich as the site of Suffolk's cathedral church was a direct result of the town's ecclesiastical importance in the Middle Ages.

The site of the Abbey

The site of the Abbey of Bury St Edmunds, perhaps to a greater extent than any other important medieval monastic ruin, is challenging to interpret. Compared with the ruins of other great English abbeys, such as Glastonbury, Fountains or Rievaulx, the ruins of the Abbey of Bury St Edmunds seem distinctly unimpressive. Some great monastic churches survived by being transformed into cathedrals, like Peterborough, Gloucester, Bristol and (eventually) St Albans; others, like Tewkesbury, Malmesbury and Sherborne, survived as large parish churches. Bury was distinctly unlucky in this regard, and its location at the heart of an urban centre meant that the site was quickly stripped of anything of value. It is very difficult to visualise the church from what is left of it, and as the author of one guide to Britain puts it, 'The abbey ruins … are like nothing so much as petrified porridge, with little to remind you of the grandiose Norman complex that dominated the town.'[6] Yet,

---

4 Sarah Foot, 'The Abbey's Armoury of Charters', in Tom Licence (ed.), *Bury St Edmunds and the Norman Conquest* (Woodbridge: Boydell Press, 2014), pp. 31–52, at p. 32.
5 Margaret Statham, *The Book of Bury St Edmunds*, 2nd edn (Whittlebury: Baron Birch, 1996), p. 11.
6 Robert Andrews, *The Rough Guide to Britain* (London: Rough Guides, 2001), p. 439.

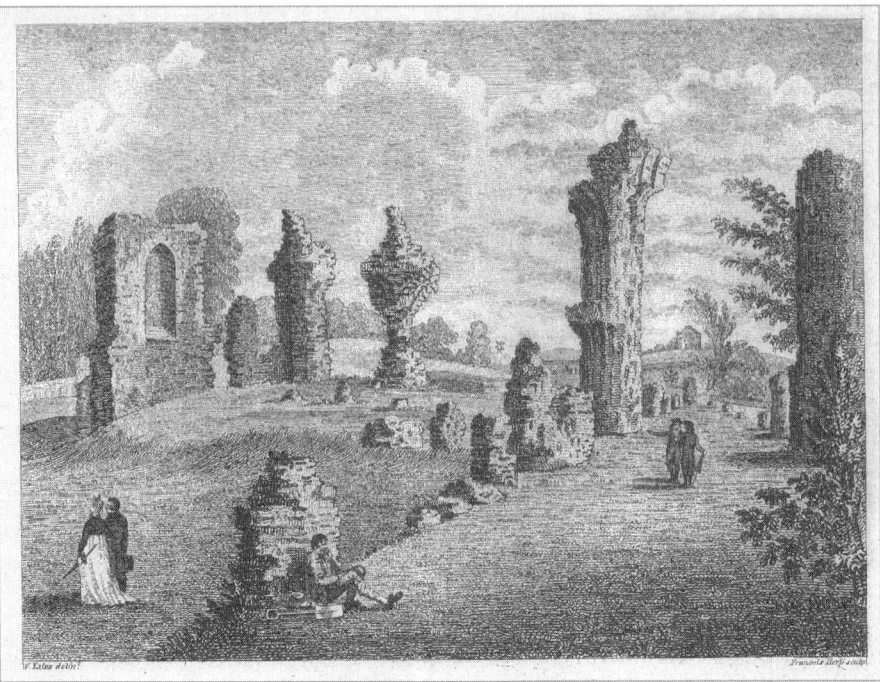

Figure 5 The ruins of the Abbey Church, looking east (1804). Engraving from Richard Yates, *An Illustration of the Monastic Antiquities of the Town and Abbey of St Edmund's Bury* (1843), plate facing p. 28.

as Eric Fernie has observed, '[Abbot] Baldwin's church must have been one of the most impressive buildings not just of the eleventh century but of the entire Middle Ages.'[7]

From a historical point of view, the Abbey is one of the best documented of England's pre-Reformation religious houses. Few inhabitants of Bury St Edmunds – and even fewer visitors to the town – are aware of the rich documentary evidence and the wealth of historical research that has been undertaken into the Abbey, especially in recent years. However, the ruins are too monumental to make much sense of on the ground, and it is easiest to appreciate them from the air. Nevertheless, the survival of two of the gateways to the monastic precinct, the fourteenth-century Abbey Gateway and the so-called Norman Tower, along with the churches of St Mary and St James (now St Edmundsbury Cathedral), does make it possible to imagine some of the grandeur of the monastic precinct, if not the Abbey Church itself. Leland's impression that the Abbey was a city in itself is borne out by the ground plan of the monastic complex as reconstructed in the 1950s by Arthur Whittingham.

More survives of the Abbey Church than at first appears; in the crypt at the east end there are even traces of plaster remaining, and the chapel of St Robert still retains its stone altar. The basic form of the entirely unique west front of the Abbey has survived owing to

---

7   Eric Fernie, 'Baldwin's church and the effects of the Conquest' in Licence (2014), pp. 74–93, at p. 81.

the houses incorporated into it in the seventeenth century, and the octagonal 'Samson's Tower' at the south-east corner still retains some grandeur. The ruins may be rough and undressed, but they still have much to reveal to the determined interpreter. The boundary of the Abbey precincts remains clear and well preserved. On the north side of the Abbey Gardens the northern boundary wall of the Abbey still stands, running behind the houses on the south side of Mustow Street. The western boundary wall is partially preserved on either side of the Abbey Gate, and would originally have followed the line of the railings of the Great Churchyard running southwards towards St Mary's Church, which stood at the south-easternmost corner of the precincts. The eastern boundary of the precincts was simply marked by the River Lark itself.

Within this large precinct, the Abbey in its developed state can roughly be divided into a 'temporal' zone (the north side) and a 'spiritual' zone (the south side). On the south side St James's Gate (misleadingly called the 'Norman Tower') was the ceremonial entrance to the Abbey Church; south of the Church was the large and ancient cemetery, which dated back to the days before the Abbey. North of the Abbey Church lay the cloister, and beyond that the 'temporal' buildings of the Abbey: the guesthouse was on the south side of a great courtyard which occupied the space where a cruciform path now divides the flowerbeds of the Abbey Gardens, with the fourteenth-century Abbey Gate to the west. To the east lay the principal temporal building of the complex, the Abbot's Palace, which was converted to secular use after the dissolution and was still standing in 1720. The small octagonal tower (or dovecote) that the visitor now sees standing between the ruins of the Abbot's Palace and the river was part of a precinct wall that ran along the riverbank, and may have been built after the riots of 1327 in order to give the Abbey added protection from the townsfolk.

Apart from the Norman Tower and Abbey Gate, which survive in their entirety, the best preserved parts of the complex are the north and west precinct walls and the west front of the Abbey, although this is not immediately apparent on account of the houses built into the west front. Of the body of the Abbey Church, more survives of the north transept than any other part above ground, and the crypt is comparatively well preserved because it was only excavated in the late 1950s. Another well-preserved monument is the Abbot's Bridge at the north-east corner of the precinct. However, there is barely a trace now remaining of many important buildings in the complex, including the Prior's House, the Infirmary, the Abbot's Palace and the Chapel of St Margaret, which stood near or beneath the present Shire Hall.

The organisation of the Abbey

The Abbey of Bury St Edmunds was a complex organisation that is best imagined as a series of concentric circles of influence and property. The Abbot ruled over the monastery, of course, but he also ruled 'a kind of statelet endorsed by St Edmund's protection',[8] which consisted of the territory inside the four crosses of the *banleuca* of Bury St Edmunds. This territory was later known as the Liberty of Bury St Edmunds. It should not be confused with the Liberty of St Edmund, which consisted of the eight-and-a-half hundreds given to

---

8   Anthony Bale, 'Introduction', in Anthony Bale (ed.), *St Edmund, King and Martyr: Changing Images of a Medieval Saint* (York: York Medieval Press, 2009), pp. 1–25, at p. 7.

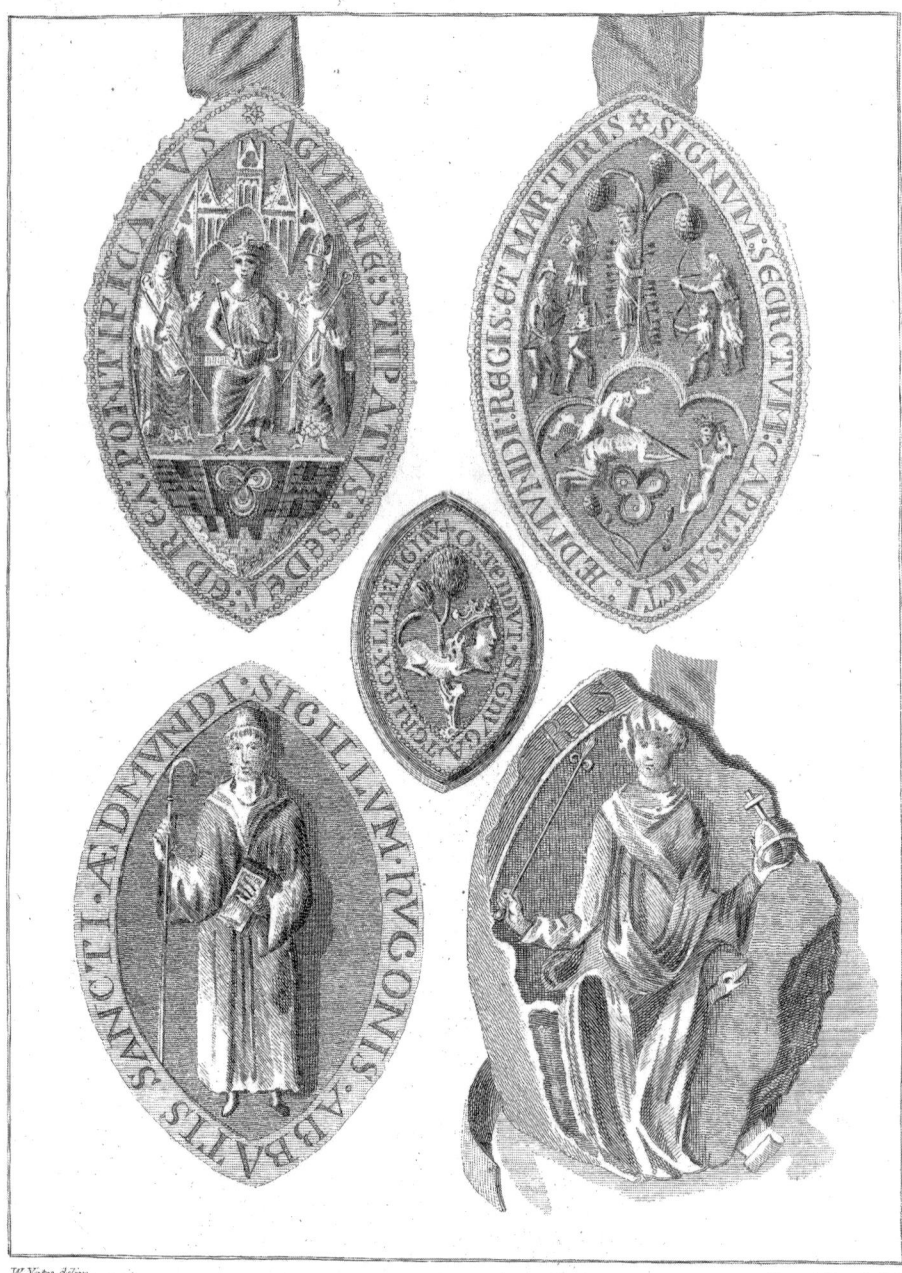

Figure 6 Seals of the Abbey and of individual Abbots. Engraving from Richard Yates, *An Illustration of the Monastic Antiquities of the Town and Abbey of St Edmund's Bury* (1843), plate facing p. 37.

St Edmund by Edward the Confessor in 1043. Whereas the Abbot enjoyed the fullness of royal jurisdiction within the *banleuca* itself, his jurisdiction over the Liberty of St Edmund was more limited; nevertheless, he acted as sheriff and had complete judicial authority over the eight-and-a-half hundreds. The Abbot's ecclesiastical jurisdiction was even more extensive, and he exercised the authority of a bishop over the entire territory.

However, the Abbey of Bury St Edmunds also owned lands beyond west Suffolk, as far away as Warkton in Northamptonshire, and at one stage even in Normandy. The Abbots maintained palaces at London and Colchester in order to facilitate journeys to and from the capital and participation in court life as peers of the realm. The majority of the manors owned by the Abbey were, in fact, owned by the Abbot and, on his death, the temporal 'barony' of Bury St Edmunds reverted to the crown. This was because the Liberty of St Edmund had been granted by a charter of Edward the Confessor and each subsequent monarch was expected to renew it. As pious devotees of St Edmund they invariably did so, but not before farming the revenues of the Abbey during the vacancy that preceded the election of a new Abbot. In addition to being elected by the Chapter of monks, Abbots had to be confirmed both by the king and the pope, making the appointment of a new Abbot a lengthy process.

By the time of Abbot Samson (1182–1211) the organisation of the Abbey was well developed. The Abbey was governed, at least in theory, by a Chapter which, by the late Middle Ages, incorporated lay members as well as monks. However, the Abbot possessed ultimate power and could overrule decisions of the Chapter. The Abbot's office was distinct from the Convent, which was led by the prior and sub-prior. This was a crucial legal distinction, because whereas the Abbot's possessions were taken over by the crown on his death, those of the Convent were not. The sacrist and the cellarer (known collectively as the 'obedientaries') administered the Abbey's wider possessions on behalf of the Abbot, although their separate spheres of jurisdiction were not always well defined. In theory, the sacrist exercised ecclesiastical authority over the town of Bury St Edmunds as archdeacon, while the cellarer held the rights of lord of the manor within the town. However, the town was also said to belong to the sacrist, and during Samson's reign the courts of the sacrist ('portmann-moot') and the cellarer (held at Eastgate Barns) sometimes came into conflict.[9] The subsacrist was in charge of the Abbey buildings.

Within the monastery, the sacrist was ultimately responsible for the wealth of the house (a development of his original role as custodian of the treasures of the church in the sacristy), for building work, and for commissioning works of art to adorn the churches and chapels. The cellarer was responsible for providing food for the monks and guests, which was why he was placed in charge of agricultural lands belonging to the Convent and served as lord of the manor. At Bury, unusually, the sacrist rather than the cellarer was always considered the senior obedientary – probably because he exercised archidiaconal jurisdiction as a consequence of the Abbot's special powers. The guestmaster was responsible for receiving guests, many of whom, at an Abbey as prestigious as St Edmunds, were of high rank and required luxurious hospitality. The almoner was responsible for the Abbey's distribution of alms to the poor, which was expected not just because St Edmunds was a monastery but also because the Abbot was a great lord and expected to display largesse and benevolence to the unfortunate. The pittancer was responsible for managing

---

9   Antonia Gransden, *A History of the Abbey of Bury St Edmunds 1182–1256* (Woodbridge: Boydell, 2009), p. 44–6.

the finances of the monks themselves and ensuring that the monks received the 'pittances' (small stipends) granted by successive donors and patrons.

The infirmarian was responsible for the care of sick monks as well as for the regular bloodletting which was a feature of medieval English monasticism. However, several of the infirmarians of St Edmunds were not mere monk-healers but learned physicians who had studied at the leading medical schools of the Middle Ages. The librarian was responsible for the care of the Abbey's immensely important archive and book collection, which was probably kept somewhere above the cloister. Other monks were shrine-keepers, entrusted with the particular care of the shrine of St Edmund, and presumably with the business of managing the flow of pilgrims and collecting offerings from them.

In addition to these monk-officials (of which this is by no means an exhaustive list), many men worked in the Abbey who were not monks. Indeed, Samson began life as a secular clerk in the service of the Abbey. The Abbot employed his own clerks, who were not usually monks, and had his own chancery for the administration of his estates in the Abbot's Palace, playing as he did a dual role as the head of a monastic house and a vastly wealthy temporal lord. There were also secular chaplains attached to specific saints' cults within the Abbey Church, whose task it was to say the masses required by the endowments of those chapels – something the monks could not do, because their principal task was celebrating the monastic offices. Furthermore, the monastery employed large numbers of lay servants. For most of their existence, the Abbey precincts must have seemed like a small town in their own right.

Town and Abbey

The town of Bury St Edmunds virtually owes its existence, and certainly its name, to a now vanished monastery. Strictly speaking, there was no such thing as the 'Abbey of Bury St Edmunds'; there was the Abbey of St Edmund, or St Edmunds Abbey (conventionally written without the apostrophe), and its adjacent town, St Edmunds Bury or Bury St Edmunds. The town belonged to the Abbey rather than the Abbey to the town, and although the town predated the Benedictine Abbey (under its original name of Beodricsworth), the change of name in the mid-eleventh century indicated the Abbey's definitive domination of the place. In fact, as medieval documents such as Domesday Book frequently attest, the town did not so much belong to the Abbey as it did to St Edmund himself, the incorrupt martyr who was spoken of in legal documents as a living person.

The medieval history of Bury St Edmunds is conventionally told as a conflict between the Abbey and the townsfolk in which the townsfolk, by means of the historical accident of the dissolution, were eventually victorious. It is undeniable that many of the Abbots were thoroughly insensitive to the aspirations of the townsfolk and treated them harshly and unjustly, but the relationship between Abbey and town was more than just one of conflict. The townsfolk took great pride in the Abbey, participating in (and benefiting from) lucrative royal visits, and on more than one occasion the people desperately tried to save the Abbey Church from fire. However, more often than not the Abbey saw the town as little more than a source of revenue, and this had disastrous consequences in 1327 and 1381 when rioters ransacked the Abbey.

There is no evidence for the idea that the townsfolk were glad when the Abbey was dissolved; they certainly reaped no benefits from the dissolution, as I shall explain in

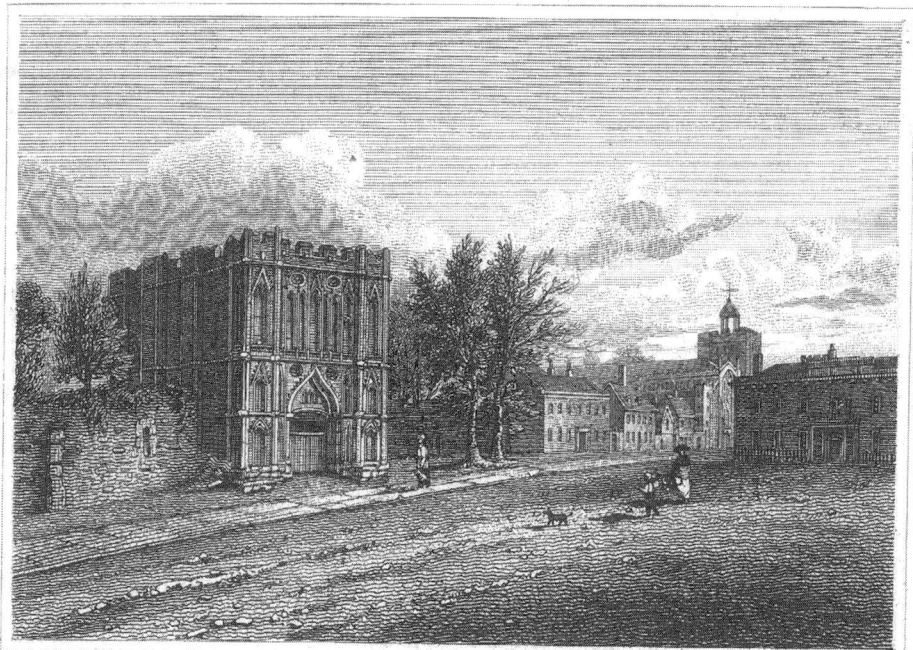

Figure 7 The Abbey precincts viewed from Angel Hill. Engraving from Thomas Higham, *Excursions in the County of Suffolk* (1818–19), plate facing p. 17.

Chapter 7. For better or worse, Abbey and town lived in a symbiotic relationship throughout the Middle Ages, although it was most certainly an unequal partnership. The Abbey allowed the burgesses (leading men) of the town to have a guild, led by an alderman; the alderman was elected by the burgesses, and he had many responsibilities (such as providing watchmen for the town gates) but virtually no authority. The alderman was compelled to pay homage to the Abbot, and the choice of the burgesses was subject to the Abbot's approval. From the point of view of the townsfolk the Abbey's governance of the town was an anachronism, but the Abbots did not see it this way. As far as they were concerned, the townsfolk were 'men of St Edmunds' who owed feudal obedience to the Abbot, and in return enjoyed privileges such as exemption from royal taxation.

According to one of the most popular legends about St Edmund, King Sweyn was killed by an apparition of the martyr when he tried to impose taxation on the men of St Edmunds, and Abbot Baldwin successfully fought off attempts by Norman nobles to impose their will on the *banleuca*. In the eleventh and twelfth centuries, the people of Bury St Edmunds may well have considered the Abbey's privileges to be advantageous to them. However, as the townsfolk aspired to self-government and found themselves unable to consolidate their economic successes, Anglo-Saxon and Norman exemptions and privileges meant increasingly little. The Abbey operated on the basis of an eleventh-century understanding of 'liberties', seeing them as large-scale institutional exemptions obtained from the crown: by the late Middle Ages, 'liberties' meant such things as the ability to elect local government and freedom from interference from monastic officials.

Histories of Bury St Edmunds

Bury St Edmunds is well served by detailed studies of a number of different periods and aspects of the Abbey's history. The first historian of the Abbey, John Battely (1647–1708), never lived to see his research published, and it was finally edited by his nephew Oliver in 1745. Battely wrote in Latin, and the authors of eighteenth-century guides for the gentleman traveller largely paraphrased his work rather than conducting any new research of their own. In 1840, the antiquary John Gage Rokewode of Hengrave Hall produced an edition of the *Chronicle* of Jocelin de Brakelond which attracted the attention of the essayist Thomas Carlyle. Carlyle's *Past and Present* (1843) made Jocelin and Abbot Samson nationally famous.[10] In the same year an expanded edition of Richard Yates's *Illustration of the Monastic Antiquities of the Town and Abbey of St Edmund's Bury* – which originally appeared in truncated form in 1805 – completed Battely's work by supplying a complete antiquarian survey of Bury's monastic history.

A shortcoming of the work of Battely and Yates was that they relied almost entirely on textual evidence, although Yates also had a good knowledge of the site, having been brought up in the Abbey ruins. In 1865 Graham Hills attempted the first true archaeological survey of the ruins for the British Archaeological Association.[11] Then, between 1890 and 1896 Thomas Arnold's three volumes of *Memorials of St Edmund's Abbey* made available to scholars some of the key historical documents, and this remains a standard work.[12] In 1895 the great Cambridge antiquary Montague Rhodes (M. R.) James turned his attention to the Abbey, a building he had been interested in since he was a child growing up at the rectory in Great Livermere.[13] James's reconstruction of the monastic library and interior furnishings of the Abbey Church were revolutionary, and informed all subsequent scholarship. James was also successful in identifying the tombs of Samson and five other abbots in the Chapter House, which was excavated by Sir Ernest Clarke, under James's supervision, in 1902–3.

A good summary history of the Abbey appeared in the second volume of the *Victoria County History of Suffolk*, edited by William Page in 1907.[14] A more thorough treatment was Albert Goodwin's Gladstone Memorial Prize Essay of 1926, which appeared in print in 1931 as *The Abbey of St. Edmundsbury*. This was hitherto the closest thing to a complete history of the Abbey, but at 84 pages it was necessarily a brief study.[15] Goodwin's approach was chronological, and he divided the history of the Abbey into four periods: the origins of the monastery and the development of the shrine of St Edmund (870–1182), the development of the Abbots as administrators (1182–1263), the conflict between Abbey and town (1263–1390), and what Goodwin saw as the revival of the Abbey in the late Middle Ages (1390–1539). In 1935 Mary Lobel produced a detailed study of the relations between

---

10   Jocelin de Brakelond, *Chronica Jocelini de Brakelond*, ed. J. Gage Rokewode (London: Camden Society, 1840); Thomas Carlyle, *Past and Present* (London: Chapman and Hall, 1843).
11   Graham M. Hills, 'The antiquities of Bury St. Edmunds', *Journal of the British Archaeological Association* 21 (1865), pp. 32–56, 104–40.
12   Thomas Arnold (ed.), *Memorials of St Edmund's Abbey* (London: HMSO, 1890–96), 3 vols.
13   M. R. James, *On the Abbey of S. Edmund at Bury* (Cambridge: Cambridge Antiquarian Society, 1895), 2 vols.
14   William Page (ed.), *The Victoria History of the County of Suffolk* (London: Archibald Constable and Co., 1907), vol. 2, pp. 56–72.
15   Albert Goodwin, *The Abbey of St. Edmundsbury* (Oxford: Blackwell, 1931).

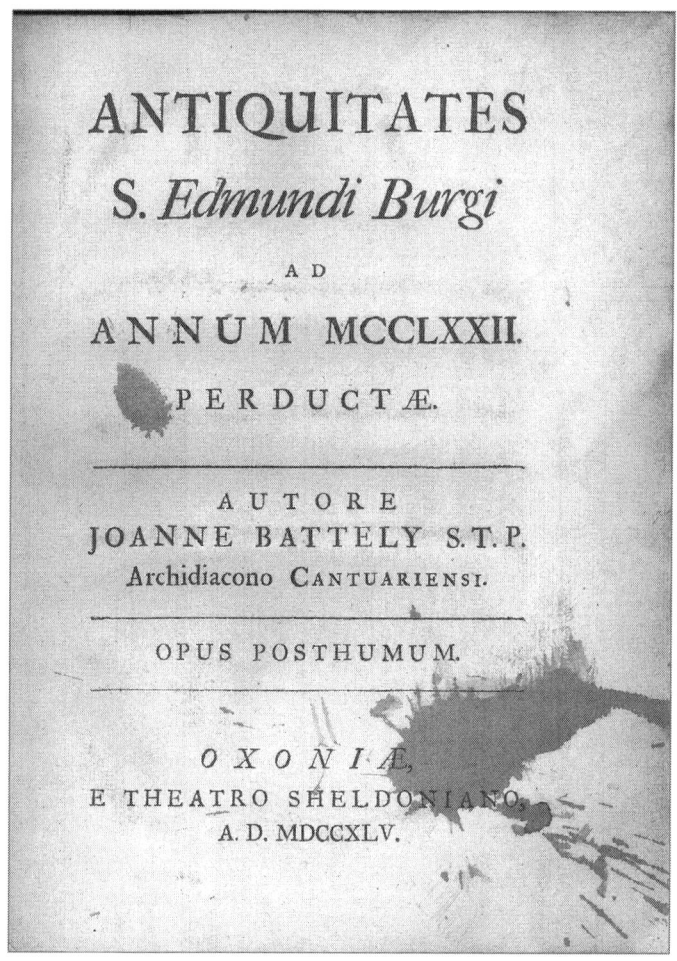

Figure 8 Title page of the first published history of Bury St Edmunds, John Battely's *Antiquitates Sancti Edmundi* (1745)

town and Abbey in the Middle Ages,[16] and a steady stream of editions of important original texts relating to the Abbey appeared throughout the twentieth century.[17]

In 1952 the archaeologist Arthur Whittingham undertook what is still the definitive

---

16 Mary D. Lobel, *The Borough of Bury St. Edmunds: A Study in the Government and Development of a Monastic Town* (Oxford: Clarendon Press, 1935).
17 D. C. Douglas (ed.), *Feudal Documents from the Abbey of Bury St. Edmunds* (Oxford University Press: Oxford, 1932); Jocelin of Brakelond, *The Chronicle of Jocelin of Brakelond*, ed. H. E. Butler (Oxford: Oxford University Press, 1949); R. H. C. Davis (ed.), *The Kalendar of Abbot Samson and related Documents* (London: Camden Society, 1954); Rodney M. Thomson (ed.), *The Chronicle of the Election of Hugh, Abbot of Bury St Edmunds and later Bishop of Ely* (Oxford: Oxford University Press, 1974).

survey of the Abbey ruins,[18] and all subsequent historians are indebted to the plans of the Abbey Church and convent he produced. The current English Heritage guidebook to the Abbey of Bury St Edmunds, first published in 1971 and last reprinted in 2012, is still based on Whittingham's article of 1952.[19] This is an indication of the quality of Whittingham's work, but also of the relative lack of attention paid to the Abbey ruins since the last major archaeological investigation of 1959–64. Significant areas of the ruins have never been excavated or surveyed using the non-invasive technology that is now available to archaeologists. By contrast, the library, archives and artistic treasures of the Abbey have been well served by scholarship.[20]

No contemporary historian has made a more significant contribution to the history of the Abbey than Antonia Gransden. After completing a PhD thesis at the University of London in 1956 on the *Bury St Edmunds Chronicle*, Gransden's edition of the *The Letter-Book of William of Hoo* appeared in 1963, followed by an edition of the *Chronicle* the following year.[21] Gransden produced a steady stream of editions of original documents and articles on different aspects of St Edmunds which culminated in a two-volume history of the Abbey in the period 1182–1301, published between 2009 and 2015.[22] Other scholars also made important contributions. Robert Gottfried's *Bury St Edmunds and the Urban Crisis* (1982) returned to the theme of the relations between Abbey and town between 1290 and the dissolution,[23] building on Lobel's earlier work, and Diarmaid MacCulloch shed much light on the dissolution period in his *Suffolk and the Tudors* (1986).[24]

In 1998 the proceedings of a meeting of the British Archaeological Association held at Culford Hall in 1994 were published under Gransden's editorship as *Bury St Edmunds: Medieval Art, Architecture and Economy*. This seminal volume contained a number of authoritative chapters on the history of the Abbey, focusing primarily on the twelfth century.[25] Further important edited collections followed in 2009 (on the cult of St Edmund) and 2014 (on Bury St Edmunds during the period of the Norman Conquest).[26]

---

18 Arthur B. Whittingham, 'Bury St. Edmunds Abbey and the churches of St Mary and St James', *Archaeological Journal* 108 (1952), pp. 168–89.
19 Arthur B. Whittingham, *Bury St Edmunds Abbey* (London: HMSO, 1971).
20 Henry of Kirkstead, *Catalogus de libris autenticis et apocrifis*, ed. R. H. and M. A. Rouse (London: British Library and British Academy, 2004); R. M. Thomson (ed.), *The Archives of the Abbey of Bury St Edmunds*, SRS 21 (Woodbridge: Suffolk Records Society, 1980); Dee Dyas and Rodney M. Thomson, *The Bury Bible* (Woodbridge: Boydell & Brewer, 2008).
21 Antonia Gransden (ed.), *The Letter-Book of William of Hoo 1280–1294*, SRS5 (Ipswich: Suffolk Records Society, 1963); Antonia Gransden (ed.), *The Chronicle of Bury St. Edmunds 1212–1301* (London: Nelson, 1964).
22 Gransden (2009); Antonia Gransden, *A History of the Abbey of Bury St Edmunds 1257–1301* (Woodbridge: Boydell, 2015).
23 Robert S. Gottfried, *Bury St Edmunds and the Urban Crisis: 1290–1539* (Princeton, NJ: Princeton University Press, 1982).
24 Diarmaid MacCulloch, *Suffolk and the Tudors: Politics and Religion in an English County 1500–1600* (Oxford: Clarendon Press, 1986).
25 Antonia Gransden (ed.), *Bury St Edmunds: Medieval Art, Architecture and Economy* (London: British Archaeological Association, 1998).
26 Bale (2009); Tom Licence (ed.), *Bury St Edmunds and the Norman Conquest* (Woodbridge: Boydell Press, 2014).

The medieval cult of St Edmund has also been the subject of a recent book by Rebecca Pinner,[27] while my own previous research has concentrated on the post-medieval interest in St Edmund, early antiquarian interest in the Abbey in the seventeenth century and the post-medieval use of the Abbot's Palace.[28]

Over the past few decades, most of the energy of local historians has been directed at producing histories of the town of Bury St Edmunds, many of which are excellent, such as those by Elsie McCutcheon, Margaret Statham and Frank Meeres.[29] However, of necessity these studies provide only a cursory survey of the history of the Abbey, which is not their main subject. Likewise, Robin Eaglen's two-volume history of the Bury St Edmunds mint is a specialist work most likely to be of interest to numismatists, although it contains valuable research on the Abbey.[30] It is indicative that a recently published guidebook to the legend of St Edmund and St Edmundsbury Cathedral contains scarcely any information on the Abbey at all, and certainly no interpretative guide to the ruins.[31]

The Abbey of Bury St Edmunds, which played a key role in English history as well as the surrounding region, deserves a history in its own right. The history of the Abbey cannot merely be treated as an adjunct to the history of the town, since there were many aspects of the life of the Abbey in which the townsfolk played no part and which had little effect on them. History is written by the victors – or in this case about the victors – and since the town of Bury St Edmunds was (by default) the victor in its long struggle with the Abbey, the town has tended to command more historical attention. An accessible narrative account of the Abbey's story, taking into account recent historical work, is much overdue. Nothing in this book can be considered original research, and that is not the intention: it is, rather, an account of the Abbey's history from foundation to dissolution, based on secondary sources, and synthesising the insights of medieval historians, archaeologists, and historians of art and architecture. The aim is to introduce the vast historical subject that is the Abbey of Bury St Edmunds, and to stimulate the reader to explore the subject in more detail in the scholarly works referred to throughout the text.

The telling of monastic history is attended by particular challenges that are not encountered by the biographer of an individual person or the historian of a period or dynasty. These challenges are very evident in Gransden's two volumes on the Abbey in the period 1182–1301. Gransden began with a broadly chronological approach in the first volume but abandoned this entirely in the second, on the grounds that an institutional history does

---

27 Rebecca Pinner, *The Cult of St Edmund in Medieval East Anglia* (Woodbridge: Boydell, 2015).
28 Francis Young, *Where is St Edmund? The search for East Anglia's martyr king* (Ely: East Anglian Catholic History Centre, 2014); Francis Young, 'St Edmund, king and martyr in popular memory since the Reformation', *Folklore* 126 (2015) pp. 159–76; Francis Young, 'John Battely's *Antiquitates S. Edmundi Burgi* and its editors', *PSIAH* 41 (2008) pp. 467–79; Francis Young, '"An Horrid Popish Plot": the failure of Catholic aspirations in Bury St Edmunds, 1685–88', *PSIAH* 41 (2006), pp. 209–55.
29 Elsie McCutcheon, *Bury St Edmunds: Historic Town* (Bury St Edmunds: Alastair Press, 1987); Statham (1996); Margaret Statham, *Yesterday's Town: Bury St Edmunds* (Whittlebury: Baron Birch, 1992); Frank Meeres, *A History of Bury St Edmunds* (Stroud: History Press, 2010).
30 Robin J. Eaglen, *The Abbey and Mint of Bury St Edmunds to 1279* (London: British Numismatic Society, 2006); Robin J. Eaglen, *The Abbey and Mint of Bury St Edmunds from 1279* (London: British Numismatic Society, 2014).
31 Martyn Taylor, *St Edmundsbury Cathedral* (Bury St Edmunds: Jarrold, 2013).

not lend itself to a chronological narrative. As early as 1805, Richard Yates eschewed John Battely's abbot-by-abbot approach to the history of the Abbey and opted for a thematic treatment, which better illustrated the development of the Abbey as an institution and the extent of its influence. Although some of the Abbots left the mark of their personality on the institution, such as Baldwin, Anselm, Samson and William Curteys, others were lesser figures who served the Abbey rather than leading it in new directions. The history of the Abbey is the history of a large, complex and continuously evolving monastic house, and cannot be reduced to a succession of 'great men'.

In spite of these difficulties, I have nevertheless opted for a chronological approach in this book, primarily because narrative history remains the most accessible form of non-fiction to the non-specialist reader. The Abbots occupy an important – but not exclusive – place in the narrative, and it is worth noting that the Abbots were far more involved in the day-to-day running of their monastery than many medieval bishops were in the running of their sees. There was a strong tradition of residence at Bury that contrasted with the absenteeism of bishops. However, I am mindful of the need to devote due attention to the parallel evolution of the monastic buildings, the library and the intellectual life of the monks in each chapter. Decisions concerning the chronological scope of each chapter have not always been straightforward. The period 869–1065 seems a natural one, since it witnessed the early development of the cult of St Edmund in an Anglo-Saxon context, and the appointment of Baldwin was a decisive transitional moment in the life of the Abbey just as the Norman Conquest was a watershed in English history. The decision to group Baldwin and Anselm together can be justified on the grounds that both men are famed for fostering the intellectual and cultural life of the Abbey and for erecting most of the main buildings.

My decision to combine the reigns of Abbot Samson (1182–1211) and Hugh of Northwold (1214–1229) may be more controversial, given Samson's fame, but I believe it to be justified on the grounds that recent scholarship on Magna Carta has established the true stature of Hugh II. Less well recorded than Samson, as the man who stood up to King John and made Magna Carta possible, Hugh certainly stands comparison with him. The century 1229–1329 is treated in a single chapter because although the Abbey faced a diverse range of sometimes unrelated challenges during these years, I argue that the disastrous revolt of 1327–29 ought to be seen as the culmination of popular dissent reaching back to conflict with the friars rather than a harbinger of the Peasants' Revolt of 1381. The events of 1381 had their own distinct causes, rooted in the disputed abbacy of Edmund Bromefield, and they were considerably less serious for Bury in the long term. Chapter 5 takes the weakening of the Abbey by the Black Death as the starting point of its exploration of the Abbey's changing fortunes in the fourteenth and fifteenth centuries. The restorations following the great fire of 1465, which very nearly destroyed the Abbey Church, seem to provide a natural starting point for Chapter 6's exploration of the final decades of the Abbey's existence.

The existing historical literature on the history of the Abbey is inordinately focused on the period from the appointment of Abbot Baldwin to the death of Abbot John of Northwold (1065–1301). There is little scholarship on the later history of the Abbey, and none of recent date other than Gransden's lives of later Abbots contributed to the *Oxford Dictionary of National Biography* (2004). The Abbey's fourteenth and fifteenth-century history is well overdue a re-evaluation, but it seems unlikely that Gransden will now undertake this task and add further volumes to her history of the Abbey. The one area of the Abbey's life in the later Middle Ages that is receiving extensive treatment is the life and poetry of John Lydgate (c. 1370–1449). It is very much to be hoped that at some future point the registers of Abbots Curteys and Reeve will receive editorial attention, and it will become possible to explore the later history of the Abbey in more depth.

In addition to telling the story of the Abbey as an institution from foundation to dissolution, this book completes the narrative by considering the Abbey's lingering legacy, as well as examining the men and women who, since the seventeenth century, have uncovered its history. It is hardly surprising that an institution that dominated East Anglia for over 500 years left behind considerable traces, and it is short-sighted to regard the story of the Abbey as one that ended in 1539. The Abbey's legacy took many forms, from the ghostly traces of its former jurisdictions (governmental, judicial and ecclesiastical) that lingered down to the nineteenth and twentieth centuries, to the inspiration the Abbey provided for English Benedictine monks in exile on the Continent trying to preserve and maintain their nation's ancient monastic tradition. The discovery of the Abbey is still ongoing. In comparison with other similar sites, archaeological investigation of the Abbey ruins has been very limited. Much remains to be discovered, perhaps even fragments of the shrine of St Edmund itself.[32] The story of the Abbey of Bury St Edmunds is very far from over.

The book's two appendices are a list of Abbots, priors and sacrists and an imaginary tour of the Abbey Church on the eve of the fire of 1465. The names of the Abbots of St Edmunds are well known, but the reader will find it helpful to have the names of the priors as well, since these men ruled the Convent and were responsible for the everyday running of the monastery. Strictly speaking, the sub-prior came next in importance after the prior, but in practice it was the sacrists, to whom the town of Bury St Edmunds belonged and who were in charge of the Abbey's physical fabric, who were the Abbey's most important officials. The sacrists also exercised the ecclesiastical powers of an archdeacon within the *banleuca*.

In including an imaginary tour of the Abbey Church in 1465 I have followed the same historical method as M. R. James, who concluded in 1895 that the best and simplest way to provide a complete description of the building was to lead the reader through it, step by step. Since James wrote, further light has been thrown on the physical arrangement of the church by Arthur Whittingham, John Crook and Rebecca Pinner, and my description takes account of these developments. The physical fabric of the Abbey Church looms large in the story, and the reader may choose to read Appendix II first in order to have a clear idea of the setting of many of the events described.

---

32 John Crook, 'The architectural setting of the cult of St Edmund at Bury 1095–1539', in Antonia Gransden (ed.), *Bury St Edmunds: Medieval Art, Architecture and Economy* (London: British Archaeological Association, 1998), pp. 34–44, at pp. 42, 44n.

Chapter 1
Origins, 869–1065

The Abbey of Bury St Edmunds has no straightforward, universally accepted foundation story. The story that lies *behind* the foundation of the Abbey is, of course, well known to anyone acquainted with the history of East Anglia. It is the tale of the final struggle between Eadmund, last King of the East Angles, and the invading 'Great Army' of Danes, who clashed at Thetford in the winter of 869. Eadmund was killed, either in battle or away from the battlefield, and within thirty years of his death he was being venerated as a Christian martyr by the very Danes who had caused his death. Not for nothing did the historian of Suffolk Norman Scarfe entitle his important article on the body of St Edmund 'Defeat into victory'; the same motto could be applied to the Abbey itself, a foundation that, like the Christian religion itself, turned a martyred leader into a symbol of victory. The victory, in this case, was the triumph of the English people, and English culture and religion, over the invaders. If Glastonbury Abbey, the supposed resting place of King Arthur, was the custodian of British identity, St Edmunds had a strong claim to be considered the custodian of English identity.

Until 1032, the year in which a round church was consecrated at Bury St Edmunds in honour of St Mary and St Edmund, the history of the Abbey and its predecessor, the Church of St Mary with its college of secular priests, is distinctly murky. However, it is clear that Bury became a Benedictine foundation in the first quarter of the eleventh century, and by the middle of the century we have good evidence of royal grants of land

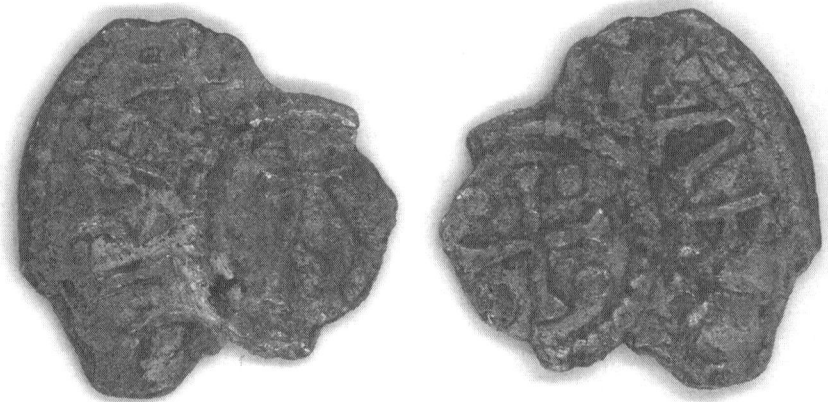

Figure 9 Contemporary documentary evidence for Eadmund: a fragmentary penny of the last king of the East Angles, minted c. 855–69 by the moneyer Beornhæh. Photo by the author.

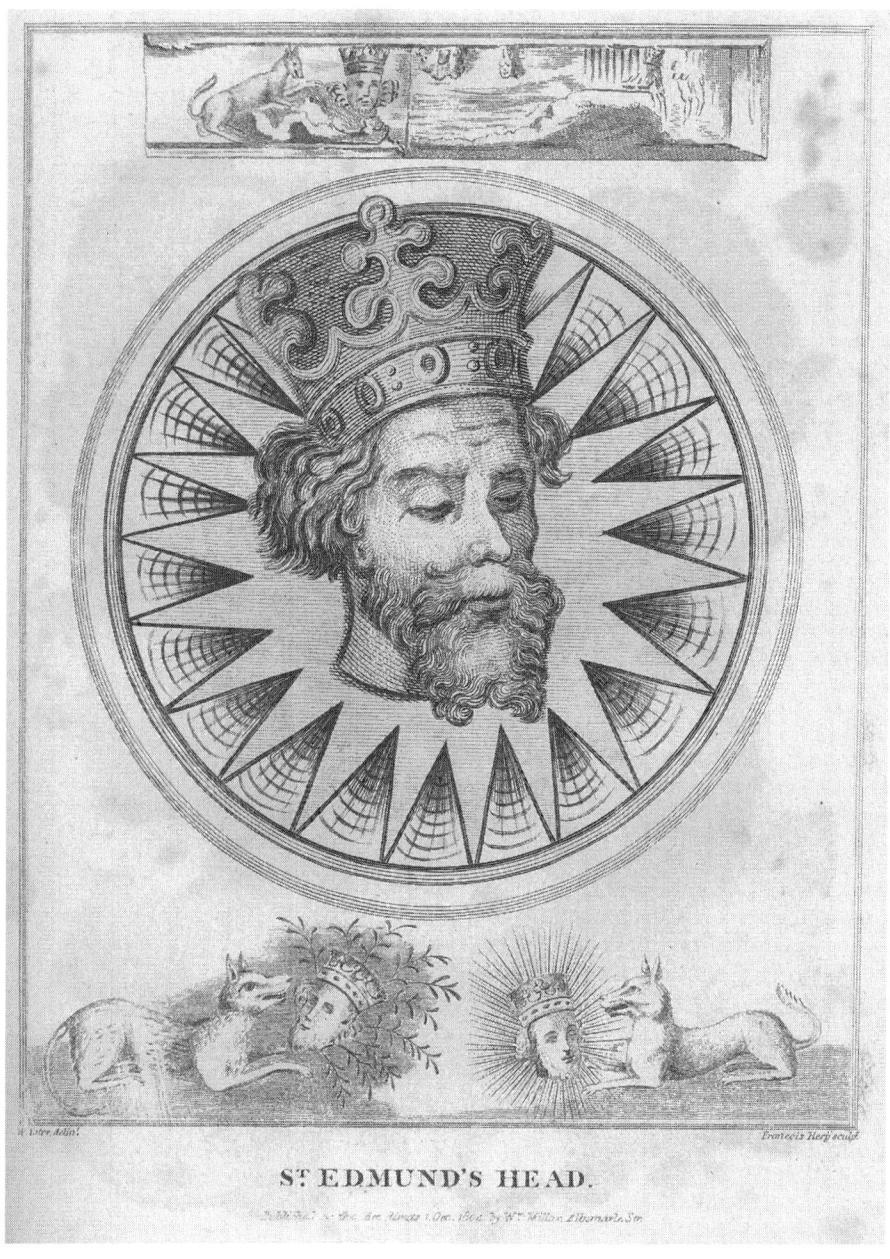

Figure 10 St Edmund's head. Engraving from Richard Yates, *An Illustration of the Monastic Antiquities of the Town and Abbey of St Edmund's Bury* (1843), plate facing p. 44 (depicting a surviving fragment of stained glass from the Abbey).

and privileges in the reign of Edward the Confessor. This chapter examines the historicity of St Edmund and his cult, the early years of the Anglo-Saxon monastery, and the evidence for the first two Abbots of St Edmunds, Ufi (reigned 1020–43) and Leofstan (reigned 1043–65).

St Edmund

Eadmund, King of the East Angles, certainly existed as a historical person – which is more than can be said for some of the saints venerated in medieval monasteries. The sole contemporary evidence for his existence is a series of coins bearing his name and clearly dating, on the basis of style, from the 850s or 860s.[1] A near-contemporary source recording his death was the *Anglo-Saxon Chronicle*, compiled in around 890 (two decades after the events), which simply recorded for the year 870:

> In this year the raiding army rode across Mercia into East Anglia, and took up winter quarters at Thetford. And that winter King Edmund fought against them, and the Danes had the victory, and killed the king and conquered all the land.[2]

The *Anglo-Saxon Chronicle*'s account is so straightforward and without elaboration that most historians accept it as factual.[3] Eadmund died in battle fighting the Danes at Thetford (a strategic location that makes a lot of sense).[4] Rebecca Pinner draws a distinction between the 'chronicle tradition' of St Edmund, which remained more or less unchanged in subsequent chronicles, and the more elaborate hagiographical tradition, which described St Edmund's passion and holy life.[5] On the face of it, it seems more likely that the simple chronicle tradition, recorded nearer in time to the event of Edmund's death, comes closer to the truth. However, St Edmund's earliest hagiographer, Abbo of Fleury, also made strong claims in favour of the historicity of his martyrdom narrative which have been accepted by many historians.[6]

A significant historical gulf separates Eadmund's East Anglia from the world in which the Abbey of Bury St Edmunds came into being. In spite of its status as the symbolic custodian of English national identity, in reality the Abbey depended on the Norse rulers

---

1　Francis Hervey (ed.), *Corolla Sancti Eadmundi: The Garland of Saint Edmund King and Martyr* (London: John Murray, 1907), pp. xiii–xvi.
2　Quoted in Susan J. Ridyard, *The Royal Saints of Anglo-Saxon England: A Study of West Saxon and East Anglian Cults* (Cambridge: Cambridge University Press, 1988), p. 61.
3　On the accuracy of the *Anglo-Saxon Chronicle* see Antonia Gransden, *Historical Writing in England c. 550 to c. 1307* (London: Routledge & Kegan Paul, 1974), vol. 1, p. 39. On the evidence for the historical Eadmund see Dorothy Whitelock, 'Fact and fiction in the legend of St Edmund', *PSIAH* 31 (1970), pp. 217–33; Ridyard (1988), pp. 61–2; Antonia Gransden, 'St Edmund' in *ODNB*, vol. 17, pp. 754–5; Steven Plunkett, *Suffolk in Anglo-Saxon Times* (Stroud: Tempus, 2005), pp. 202–10.
4　The early tradition that Eadmund was killed in battle is also repeated by Asser, the biographer of Alfred the Great, early in the tenth century (Asser, *De Rebus Gestis Alfredi*, extract quoted in Hervey (1907), p. 4).
5　Pinner (2015), p. 5.
6　For a discussion of the evidence for the early hagiographic tradition see ibid., pp. 33–47.

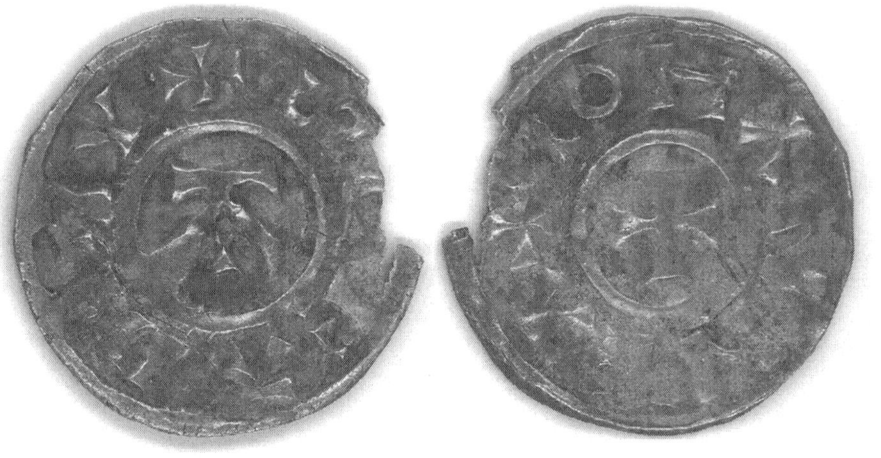

Figure 11 The earliest evidence for a cult of St Edmund: a Danish 'memorial penny' minted c. 890 by the moneyer Iohannea. Photo by the author.

of England – the descendants of Eadmund's slayers – for its very existence. In fact if not in theory, the Abbey was a celebration of the composite identity of the East Anglian people as Anglo-Danes. For at least a century after the Danish defeat of Eadmund's army, monastic life – then the underpinning of a literate culture – was disrupted throughout those areas of England that were part of the Danelaw. The Danish invaders progressively became more English, and even adopted Christianity, yet the founding of monasteries was a major undertaking: it was the business of kings and archbishops, not local communities, and England was still in a period of transition. The age of the seven ancient English kingdoms (the Heptarchy) was over, but England was not yet a unified country.

The intervening period between St Edmund's death and the unification of England by Edward the Elder was truly a 'dark age' as far as East Anglia was concerned. Although we have written sources from Wessex from this period (such as the *Anglo-Saxon Chronicle*), scarcely any sources survive from East Anglia. Again, we are forced to fall back on numismatic evidence in the form of the so-called 'St Edmund memorial coinage', silver pennies deliberately copied from coins issued in Edmund's reign from Danish mints in East Anglia. These (often crude) imitations offer an indication that the Danes had not only accepted Christianity within a few years of St Edmund's death but also felt the need to make some sort of symbolic reparation by venerating the East Anglian king. The coins were certainly minted before 900.[7]

Moving into the tenth century, it seems highly likely that an account by Abbo of Fleury (writing in around 985) recounting how Theodred, bishop of London 942–51,

---

7   On the St Edmund memorial coinage see Eaglen (2006), pp. 13–16; Bale (2009), p. 2; A. Finlay, 'Chronology, genealogy and conversion: the afterlife of St Edmund in the north', in Bale (2009), pp. 45–62, at p. 55.

inspected the incorrupt body of St Edmund, is accurate.[8] Theodred's authentic will, in which the bishop left lands to St Edmund in Norfolk and Suffolk, has survived and proves his interest in the saint. It is hardly surprising that the idea that the body of St Edmund was incorrupt was an early feature of his cult, since two other great Anglian saints were credited with incorruption: St Cuthbert in the Anglian kingdom of Northumbria and the East Anglian princess Æthelthryth (St Etheldreda) at Ely in the Fens. In fact, these three were the only incorrupt Anglo-Saxon saints. In a ninth-century East Anglian world of 'folk Christianity', without literacy or monasteries, the surviving body of the saint was a text that spoke for itself.

There are conflicting accounts of the conditions under which St Edmund's body was preserved and venerated, however. In around 985 Abbo, a monk of the French Abbey of St Denis, visited Ramsey Abbey, where the monks commissioned him to write a life of St Edmund, the *Passio Sancti Edmundi* ('Passion of St Edmund'). This seems to have been the first attempt at a life of the saint, and Abbo provided an impressive pedigree for his story in an effort to make it sound convincing. The account derived from St Dunstan (909–88), Archbishop of Canterbury, to whom it was also dedicated. Dunstan claimed in turn to have heard the story of St Edmund's death from the king's armour bearer, an aged man at the court of King Æthelstan of Wessex, in around 925. Abbo provided a distinctive martyrdom story for St Edmund that remains to this day an inspiration for poets and artists. Whether it has any foundation in fact is another matter.

Abbo gives a brief account of East Anglia before offering a highly conventional description of Edmund's reign that strongly suggests he knew nothing whatsoever about it.[9] He identifies the Danish leaders who invaded East Anglia in 869 as Hinguar and Hubba, who send a messenger to Edmund at a place called Hægelisdun, demanding that the king submit to the invaders. After a lengthy dialogue with an unnamed bishop, in which the bishop argues that Edmund should accept the Danes' terms but Edmund himself declares that he would rather die for his country, Edmund sends a message back to Hinguar in which he refuses to submit unless Hinguar first converts to Christianity.[10] Hinguar, however, is already on the way to Hægelisdun and surrounds the king's house with his guards, taking Edmund prisoner. The king is bound, scourged, tied to a tree and shot with arrows 'like a prickly hedgehog' (*velut asper hericius*); then, when it is discovered that he is still alive, Edmund is beheaded and 'his ribs laid bare by numberless gashes' (*retectis costarum latebris prae punctionibus crebris*).[11] Abbo identified the date of St Edmund's death as 20 November.

After the king's death, the Danes deliberately hide his head in a nearby wood so that his whole body will be denied Christian burial. Sometime later, local Christians return searching for the king's head, and find it when the head itself miraculously calls out 'Here! Here! Here!', guiding them to its true location. The searchers find the head being guarded between the paws of a wolf,[12] and when the head is reunited with the body the two miraculously re-join, leaving only a small red crease on the king's neck. Abbo informs his

---

8   Abbo of Fleury, *Passio Sancti Eadmundi* in Hervey (1907), pp. 6–59, at p. 8.
9   Ibid., pp. 15–17.
10 Ibid., pp. 22–33.
11 Ibid., pp. 33–5.
12 Ibid., pp. 35–43.

readers that St Edmund's body was placed in a 'church built of simple work' (*aedificata vili opera ... basilica*) at the site of his martyrdom, in which the body lay buried for many years (*multis annis requievit humatum*). However, the proliferation of miracles at St Edmund's shrine led the inhabitants to move Edmund to a more prominent location. Accordingly, 'in the royal town that is called in the language of the English *Bedrices-gueord*, and in Latin is called *Bedrici-curtis* they built a very great church, with wood wondrously storeyed'.[13]

Scholars are divided on the truthfulness of Abbo's account. Dorothy Whitelock thought that 'the main facts of the martyrdom are likely to be true'.[14] Norman Scarfe was more cautious in accepting the story of the martyrdom by archers, but thought that 'we need not deny [Edmund] the wounded body and severed head specified by Abbo'.[15] Antonia Gransden has been the most critical of Abbo's story, describing it as 'little more than a hotchpotch of hagiographical commonplaces' and rejecting its historical usefulness entirely.[16] Abbo himself makes clear that he is telling the story at third hand, and there are certain aspects of the story that are clearly the result of the author's elaboration, such as the lengthy exchange between Edmund and the bishop. Elaborations of this kind were acceptable and expected in medieval hagiography.

Abbo's *Passio* is clearly a literary production and needs to be treated as such, and it may well be that one of Abbo's main reasons for writing was to make St Edmund a 'respectable' martyr for a late-tenth-century audience, for whom a heroic death in battle fighting pagans was no longer a guarantee of sanctity in and of itself.[17] Both St Oswald of Northumbria and one of Edmund's own ancestors, St Sigebert of East Anglia, had been venerated as saints after dying in battle, but Abbo grants Edmund a 'set-piece' martyrdom in which the saint has the opportunity to save his life by renouncing Christianity and explicitly refuses this offer. This is perhaps the least historically plausible part of the *Passio*, because there is no evidence that the pagan Danes persecuted Christians for their faith or put pressure on them to renounce Christianity. Rather, they were simply indifferent to Christianity and showed no respect for monasteries, monks and nuns.

On the other hand Abbo does supply some precise pieces of information: the place of St Edmund's martyrdom, for instance, which was also the place where a small chapel was initially built, and a description of the first church at Beodricsworth (the ancient name for Bury St Edmunds) as 'wondrously storeyed in wood'. It seems unlikely that, even if the place where St Edmund died had been forgotten by 985, the site where his body was venerated had been. Abbo was writing over a century after Edmund's death, but probably within living memory of the saint's body being removed to Beodricsworth. Even if Edmund did not really

---

13   Ibid., pp. 42–4: *in villa regia quae lingua Anglorum Bedrices-gueord dicitur, Latina vero Bedrici-curtis vocatur, construxit permaximam miro ligneo tabulatu ecclesiam*. Richard Gem and Laurence Keen translate *permaximam miro ligneo tabulatu ecclesiam* as 'a very large church of wonderful wooden plankwork' ('Late Anglo-Saxon finds from the site of St Edmund's Abbey', *PSIAH* 35 (1981), pp. 1–30, at p. 1).
14   Whitelock (1970), pp. 221–2.
15   Norman Scarfe, 'St Edmund's corpse: defeat into victory', in *Suffolk in the Middle Ages* (Woodbridge: Boydell, 1986), pp. 55–72.
16   Antonia Gransden, 'The legends and traditions concerning the origins of the Abbey of St Edmund', *English Historical Review* 100 (1985), pp. 1–24, at p. 6.
17   On this issue see Carl Phelpstead, 'King, martyr and virgin: *Imitatio Christi* in Ælfric's *Life of St Edmund*', in Bale (2009), pp. 27–44.

die at Hægelisdun, it seems likely that his body was venerated there at some point and a story told of his martyrdom there – why else would Abbo mention this place, otherwise unknown to history? Furthermore, although it may seem implausible that Abbo's account really is based on the eyewitness testimony of Edmund's armour bearer, this does not mean that Dunstan did not really meet the old man at King Æthelstan's court. Dunstan, rather than Abbo, may be the one who was guilty of elaborating the story – something he may have done consciously or unconsciously in the years following his encounter with the armour bearer.[18]

In truth Abbo's *Passio* probably has little to tell us historically about St Edmund himself, but it is informative on the early cult of St Edmund, and therefore on the origins of the monastic community at Beodricsworth. Unfortunately, an alternative account of the disposal of the martyr's body exists in the *De miraculis Sancti Eadmundi* ('On the miracles of St Edmund') written by Hermann the Archdeacon in the late eleventh century.[19] Hermann agreed with Abbo that the place of Edmund's martyrdom was Hægelisdun but identified Edmund's first resting place as Suthtune rather than Hægelisdun itself.[20] This suggests that more than one place may have claimed the distinction of St Edmund's resting-place before Beodricsworth staked its claim. Both Abbo and Hermann agreed, however, that the body soon came to Beodricsworth; when this took place is difficult to pinpoint with any accuracy, but Hermann seems to suggest that it was in the reign of Æthelstan (925–39). Gransden believed that the Feast of the Translation of St Edmund later celebrated in the Abbey on 30 March commemorated the transfer of the martyr's body to Beodricsworth.[21]

The community at Beodricsworth

According to the *Liber Eliensis*, an ancient chronicle of the monastery at Ely, Beodricsworth was the site of a monastery predating the Danish conquest. The *Liber Eliensis* records that some time after his accession (in around 629), St Sigebert, one of the sons of King Rædwald, founded a monastery at 'Betrichesworde' and handed over the government of the kingdom to a relative called Ecgric, while he withdrew to his own foundation.[22] In around 640 the kingdom was menaced by the pagan king of Mercia, Penda, and popular pressure forced Sigebert to leave his monastery and lead his men in battle, but he refused to carry any weapon other than a wooden staff, and was killed. There is no archaeological evidence for a pre-Viking age monastic complex at Bury St Edmunds, but the story of Sigebert's foundation of Beodricsworth is given some support by the existence of a church of St Mary at the time when the body of St Edmund was brought there, as well as by the

---

18 It is also possible, of course, that the armour bearer himself chose to elaborate his tale over the years, or that he was simply lying about being there.
19 Antonia Gransden, 'The cult of St Mary at Beodericsworth and then in Bury St Edmunds Abbey to c. 1150', *Journal of Ecclesiastical History* 55 (2004), pp. 627–53, at p. 627. Gransden argued in 'The composition and authorship of the *De miraculis Sancti Eadmundi* attributed to "Hermann the archdeacon"', *Journal of Medieval Latin* 5 (1995), pp. 33–9 that Hermann was not the author, but this is not universally accepted.
20 Gransden (1974), p. 125. For a version of Hermann's narrative see Hervey (1907), pp. 90–5.
21 Gransden (2004), p. 636.
22 E. O. Blake (ed.), *Liber Eliensis*, Camden 3rd Series 92 (London: Camden Society, 1962), p. 11.

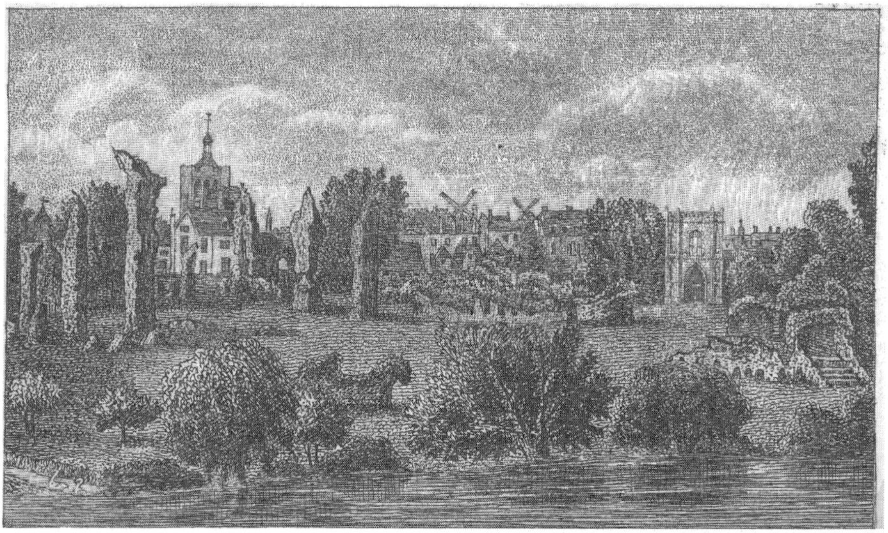

Figure 12 The site of the Abbey viewed from the River Lark. Engraving from Edmund Gillingwater, *An Historical and Descriptive Study of St. Edmund's Bury, in the County of Suffolk* (1804), facing p. 66.

fact that St Mary remained part of the dedication of the Abbey and the cult of the Virgin Mary continued there, suggesting an earlier stratum of Christian cult predating the arrival of St Edmund.[23] Abbo himself described Beodricsworth as a *villa regia*, a term used for sites with a personal association with the East Anglian Wuffing dynasty. The discovery of a fragment of Ipswich ware from the seventh to ninth centuries in the Abbey precincts lends some support to the Sigebert legend.[24]

There is a consensus amongst archaeologists that St Mary's Square (formerly the horsemarket, but referred to as the 'old market' in some fourteenth-century documents) probably represented the centre of an older settlement which was connected to Mustow Street by a road running north–south through the later site of the Abbey. This was the so-called 'great axis', uncovered by Stanley West in excavations of the bowling green behind St Edmundsbury Cathedral in the 1980s, and its existence suggests that Angel Hill and Cornhill developed as central market areas only later.[25] There is some reason, therefore, to suppose that the place to which Edmund's body was brought in the reign of Æthelstan was already hallowed by monastic life in the pre-Viking period, although the original community could not have survived the Danish invasion. Indeed, the very fact that the martyr's body was brought to Beodricsworth could be seen as supporting the idea

---

23 See Gransden (2004), pp. 627–53. Sarah Foot, in *Monastic Life in Anglo-Saxon England, c. 600–900* (Cambridge: Cambridge University Press, 2006), p. 149 suggests Burgh Castle as the site of Sigebert's monastery.
24 Margaret Statham, 'The medieval town of Bury St Edmunds' in Gransden (1998), pp. 98–110, at p. 98.
25 James Bond, *Monastic Landscapes* (Stroud: Tempus, 2003), p. 281. See also Statham (1998), p. 99.

that St Sigebert had already founded a monastery there, apart from the fact that this would be circular reasoning. The location of Hægelisdun remains unknown, but if, as Stanley West argued in the 1980s, it was indeed in the present day parish of Bradfield St George, this was a short and convenient distance from Beodricsworth.[26]

The church of St Mary, of which the present St Mary's church is the symbolic successor even if it does not stand on the original site, would have been a simple wooden structure when St Edmund's body was brought there. The original site of St Mary's church seems to have been under the north transept of the later Abbey Church, since it had to be demolished for Abbot Anselm's expansion of the building in the twelfth century.[27] Abbo tells us that in the early years, the body of St Edmund was attended by a devout woman named Oswin, who trimmed the still-growing hair and fingernails of the martyr, while the church was served by a sort of college of priests. The latter is unsurprising, given the disruption to monastic life during the Danish invasion and the hiatus in ecclesiastical authority.

The intimate involvement of a woman in the early days of the cult of St Edmund is striking, especially since the only other incorrupt Anglo-Saxon male saint (Cuthbert) was notoriously misogynistic, excluding women from the monastic church at Durham altogether. Although Gransden has argued that the motif of a devout woman tending the body of a saint was stereotypical,[28] Abbo makes clear that Oswin was still doing this only a little while before the time when he was writing. It seems unlikely, therefore, that Abbo would have invented a detail that could easily have been confirmed by people still living in the 980s. In the eleventh century, Hermann the Archdeacon reinforced St Edmund's special relationship with women, in contrast to St Cuthbert; some of St Edmund's most famous healings were of women, and he appeared in visions to them as well as to men.[29] There is no reason to suppose that the clerics who originally served the shrine were not married, and even in the monastic period some women lived within the monastic precinct under vows (they were not nuns in the strict sense).[30]

In the late ninth and early tenth centuries a new England was steadily emerging from the chaos of the Danish invasions, dominated by the House of Wessex, the sole surviving English royal dynasty. Furthermore, under the leadership of Dunstan the church was moving towards reform, and Dunstan favoured the proliferation of ordered monastic communities under the Rule of St Benedict which could replace unregulated clergy, such as the priests who cared for the body of St Edmund. In later centuries, the Abbey claimed that Edmund I of England (921–46) granted a charter to the community at Beodricsworth in 945, and historical opinion is divided on whether the charter of King Edmund preserved in the Abbey was a forgery or not. Gransden, while not committing herself to the authenticity of the charter, considered that 'Possibly the earliest royal benefactor of the community at Beodricesworth was King Edmund.'[31] The charter

---

26 Stanley West, 'A new site for the martyrdom of St Edmund', *PSIAH* 35 (1983), pp. 223–5.
27 Statham (1998), pp. 99–100.
28 Gransden (1985), p. 7.
29 Antonia Gransden, 'Baldwin, Abbot of Bury St Edmunds, 1065–1097', *Proceedings of the Battle Conference on Anglo-Norman Studies* 4 (1981), pp. 65–76, at pp. 73–4.
30 Elisabeth van Houts, 'The women of Bury St Edmunds', in Tom Licence (ed.), *Bury St Edmunds and the Norman Conquest* (Woodbridge: Boydell Press, 2014), pp. 53–73, at p. 53.
31 Gransden (1985), p. 12.

was probably fabricated, but it may have grown out of an authentic tradition of royal patronage.³²

Cyril Hart and Anthony Syme considered the 945 charter genuine, partly on the grounds that it correctly specified the later boundaries of the *banleuca* of the Abbey.³³ The *banleuca* (literally 'suburbs') was a territory surrounding the town, demarcated by four crosses on the roads in and out of Bury, within which the Abbot later exercised 'regalian rights' – full sovereign authority, in modern terms. No official of the king or the bishop of Norwich could enter the *banleuca* without the Abbot's consent, and when one did so he was compelled to surrender his royal or episcopal marks of authority. Until 1934, when Bury began to expand into the parishes of Fornham All Saints and Westley, the *banleuca* marked the boundary of the modern town as well.³⁴ Unfortunately the presence of the *banleuca* in King Edmund's charter may serve to demonstrate the opposite of what Hart and Syme intended, because it suggests that a monastic forger was projecting back onto the tenth century a territory that existed in the eleventh.

Nevertheless, it seems likely that lesser grants of land to the collegiate community at Beodricsworth (although technically the grants are directly to St Edmund himself) from the tenth century are genuine. The will of Theodred, bishop of London has already been mentioned; other grants included the gift of Cockfield by Ælfgar, the father of King Edmund's queen Æthelflæd, and Edmund's son Eadwig's grant of Beccles and Elmswell in 955–57.³⁵ In her will, Æthelflæd left Chelsworth to St Edmund, and the community received the bequest in 1002.³⁶ Hart and Syme argued that the preservation of charters at Beodricsworth in the tenth century shows that the foundation there was already monastic in some sense, and that the community at Beodricsworth may have become a 'satellite' of Ramsey Abbey by the end of the tenth century. Ramsey was known for 'its propensity for collecting together a small empire of satellite houses', and Ramsey's acquisition of four estates very close to the *banleuca* – Horningsheath, Lawshall, Risby and Hawstead – suggested to Hart and Syme that Ramsey took over Beodricsworth. Furthermore, the wills of both Æthelflæd and her father Ælfgar show that the family intended to found a monastery at Stoke-by-Nayland,³⁷ which would make more sense if Benedictine monks were already established at nearby Beodricsworth who could staff the new monastery.

The last years of the tenth century and the early years of the eleventh were a time of almost unimaginable instability and chaos throughout England. It began in 991 with the defeat of Ealdorman Byrhtnoth by a Danish army at Maldon in Essex; regular Danish raids continued thereafter, and in 1002 King Æthelræd (known to history as 'Ethelred the Unready') ordered the slaughter of all Danes in the kingdom in what became known as the St Brice's Day Massacre. The Danish king Sweyn Forkbeard replied with an invasion of England, focusing on East Anglia, in 1003. Even though the Danes were Christians by

---

32 For a discussion of this charter see Foot (2014), pp. 47–8.
33 Cyril Hart and Anthony Syme, 'The earliest Suffolk charter', *PSIAH* 36 (1987), pp. 165–81, at p. 165.
34 Statham (1996), p. 11.
35 Hart and Syme (1987), p. 169.
36 Ibid., p. 171.
37 Ibid., p. 165.

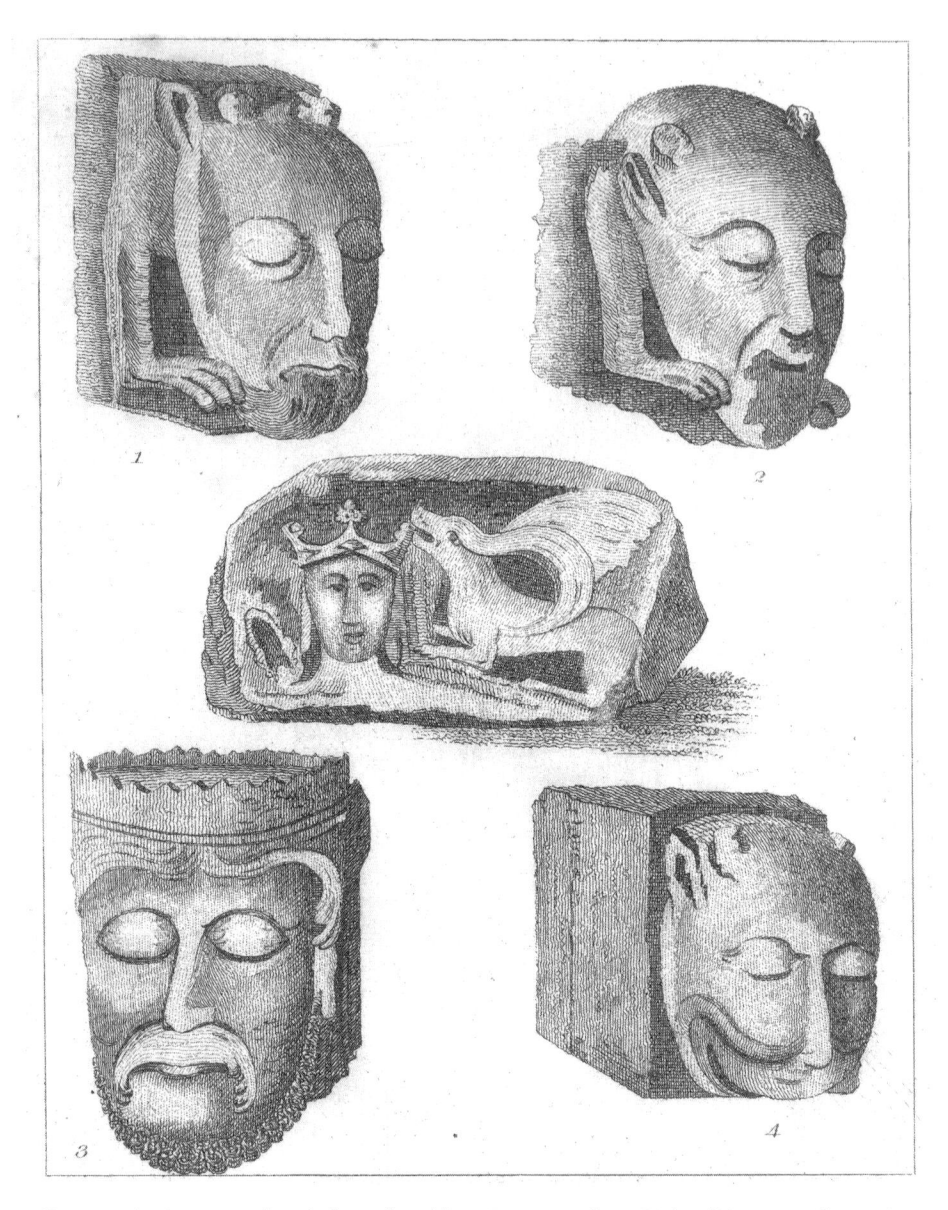

Figure 13 Ancient stone heads from the Abbey. Engraving from Richard Yates, *An Illustration of the Monastic Antiquities of the Town and Abbey of St Edmund's Bury* (1843), facing p. 43.

this date, the community at Beodricsworth would have lived on a knife edge, fearing the sacking of their church and the desecration of the shrine of the martyr at any moment. In 1010 the community made the decision to entrust the body of the saint to the sacrist Æthelwine (called Aylwin or Egelwin in later sources), the first named member of the community at Bury St Edmunds to enter history. Æthelwine was to take the body to London for safekeeping, where it lay for three years in the church of St Gregory, next to

St Paul's Cathedral, until its return in 1013.[38] It was during this peregrination of the body that St Edmund lay at Greenstead in Essex.

The turmoil of raids and invasions showed no sign of abatement, however, and in 1013 Sweyn invaded England for a second time. The Danish king seemed unstoppable, but it was Sweyn's second invasion that gave rise to what was probably the most famous – and frightening – of all the miracles attributed to St Edmund. Sweyn heard that the men of Beodricsworth, on account of the privileges of St Edmund, were exempt from taxation. He swore to impose his taxes on them, and shortly thereafter, while sitting down to eat in front of his thegns, he saw the apparition of St Edmund advancing towards him with a spear that pierced his heart. Sweyn died on 3 February 1014, supposedly a victim of the wrath of the saint and his jealous guardianship of his privileges.[39]

Sweyn's death resulted in a short-lived restoration of Æthelræd, but Sweyn's son Cnut (better known to history by his Latinised name Canute) invaded in 1015. On 18 October 1016 Æthelræd's son, Edmund Ironside, engaged Cnut in battle at Assandun in Essex. Edmund was defeated, and Cnut was crowned King of the English at Christmas 1016. A Dane was finally on the throne of England, but Cnut was a Christian keen to expiate the misdeeds of his pagan forebears and to forge a common Anglo-Danish identity, especially in the old Danelaw. According to tradition, within a few years of his successful conquest Cnut turned his attention to the foundation of a Benedictine monastery at the shrine of his father's supernatural enemy, St Edmund.

The 'foundation' of the Benedictine Abbey

Exactly how the church housing the body of St Edmund became a Benedictine monastery in the first quarter of the eleventh century remains obscure. Even the foremost historical authority on the Abbey, Antonia Gransden, changed her mind on the subject at least once. According to the traditional account, which was universally believed by the monks themselves throughout the Middle Ages, in the year 1020 King Cnut refounded St Edmunds as an abbey of Benedictine monks by royal charter, on the advice of Bishop Ælfwine of Elmham, a former monk of Ely. However, the earliest source for this story is an account by Hermann the Archdeacon, writing at the very end of the eleventh century, and the surviving 'copy' of the charter from Cnut preserved by the Abbey contains a suspicious clause exempting the Abbey from the jurisdiction of the bishop. It is highly unlikely that a charter issued in 1020 would have contained such a clause, because a dispute over episcopal jurisdiction in relation to the Abbey only developed in the 1070s.[40]

The traditional story of the Abbey's foundation also has it that the first Abbot of St Edmunds was Ufi, Prior of St Benedict's, Holme (or Hulme) in Norfolk, and that he presided over a group of twenty-six monks taken from Hulme and Ely. Unfortunately, this story is first recorded in the fourteenth century, and Gransden thought it unlikely that a monastery as obscure as St Benedict's, Holme in the faraway Norfolk Broads would have played a founda-

---

38   Scarfe (1986), p. 59.
39   Ibid., p. 55. Gransden has argued that this story may have been invented after the Norman Conquest at the instigation of Abbot Baldwin, keen to preserve the Abbey's privileges against the Normans (Gransden (1981), p. 68).
40   Gransden (1985), pp. 10–11.

tional role in the establishment of St Edmunds. The idea of monks coming from nearby Ely (a well-established Anglo-Saxon minster) is more plausible, but Gransden argued instead that the most likely founder-monastery for St Edmunds was the Abbey of St Benedict at Ramsey, which was an extremely powerful and influential monastery in the Benedictine reform of the late tenth and early eleventh centuries. In Gransden's view, the attribution of the foundation to St Benedict's, Holme was a mistake (perhaps deliberate) for St Benedict's, Ramsey.[41]

Gransden's case for identifying Ramsey as the founder-monastery of St Edmunds rested on circumstantial rather than direct evidence. In the first place, we know that the monks of Ramsey commissioned Abbo of Fleury to compose his *Passio Sancti Eadmundi*, the single most important hagiography of the saint, during his visit to Ramsey in the 980s. It is unclear why Ramsey would have been so concerned to ensure the veneration of a saint whose shrine was located so far away – unless, of course, St Edmunds was already a dependent priory of Ramsey Abbey at that date. On this interpretation the secular priests at Beodricsworth were replaced by monks at an early date, and the real significance of the eleventh-century 'foundation' was that St Edmunds went from the status of a dependent priory to that of a powerful independent abbey. Gransden theorised that this transformation was brought about, at least in part, by the disruption of religious life by Danish invasions in the early tenth century. The Abbot of Ramsey was killed at the Battle of Assandun in 1016, and the umbilical cord between Ramsey and St Edmunds was broken. Relying on the reputation of St Edmund alone, St Edmunds was able to make its own way as a significant pilgrimage centre and abbey.

Gransden held this view in the 1980s, but by 2004, apparently persuaded by the arguments of Simon Keynes, she had shifted to believing that the association with St Benedict's, Holme might have some basis in fact. She noted that the Bury St Edmunds Psalter in the Vatican Library (MS Reg. Lat. 12) which may date from as early as 1050, contains a note next to a liturgical table for the years 1020–24 to the effect that 'Bishop Ælfwine, under Earl Thorkil and at the wish and with the permission of King Cnut established the regular rule in St Edmund's monastery'.[42] Although this throws no further light on where the monks came from it, it does show that the bishop of Elmham was involved in the foundation, and therefore makes a transplantation of monks from St Benedict's, Holme more likely. However, Gransden continued to maintain that Ramsey was involved in the foundation, on the grounds that the aged abbot of Ramsey, Ælfwine (1043–80), was called upon in 1070 to testify that St Edmunds had enjoyed its special privileges in the reign of Cnut.[43] It also seems unlikely that the first Abbot, Ufi, was entirely a fictional creation, as his tomb was located in front of the altar of St Benedict in the infirmary – which was the site of the Anglo-Saxon church of St Benedict.[44]

The charter of Cnut allegedly founding the Abbey in 1020 may not be altogether fabricated, and Gransden suggested that one part of the document, containing 'the grant of fish due annually to Canute, a fishery, and all rights from pleas in the vills owned by St

---

41 Ibid., pp. 15–19.
42 Gransden (2004), pp. 632–3. On the Bury St Edmunds Psalter see William Noel, 'The lost Canterbury prototype of the 11th-century Bury St Edmunds Psalter' in Gransden (1998), pp. 161–71.
43 Gransden (2004), p. 632.
44 James (1895), p. 147.

Edmund's, and the confirmation of Queen Emma's gift of 4000 eels a year' may be genuine.[45] In other words, Cnut did grant some sort of charter to St Edmunds, but whether this was truly a foundation charter or a more limited confirmation of grants and liberties is unclear. Part of the problem may be that canon law (the law of the church) was highly developed in the later Middle Ages and therefore the monks read back on a much earlier period the legal expectations of their own age. A monastery as great as St Edmunds could not afford to be without a clear history, and as the example of Abbot Baldwin will show, the medieval clergy adopted a liberal attitude to the systematic forgery of documents.

The first Abbey buildings

The first event associated with the Abbey that can be dated with certainty is the consecration of the church of St Mary and St Edmund by Bishop Æthelnoth of Elmham on 18 October 1032, although the monks actually celebrated the Feast of the Minster of St Edmund annually on 11 October.[46] This new stone church replaced the church of St Mary, 'wondrously storeyed in wood', in which the body of St Edmund had been placed in the reign of Æthelstan. It is possible that the old church burned down or was somehow destroyed by accident, because it did not need to be demolished in order to make way for the new church. The language used in the key document describing the events is ambiguous: *destructa basilica antiqua et lignea clericorum, coepit idem episcopus construere nouam* ('with the old wooden basilica of the clerics having been destroyed, the same bishop [i.e. Ælfric] began a new one').[47] Eric Fernie, however, has argued that the wooden church might have continued to exist, with the new stone rotunda attached, since according to the *Gesta sacristarum* a wooden church had to be knocked down when work began on Baldwin's minster in the 1090s.[48]

Gransden believed that the stone church was begun under the auspices of Ælfric, bishop of Elmham, the immediate founder of the Abbey according to the Bury St Edmunds Psalter in the Vatican Library. This new church was a circular *martyrium* or rotunda surrounded by an ambulatory. Suffolk's Anglo-Saxon round-towered churches are well known, but no round churches from this period now survive, although other examples once existed at Abingdon and Canterbury. Gransden has argued that the rotunda at Bury was inspired by three models: the round church outside Jerusalem supposed to contain the tomb of the Virgin Mary, the mausoleum-church of the Emperor Charlemagne at Aachen, and above all, the Church of the Holy Sepulchre in Jerusalem.[49]

Round churches were associated with tombs of the saints and of Christ himself, but they were also associated with imperial power. Charlemagne's rotunda at Aachen was as much inspired by the Emperor Constantine's round church of the Holy Apostles in Constantinople as it was by the Holy Sepulchre.[50] It is possible that the decision to translate St Edmund to

---

45 Gransden (1985), p. 11.
46 Hervey (1907), p. 642.
47 Oxford, Bodleian Library, MS Bodley 240 quoted in Eric Fernie, 'Baldwin's church and the effects of the Conquest', in Licence (2014), pp. 74–93, at p. 74.
48 Fernie (2014), p. 75.
49 Gransden (2004), pp. 637–8.
50 John Freely and Ahmet S. Çakmak, *Byzantine Monuments of Istanbul* (Cambridge: Cambridge

a round basilica was influenced by the longstanding pretensions of the East Anglian royal house to *Romanitas*, as suggested in the seventh and eighth centuries by the appearance of Romulus and Remus on the coins of Æthelberht II, the design of the Larling Plaque, and the inclusion of Byzantine artefacts in the Sutton Hoo ship burial. The rotunda could have symbolically served the dual purposes of *martyrium* and royal mausoleum of the East Anglian royal house, effectively supplanting the old pagan barrows of Sutton Hoo.

Fragments of stonework that may have been from the rotunda were discovered during excavations by the Ministry of Works in 1959–64, which cleared out Abbot Baldwin's crypt. This was full of rubble from parts of the choir that collapsed into the crypt after 1539, and contained even more ancient stonework which had been used as 'core material' (rubble infill that was then faced with stone). The reason that the Abbey ruins look as they do today is because the facing stone was stripped away, leaving the rubble core as a free-standing structure. Amongst the rubble was found a series of small 'moulded balusters', miniature columns crudely copied from Roman models which are characteristic of Anglo-Saxon architecture. Although it is impossible to determine exactly where these came from, they are certainly of eleventh-century date and we would expect to find the rotunda decorated with balusters, perhaps framing the windows or even supporting the shrine of St Edmund itself.[51] My own view is that if the balusters were part of the infill used in the choir, they were rubble from the demolition of the outer ambulatory of the rotunda, which had to be knocked down to accommodate Baldwin's huge minster.

Gransden theorised that, since the Abbey celebrated the Feast of the Translation of St Edmund to the new church on 31 March, the martyr's body may have been relocated to the rotunda on 31 March 1034, which was a Sunday.[52] Within a few years, the church of St Mary and St Edmund was joined by the basilica of St Benedict, which lay 30 metres north-east of the rotunda, closer to the river. St Benedict's comprised a 'great tower' and a portico, and consisted of bays divided by stone piers. Its primary function seems to have been as a mausoleum for the abbots, although the infirm son of the donor of the building, Ælfric, lived for a while in the tower.[53]

During this period it is likely that the high street of the town still passed through the Abbey precincts, linking the present Sparhawk Street to Northgate Street on the other side of the Abbey.[54] There were two churches on the east side of the street with the river behind them: the rotunda of St Mary and St Edmund, and St Benedict to the north-east. Perhaps we should imagine the Abbey in its earliest phase as a rather ramshackle collection of buildings, not strictly separated by a precinct wall from the straggle of houses along the River Lark (then called Ulnoth's River) which was Beodricsworth/Bury St Edmunds. The multiplication of smaller churches around a monastic centre was unusual in both England and France, and the continuation of this pattern under Abbot Baldwin suggested to David Bates a conscious imitation of St Denis.[55]

University Press, 2004), pp. 32–5.
51 Gem and Keen (1981), pp. 3–26.
52 Gransden (2004), p. 637.
53 Gem and Keen (1981), p. 2.
54 Statham (1996), pp. 11–12.
55 David Bates, 'The Abbey and the Norman Conquest: an unusual case?' in Licence (2014), pp. 5–21, p. 10.

Abbot Leofstan, c. 1043–65

If Abbot Ufi's existence cannot be established with certainty, the first historical Abbot of St Edmunds was Leofstan, whose appointment seems to have coincided with the most important of all bequests to the Abbey, a gift so significant that it would continue to affect the history of Suffolk even long after the dissolution. In 1043 or 1044 Edward the Confessor granted eight-and-a-half hundreds of the county of Suffolk to St Edmund: Thingoe, Thedwastre, Blackbourn, Bradmore (later merged with Blackbourn), Lackford, Risbridge, Babergh (a double hundred) and Cosford (a half hundred).[56] This territory, which comprised the entire western half of Suffolk, would thenceforward be known as the Liberty of St Edmund. The charter granting this territory is generally considered authentic:

> King Edward sends friendly greetings to Bishop Grimketel and Ælfwine and Ælfric and all my thegns in Suffolk. And I inform you that the land at Mildenhall and the sokes of the eight and a half hundreds pertaining to Thingoe shall belong to St Edmund's with sake and soke as fully and completely as my mother possessed it. And I will not permit anyone to take away from them any of the things that I have already granted to them.[57]

Edward's charter fixed the political geography of Suffolk for almost a thousand years. Even after the dissolution in 1539 this territory continued to exist as a legal and administrative unit, and was often called the 'Franchise of Bury'. In 1874 it formally became an administrative county in its own right, West Suffolk. In 1974 the Local Government Act finally abolished West Suffolk, an event commemorated by Elizabeth Frink's bronze statue of St Edmund in front of the ruined west front of the Abbey.

As the charter indicated, the Liberty predated King Edward's gift and had previously belonged to his mother Emma. It may have been even older, given that the ceremonial centre of this 'little shire' was a hill within the *banleuca* of Bury St Edmunds, Thingoe Hill (now sadly cut in half by the A14). It is conceivable that a *thing* (an Anglo-Saxon parliamentary gathering) had assembled on Thingoe Hill in pre-Christian times. Edward also gave the Abbey the manors of Mildenhall, Pakenham and Coney Weston as well as Kirby Cane in Norfolk, and around the same time the nobleman Ælfric Modercope endowed the Abbey with Loddon in Norfolk.

The king exempted the Liberty of St Edmund from *heregeld* (a tax to pay for mercenaries in the army and navy) and all other direct taxation, as well as granting St Edmunds the right to 'the six forfeitures'. These were judicial privileges (pleas of the crown) usually enjoyed by the king but here enjoyed by the Abbot, and which included the right to receive outlaws.[58] In other words, outlaws in the Liberty were at the mercy of the Abbot rather than the king. This was the beginning of the judicial independence of the Abbey, which would lead eventually to the Abbot exercising the powers of sheriff within the

---

56 Gransden (1981), p. 66. A hundred was, at least in theory, an area that could provide a hundred armed men in time of war.
57 Quoted in Eaglen (2006), p. 24.
58 F. W. Maitland, *Domesday Book and Beyond: Three Essays in the Early History of England*, 2nd edn (Cambridge: Cambridge University Press, 1987), pp. 88–9.

Liberty, as well as having the right to appoint his own justices. Indeed, a chief justice of the Liberty of St Edmund continued to be appointed after the dissolution, and assizes took place at Bury until they were abolished under the Courts Act 1971.

A market already existed at Bury in 1043, but Edward granted an even more important economic privilege to the Abbey: the right to mint coins. Although no copy survives of the original grant, coins of the 'Small Flan type' of Edward the Confessor, an issue struck between 1048 and 1050, are the earliest minted at Bury. All were struck by the same moneyer (the manager of the mint), Morcere (his name was sometimes spelled Marcere, Morcare or Morcre).[59] However, since only thirty coins minted at Bury in Edward's reign survive, Robin Eaglen has concluded that 'the mint of the abbot of Bury St Edmunds was of minor significance and may well have been mainly employed for his own monetary needs'.[60] Possession of a mint meant that the king's silver was brought to the Abbey in order to be struck into coins of standard weight, but it is probable that the Abbot deducted a proportion of silver as a fee before minting began. This was balanced to some extent by a fee charged by the king every time a new die was issued to the Abbey.[61] The grant of a mint in around 1048, however small, was a mark of the great trust shown in Leofstan by the king.[62] Another mark of the Abbey's significance was the fact that in 1047 Edward chose a Bury monk named Spearhafoc ('Sparrowhawk), renowned as a craftsman in gold and silver, as abbot of Abingdon.[63]

According to one story, Leofstan once visited Rome and stopped at Lucca either on the way there or the way back. He was impressed by the *Volto Santo* ('Holy Face') of Lucca, an ancient cross in the cathedral there, and commissioned a facsimile which he brought back with him to Bury. This was later placed in the Chapel of St Peter at the far east end of the apse of Baldwin's minster, which was thereafter known as the Chapel of the Cross.[64] Another of Leofstan's supposed achievements was to have translated the bodies of St Jurmin and St Botolph to the Abbey Church. St Jurmin was discovered buried in a lead coffin at Grundisburgh, and was reputedly a brother of St Etheldreda, martyred by pagans in the seventh century. The body of St Botolph was discovered at Blythburgh, but whereas Jurmin was uniquely venerated at Bury, there were several claims on the body of St Botolph.[65] Two other local saints whose relics were reputedly held by the Abbey were Anna, the cousin and successor of King Sigebert, and Anna's son Firminus, both of whom were also translated from Blythburgh to Bury.[66]

---

59 Eaglen (2006), pp. 36–8.
60 Ibid., p. 39.
61 Ibid., p. 33.
62 The location of the mint is disputed. One suggested location is behind the guest hall, which was roughly where the garden of the Cathedral Library is now, to the south of the Abbey Gate; another suggestion is that the mint was next to the sacristy, at the south-east corner of the Abbey Church. A writ of 1329 has the mint located outside the Abbey precincts in Mustow Street (Eaglen (2006), p. 207).
63 John Blair, 'Spearhafoc (*fl.* 1047–1051), abbot of Abingdon' in *ODNB*, 51, pp. 761–2.
64 James (1895), p. 139. In reality, it is far more likely that the cross was commissioned by Baldwin, who certainly visited Lucca.
65 Gransden (2009), pp. 112–13. Richard Hoggett in *The Archaeology of the East Anglian Conversion* (Woodbridge: Boydell, 2010), p. 48 notes that, according to another tradition, Cnut ordered Botolph's body to be moved from Grundisburgh to Beodricesworth in 1020.
66 Yates (1843), p. 21. M. R. James noted that 'Firminus' was probably just a misspelling of

Edward the Confessor had a personal devotion to St Edmund, who was England's principal royal saint, and when he visited the Abbey he dismounted from his horse and walked the last mile to the monastery on foot. Edward also referred to St Edmund, inaccurately, as his 'kinsman'.[67] However, there is some evidence to suggest that the shrine of St Edmund was not as popular at this time as it would later become. According to Hermann, a dumb woman from Winchester named Ælfgeth, who had come to the shrine seeking healing, received a vision of St Edmund in which the saint complained that his tomb was covered in spiders, cobwebs and flies.[68] As a consequence of Ælfgeth's miraculous healing, and the message she had received from St Edmund, Abbot Leofstan decided to open the shrine for cleaning, but took the opportunity to check whether the body of the saint really was incorrupt. According to Hermann, a monk called 'Egelwin', who was really Æthelwine, the sacristan of the original community who had taken the body of St Edmund to London in 1010, recognised a cross around the holy body and confirmed that it really was the saint.

Leofstan then decided to test whether the body of St Edmund had miraculously united with the saint's head, as Abbo of Fleury had written. Taking the head while another monk, Thurstan, took the feet, Leofstan pulled and the body came towards him, showing that the head was indeed firmly attached. However, Leofstan was instantly paralysed as a divine punishment for his impiety, and was struck blind and dumb. The celebrated monk-physician Baldwin, who would later succeed Leofstan as Abbot, managed to cure Leofstan's deafness and blindness but his hands remained palsied, as a warning to others against sacrilege.[69]

Gransden was very suspicious of this episode. If the man who took the body of St Edmund to London in 1010 was still alive after 1043, he would have been a very young sacristan when his community entrusted him with such an important task. The fact that Abbo recorded the story of a proud thegn called Leofstan who was paralysed after demanding to see the body may have given rise to the story of Abbot Leofstan's paralysis. It is possible that this story was included by Hermann, who was writing under Baldwin, in order to portray his French patron in a good light and throw suspicion on his English predecessor.[70]

According to tradition, the reinstallation of St Edmund in his restored shrine took place on 9 June, when the monks celebrated the Feast of the Representation of St Edmund,[71] but the year of this event is impossible to determine. One document that gives a contemporary glimpse of Leofstan and his community is a note in an eleventh-century manuscript of the Rule of St Benedict at Corpus Christi College, Oxford, which is an inventory of the books and other items in the possession of Bury monks. Rather unusually, the list is in Old English rather than Latin:

Jurmin rather than a separate person (M. R. James, *Suffolk and Norfolk: A Perambulation of the Two Counties with Notices of their History and their Ancient Buildings* (London: J. M. Dent & Sons, 1930), pp. 12–13).
67 Gransden (1981), p. 66.
68 Ibid., p. 67.
69 Irina Metzler, *Disability in Medieval Europe: Thinking About Physical Impairment During the High Middle Ages, c. 1100–1400* (Abingdon: Routledge, 2006), p. 147.
70 Gransden (1981), p. 73.
71 Hervey (1907), p. 641.

Leofstan found ten books in the church, viz. four Christ's book and one mass book and one epistle book and one psalter and one gospel book and one *capitularia* and St Edmund's *vita*[72] in *madinhus* [the vestry?] twelve mass vestments etc. Also four screens, fourteen roods. Blakere has one winter reading book, Brihtric has one mass chalice and dish (i.e. paten) and one mass book and winter reading book and summer book. Smerdus has a mass chalice and a mass book and Leofstan a hand book. Ætheric has a mass book and *capitularia*, Thurstan a psalter. Oskytel has a mass chalice and a mass book and an *Ad te levavi*.[73]

The same document gives an insight into the Abbey's landholdings at this time, listing rents from farms held by the Abbey at Worlingworth, Palgrave, Redgrave, Rickinghall, Burton, Rougham, Elmswell, Cockfield, Whepstead, Horningsheath, Lackford, Culford and Fornham. At this time the Abbey gathered its rent in foodstuffs rather than money.[74]

This note, written by Leofstan himself in the third person, indicates that at this early date books were owned by individual monks rather than by the monastery. It is worth noting that the mention of a monk called Thurstan in this contemporary document supports the story of Leofstan's sacrilegious treatment of St Edmund's body, in which the monk who held St Edmund's feet had this name. Although Hermann may well have fabricated the connection between Leofstan's palsy and his punishment for sacrilege, it seems likely that Leofstan really did suffer from a disease, and that rumour or conjecture connected it with the opening of St Edmund's tomb. Although Hermann may have exaggerated Leofstan's behaviour when the tomb was opened, it is not difficult to imagine that a mixture of curiosity and piety could have motivated Leofstan to investigate the shrine and handle the body.

---

72 Presumably Abbo of Fleury's *Passio Sancti Eadmundi*, perhaps Lambeth Palace MS 362 which contains a mass of St Edmund and might therefore have been kept in the sacristy of the Abbey Church (see Gransden (2004), p. 638).
73 James (1895), p. 5.
74 D. C. Douglas, 'Fragments of an Anglo-Saxon survey from Bury St Edmunds', *English Historical Review* 43 (1928), pp. 376–83.

Chapter 2
The Golden Age: from Baldwin to Anselm, 1065–1148

The election in 1065 as Abbot of Bury St Edmunds of the French monk Baldwin, who was Edward the Confessor's personal physician, was critical to the Abbey's survival during the Norman Conquest. In comparison with other English abbeys, Bury emerged unscathed from this momentous historical change; indeed, some historians have argued that Baldwin transformed St Edmunds from a relatively obscure regional monastery into an institution of national importance. The last three decades of the century saw East Anglia's Norman bishops challenge the privileges of St Edmunds Abbey with increasing confidence, but Baldwin took them on and defeated them every time. Yet there was a price to pay. Bury St Edmunds escaped the dubious distinction of becoming East Anglia's cathedral city, but the fight over episcopal jurisdiction led the supporters of both sides to forge numerous documents relating to the Abbey's early history. In doing so, they compromised later attempts to recover that history with any certainty.

Baldwin's achievements were not only political, however; he was the most important builder in the Abbey's history, having begun the great Abbey Church that endured until the dissolution, and he may also have been responsible for the foundation of a medical school at Bury. Baldwin has also been credited with laying out the grid plan of Bury St Edmunds. He certainly extended the town westwards from Angel Hill, creating present-day Cornhill and the Buttermarket. As Bury's longest-serving Abbot (he ruled for 32 years), Baldwin has a strong claim to be considered the founder of the town of Bury St Edmunds in its present form. He was an astute manager who exploited three traditional sources of funding for a monastery – revenue from pilgrims, income from estates and royal patronage – to the fullest possible extent. By the end of Baldwin's reign, it would have been hard to guess that Bury had been a relative latecomer among eleventh-century English monasteries.

Abbot Baldwin and the Norman Conquest, 1065–97

The circumstances in which Baldwin became Abbot were most unusual for the time. Baldwin was a native of Chartres and had been a monk of the great French royal abbey of St Denis before serving as Prior of Leberau (Lièpvre), a dependent priory of St Denis in Alsace. At an unknown date Baldwin travelled to England and became the royal physician of Edward the Confessor. Edward rewarded him for his services by presenting him with the church of Deerhurst in Gloucestershire (which, as one of England's best-preserved Anglo-Saxon churches, still looks much as it did in Baldwin's day), the manor of Taynton

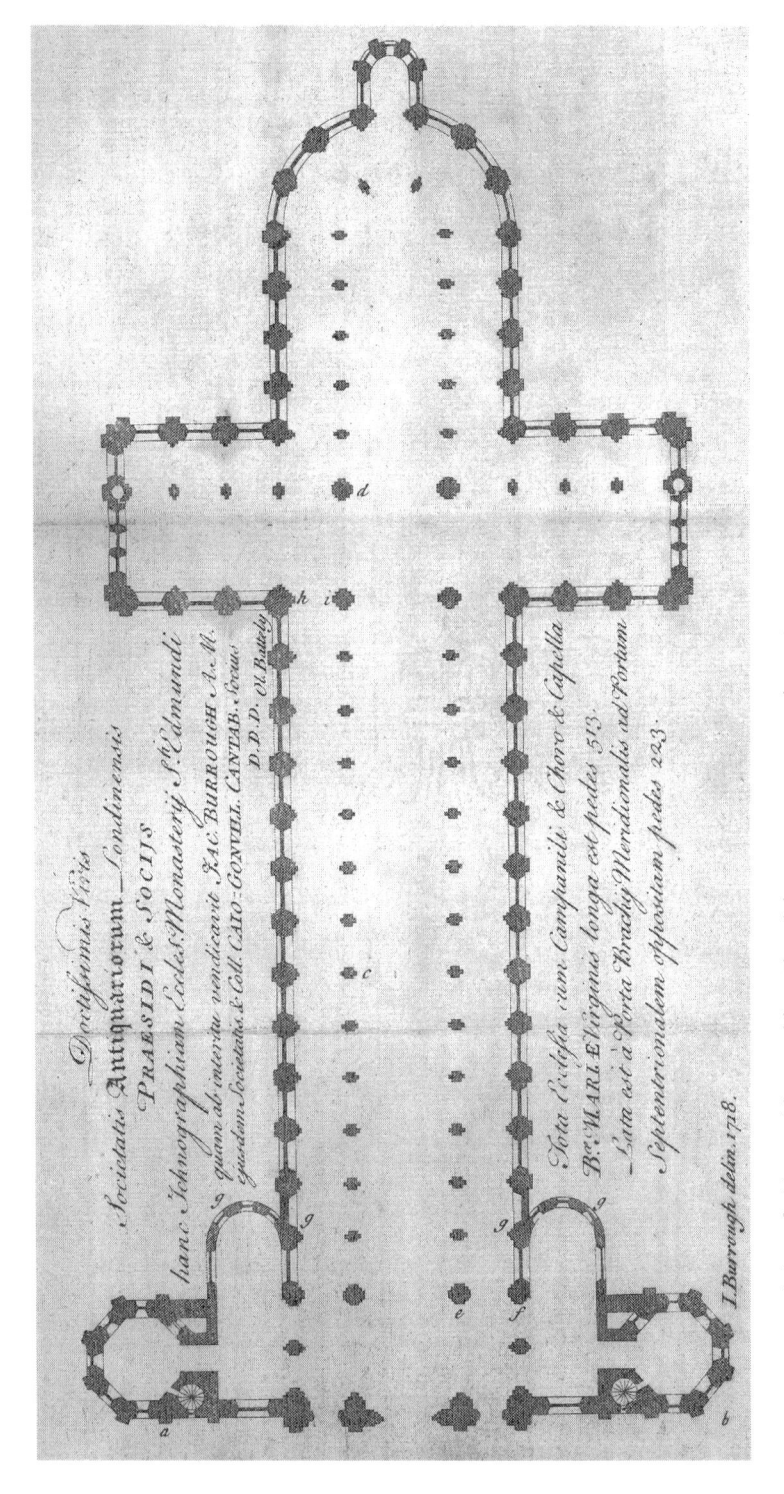

Figure 14 Ground plan of Abbot Baldwin's Abbey Church by Sir James Burrough (1718). Engraving from John Battely, *Antiquitates Sancti Edmundi* (1745), plate facing p. 164.

in Oxfordshire and, on 16 July 1065, the Abbey of St Edmunds.[1] However, as David Bates has shown, Deerhurst and Taynton were not personal gifts to Baldwin but gifts to the Abbey of St Denis, for which Baldwin acted as a sort of agent in England.[2]

Baldwin was the first foreigner to be appointed abbot of an English monastery, and at the time of the Battle of Hastings the following year he was the only senior French cleric in the country. However, within a short while the majority of the English bishops and abbots were replaced by Normans, Frenchmen and Bretons. Baldwin was therefore (albeit unwittingly) in the vanguard of a huge cultural shift that arguably occurred in Bury before it happened anywhere else. Christopher de Hamel has observed that St Edmunds was 'a relatively minor late Anglo-Saxon foundation, which benefitted enormously from the Norman Conquest', and noted that, by the time of the Domesday survey in 1081, the Abbey was the fourth richest in the land.[3] Certainly, St Edmunds was a late foundation as a Benedictine abbey in comparison with the likes of Ely and Ramsey, and Baldwin was the right man, in the right place and at the right time to ensure that St Edmunds had the best possible chance of success.

The post-Conquest success of an Abbey that housed the mortal remains of the patron saint of the English people is in some ways surprising. As Gransden pointed out, 'The Normans were not convinced that [English saints], among them St Edmund, were worthy of veneration.'[4] However, Baldwin's reputation as a physician, together with his nationality, led William I to appoint him his own royal physician.[5] It seems unlikely that this personal connection alone led William to spare Bury St Edmunds and its Liberty the experience of conquest, and the Conqueror surely realised that reverence for St Edmund had the potential to win round the English people, as well as strengthening his claim to be the chosen successor of Edward the Confessor. A more cynical theory is that Baldwin, who had been present at Edward's deathbed, witnessed his last moments and heard his last words, was in possession of knowledge that could have undermined William's position, and enjoyed the new king's special favour for this reason.[6]

A more recent theory is that both Baldwin and William made a conscious effort to forge a link between St Denis, at that time the patron saint of France, and St Edmund the patron saint of England. Both saints had in common the fact that they were martyred by decapitation, but there were few other similarities other than the fact that both saints were venerated at monasteries patronised by royalty. Bates has argued that Baldwin, a monk of St Denis, wanted to turn St Edmunds into an English version of his home monastery, and the traffic went both ways; William paid for the construction of a tower at St Denis, so tall that it collapsed, which apparently contained an altar dedicated to St Edmund.[7] Furthermore, a cycle depicting the life of St Edmund was carved on capitals around the crypt of St Denis.[8]

---

1   Gransden (1981), p. 65.
2   Bates (2014), p. 8.
3   Paul Binski and Stella Panayatova (eds), *The Cambridge Illuminations: Ten Centuries of Book Production in the Medieval West* (Turnhout, Netherlands: Brepols, 2005), p. 82.
4   Gransden (1981), p. 68.
5   Ibid., p. 66.
6   Bates (2014), p. 6.
7   Ibid,. pp. 8–9.
8   Pamela Z. Blum, 'The St Edmund cycle in the crypt at Saint-Denis', in Gransden (1998), pp. 57–68.

In Gransden's view, Baldwin 'strove to preserve the privileges, possessions and prestige which the abbey enjoyed at his succession, and to increase them ... Baldwin's greatest achievement was to ensure that the abbey emerged from the post-Conquest period richer and more powerful than it had ever been before.'[9] We know from the designs of surviving coins that a mint already existed at Bury under Leofstan, but King Edward's grant to Baldwin actually survives, which was issued between the appointment of Baldwin as Abbot on 16 July 1065 and Edward's death on 5 January 1066.[10] Since more coins of later series survive from Bury, it is likely that minting activity increased under Baldwin.

The disorder and violence of the Norman Conquest did not leave Bury entirely untouched. A Norman baron, Peter de Valognes, seized some men who belonged to St Edmunds Abbey, and another Norman courtier invaded one of St Edmund's manors. Robert de Curzun tried to obtain from Roger le Bigot the manor of Southwold to provide pasture for his horses. When he did not get what he wanted he tried to drive the horses there anyway. William gave Baldwin his full support in suppressing the disorder. A major reason for this may have been that the Liberty was of political importance to William owing to its proximity to Ely, where the major English rebellion against Norman rule was in progress until 1071. William dispossessed English tenants of St Edmunds who had fallen at Hastings, but left in possession anyone else who had held lands in Abbot Leofstan's time – including Englishmen who had fought against him.[11] In Gransden's view, William valued the Liberty as 'a loyal bloc under its French abbot'.[12]

William issued writs restoring the men taken by Peter de Valognes and, more importantly, recognised the Liberty of St Edmund as granted by King Edward. Baldwin obtained confirmation that all of the Abbey's privileges were to be held 'as in the time of King Edward'. However, William imposed a fee of forty knights on the Abbey, and had some of his own knights enfeoffed as Knights of St Edmund, who were sustained as feudal subjects of the Abbot.[13] This new knightly class changed the social structure of the Liberty and imposed a degree of 'Normanisation', even if the rights and customs of 'St Edmund's men' remained, in theory, unchanged since before the Conquest.

As royal physician to William, Baldwin spent much time in London and Normandy, but he seems nevertheless to have been a conscientious Abbot as far as obtaining written confirmation of the Abbey's privileges was concerned. Gransden has argued that Baldwin made effective and creative use of the written word in order to defend the Abbey, even stooping to overt acts of forgery in order to strengthen his position.[14] In the eleventh century, the creation of documents that we would consider today to be fakes and forgeries was not necessarily regarded as fraudulent and dishonest. In a society in which literacy was still a rarity, oral tradition played a very important part in the preservation of knowledge of rights and privileges. In some cases, the creation of fictitious charters from earlier kings may have been motivated by a desire to put into writing a tradition that such and such a

---

9   Gransden (1981), p. 67.
10 Eaglen (2006), p. 27.
11 Bates (2014), pp. 15–16.
12 Gransden (1981), p. 67.
13 Ibid., p. 68.
14 Ibid., pp. 69–72.

king bestowed this or that right or privilege. However, it is clear that Baldwin had specific political reasons to create the forgeries he did.

In 1070 Herfast, bishop of Elmham, made an attempt to relocate his see to Bury St Edmunds. This was part of a more general movement in the English church, motivated by the reforming spirit of Pope Gregory VII as well as the urbanisation that followed the Norman Conquest, to move the old Anglo-Saxon sees to major centres of population. Elmham (which may have been either North or South Elmham – both have ruins of Anglo-Saxon minsters) was a remote location, and thus unsuitable for a Norman bishop who also wished to act as a great feudal magnate. Archbishop Lanfranc of Canterbury supported the Gregorian reform but he was also a personal friend of Baldwin, who was resolutely opposed to Herfast's plan. For one thing, the re-foundation of St Edmunds as a cathedral would have relegated the Abbot to the status of a prior, and for another it would have violated the privileges granted to the Abbey by King Edward.

Faced with the threat of subordination to the bishop, Baldwin undertook the long journey to Rome to meet with the Pope. As Bates has noted, this was extremely unusual behaviour for the abbot of an English monastery at the time, and may have been a strategy he learned at St Denis.[15] According to tradition, Baldwin stopped to attend the consecration of St Martin's Cathedral in the Italian city of Lucca on the way, on 6 October 1070, where he deposited a relic of St Edmund.[16] Tom Licence has argued that Baldwin was inventive and far-sighted in adopting a deliberate policy of distributing 'contact relics' (items that had touched the saint's body) of St Edmund throughout Europe, which enhanced Edmund's reputation well beyond England.[17] Indeed, the first person to describe Edmund as *totius Angliae patronus* ('patron saint of all England') was a foreigner, Abbot Lambert of Angers.[18]

In Rome, Baldwin was received by Pope Alexander II who presented him with a ring and crozier and, on 27 October 1071, issued a bull taking the Abbey under the protection of the Roman church and forbidding its erection as an episcopal see by any temporal or spiritual power.[19] After King Edward's grant of the Liberty of St Edmund, Baldwin's Papal bull was the single most important document obtained by the Abbey, since it raised St Edmunds to the status of an exempt abbey, lying entirely outside the jurisdiction of the diocesan bishop and under direct papal authority. This was a time when the limits of papal authority were still being defined, and for an English monastery to be, in effect, a direct papal fief was unusual.

However, Baldwin seems to have felt that the bull was not enough, and Gransden argued that he also forged a diploma from William I confirming Pope Alexander's bull. On 20 November 1073 Alexander wrote to Lanfranc, chastising him for suppressing the bull, and as a result Lanfranc convened an ecclesiastical tribunal at Bury that heard both sides of the case (although Herfast did not attend) and decided in favour of Baldwin. A further

---

15 Bates (2014), p. 16.
16 Gransden (1981), p. 76. On Baldwin in Lucca see also Antonia Gransden, 'Abbo of Fleury's *Passio sancti Eadmundi*', *Revue Bénédictine* 105 (1995), pp. 20–78.
17 Tom Licence, 'The cult of St Edmund', in Licence (2014), pp. 104–30 at pp. 107–10.
18 Ibid., p. 117.
19 Gransden (1981), p. 70.

hearing in London, presided over by William himself, likewise favoured Baldwin's case.[20] Herfast removed the see to Thetford instead, but William heard the case at Winchester in 1081. Baldwin's forgeries came into their own on this occasion, as imagined by Sarah Foot:

> Baldwin displayed a veritable armour of charters to bolster his case. One imagines him pulling them out of his bag one at a time, perhaps starting with the one from the martyred king's namesake .... Next, perhaps he showed the less impressive creations in the name of the Confessor and of Harthacnut before saving until last his *pièce de resistance*: the impressive charter from Cnut.[21]

Cnut's charter was decisive because it insisted so strongly on St Edmunds' independence from episcopal jurisdiction. In the end, William sided with Baldwin. Both sides supported their case with forged documents; the bishop's party even produced an implausible story that there had once been a cathedral at Beodricsworth.[22]

Bates has connected Baldwin's prolific activity as patron of forged documents with his origins at St Denis, an abbey that adopted similar practices. Baldwin gave his forgeries sacred sanction by having them inscribed in an illuminated Gospel book that was deposited in the holiest place of all, the shrine of St Edmund.[23] Gransden has argued that Baldwin went beyond merely forging charters, and used Hermann to produce propaganda showing that those who offended against St Edmund suffered as a result. The marauding courtier received a threatening vision of St Edmund and joined the monastery; the courtier who invaded a manor was afflicted with a headache and a lump on one eye, and a candle he sent to the Abbey broke into nine pieces; Robert de Curzun ignored a thunderstorm and was afflicted with 'mental dullness', while his steward went mad.[24]

It is even possible that Baldwin interpolated Abbo of Fleury's *Passio*, adding the references to Beodricsworth.[25] Gransden was so sceptical of Abbo's account in the form it has come down to us that she dismissed most of the early history of Bury St Edmunds, arguing that 'All that is certain is that by c. 1000 a shrine containing a body, supposedly that of St Edmund, was the centre of a cult at Beodricesworth.'[26] Although this extreme scepticism may seem unwarranted, it is clear that the historical record was contaminated by Baldwin, and the weight of forged documents from the 1070s and 1080s pertaining to Bury, whether generated by Baldwin or Herfast, has distorted our perception of the pre-Norman history of the Abbey. The contest also gave rise to new and spurious traditions that later came to be accepted as fact, such as the identification of Hoxne as the site of St Edmund's martyrdom. This was a story originating with the bishop's party, owing to the superficial similarity between the names Hoxne and Hægelisdun and the fact that Hoxne's association with the bishops of East Anglia was well established.[27]

---

20 Ibid., pp. 70–1.
21 Foot (2014), p. 50.
22 Gransden (1981), p. 70.
23 Now British Library MS Harley 76; see Bates (2014), pp. 118–30.
24 Gransden (1981), p. 68.
25 Ibid., p. 72.
26 Gransden (1985), p. 9.
27 Gransden (1981), p. 70; see also Licence (2014), pp. 118–30.

Baldwin made an important contribution to the cult of St Edmund, not only by planning and beginning work on a great minster to house the shrine of the saint, but also by making the site accessible to pilgrims. This was absolutely necessary to ensure the building works could be paid for. Baldwin erected a *tabula* or painted board depicting the story of St Edmund – presumably based on Abbo's *Passio*. This was essential in an era when so few people could read or write, and the *tabula* would probably have been interpreted aloud by one of the monks in English and Norman French as the pilgrims approached the shrine. Furthermore, Bishop Walkelin of Winchester granted indulgences to anyone who visited the shrine, which meant remission of penance for pilgrims to Bury.[28] This was an attractive option at a time when severe penances were still often imposed by confessors, and failure to fulfil a penance might result in excommunication.

In around 1095 Baldwin commissioned Hermann the Archdeacon, a former supporter of Herfast who had entered the Abbey as a monk (and had therefore, in effect, changed sides) to compose the *De miraculis Sancti Eadmundi*, a comprehensive defence against the charge that St Edmund was not buried at Bury at all. This claim was being made by Norman barons as a justification for seizing the Abbey's lands.[29] Bates has argued that St Edmunds was established as a 'special abbey' during William's reign, and indeed St Edmund seems to have been the only English saint to whom the Conqueror showed special devotion. When visiting Bury he approached St Edmund's shrine with head bowed, and he granted the manors of Warkton (Northamptonshire) and Brooke (Norfolk) to the Abbey. Uniquely among English religious houses, Bury also acquired property of its own in Normandy,[30] and Bury was the only Anglo-Saxon foundation to serve as the burial site for an important member of the Norman elite. This was Alan Rufus, a descendant of Alan III of Brittany, who was buried in the Church of St Edmund in 1093.[31]

The nature of the description of Bury in Domesday Book has led historians to suspect that it was pre-prepared,[32] meaning that William's clerks never entered the town to make a survey. They seem, instead, to have been satisfied with the written evidence of the Abbey's possessions, such as the pre-Conquest gift of the manors of Culford, Wordwell and Ixworth by Thurketel (the Abbey's earliest surviving title deed).[33] Indeed, Baldwin built upon the work of his predecessor Leofstan in preparing a 'feudal book' that contained a definitive list of the Abbey's possessions and provided additional protection against the depredations of rapacious Norman barons.[34]

During Baldwin's reign the Abbot first became differentiated from the monks themselves (the Convent), in the sense that grants of land to the monastery were grants to the Abbot. This generated 'grumbling' among the monks, and Baldwin responded by issuing a charter granting two manors, Hinderclay and Newton, to the monks to keep them in clothes, as well as two ponds he had created and a fishery.[35] On the death of William

---

28   Ibid., p. 75.
29   A. F. Wareham, 'Baldwin (*d.* 1097), abbot of Bury St Edmunds', in *ODNB*, vol. 3, pp. 441–2.
30   Bates (2014), p. 12.
31   Ibid., pp. 12–13.
32   Ibid., pp. 18–19.
33   Foot (2014), p. 33.
34   Wareham (2004), pp 441–2.
35   Gransden (1981), p. 69.

the Conqueror, Baldwin arranged for ten shillings to be paid to the monks annually on his anniversary from the manor of Warkton.[36] This practice of distributing 'pittances' to the monks to compensate them for additional liturgical labours on anniversaries would continue throughout the Middle Ages. However, under Baldwin it became clear that the Abbot would become a great magnate of the kingdom rather than the Christ-like exemplar envisaged by the Rule of St Benedict.

Baldwin the physician

Abbot Baldwin owed a great deal to his medical skill; he was royal physician successively to Edward the Confessor, William I and William II. When Bishop Herfast injured his eyes in a riding accident, Baldwin threatened to withhold medical treatment until Herfast swore an oath recognising Bury's independence.[37] As Debby Banham has argued, 'the intimacy of bodily care could bring physicians to the heart of political power',[38] but Baldwin may also have been responsible for introducing a 'new', more learned medicine to England. The Anglo-Saxon medical tradition, uniquely in Europe, was a vernacular one (texts were in English rather than Latin), and consisted of fairly simple plant-based recipes accompanied by little medical theory. However, an eleventh-century manuscript that Baldwin probably brought to Bury from France (British Library Sloane MS 1621) contains more elaborate medical theory (such as the four humours) and requires the use of exotic, expensive ingredients and precise measurements.[39]

Baldwin's reign saw the transition, not only in medicine but also in legal texts, from English to Latin. The liturgy had always been in Latin, but the rich vernacular literary culture of Anglo-Saxon England gave way after the Conquest to a written culture almost entirely confined to Latin. We do not know whether Baldwin ever learned English, but it is easy to imagine that he saw no need to do so. His wealthy patients would have spoken Norman French, while the monks were expected to converse in Latin. In an age before universities, a great monastery such as Bury was the only institution with the resources and expertise to educate others, and it is possible that Bury became a centre of medical learning under Baldwin's leadership. Certainly, recent scholarship has challenged Rodney Thomson's view that in Baldwin's reign 'The climate of learning at the abbey was still Anglo-Saxon' and that 'there is no evidence that Baldwin infused it with Continental Latin culture'.[40]

Banham advances the case that one particular hand in Sloane 1621 can be identified as Baldwin's own; if the identification is correct, then Baldwin would be the first named figure associated with a surviving medical book in England. Not only that, but Baldwin would appear to have made practical use of the book (the leaves were unbound

---

36 Bates (2014), p. 12.
37 Debby Banham, 'Medicine at Bury in the time of Abbot Baldwin', in Licence (2014), pp. 226–46, at pp. 241–2.
38 Ibid., p. 226.
39 Ibid., pp. 228–9.
40 Rodney M. Thomson, 'The Library of Bury St Edmunds Abbey in the eleventh and twelfth centuries', *Speculum* 47 (1972), pp. 617–45, p. 627. See also Teresa Webber, 'The provision of books for Bury St Edmunds Abbey in the 11th and 12th centuries', in Gransden (1998), pp. 186–93.

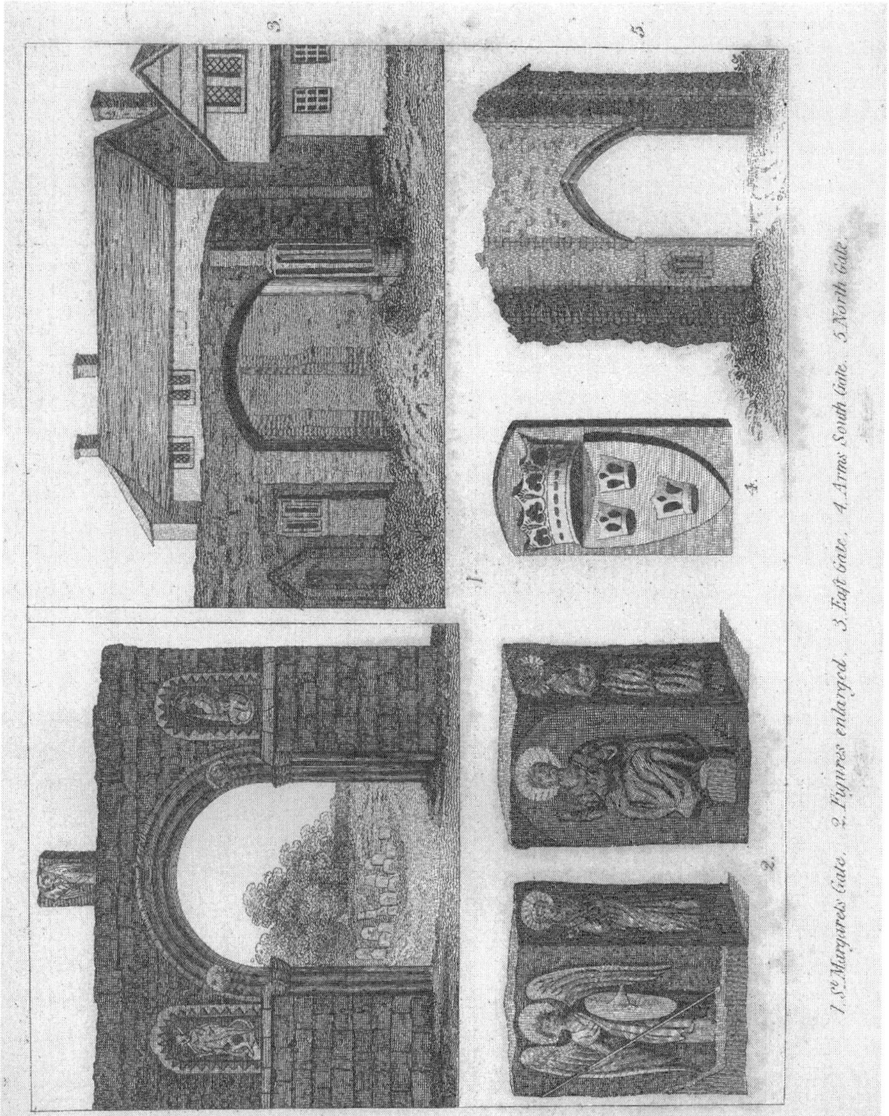

Figure 15 The town gates of Bury St Edmunds, originally built in Abbot Baldwin's time. Engraving from Richard Yates, *An Illustration of the Monastic Antiquities of the Town and Abbey of St Edmund's Bury* (1843), plate facing p. 47.

at one time, making them more portable). Banham discerned in Baldwin's medical recipes a particular concern with the welfare of the soul as well as the body, and an interest in 'exotic' recipes associated with the Holy Land, both of which were uncharacteristic of early medieval medicine.[41] It is conceivable that these were the distinctive concerns of a 'medical school' at Bury, which Banham argues for on the grounds that Hermann the Archdeacon made considerable use of technical medical terminology in his *De miraculis*. Furthermore, Hermann indicates that Baldwin had knowledge of the works of Hippocrates and Galen, which were otherwise unknown in England at the time.[42]

Another innovation that Baldwin appears to have brought into England for the first time was medical recipes involving animals killed in a certain way, such as a salve for blindness made by blinding swallow chicks in their nest.[43] This was a kind of medicine virtually indistinguishable from magic but it was supported, in the minds of early medieval doctors, by the testimony of Classical sources. Another reason to suppose that Baldwin founded a medical 'school' at Bury is the fact that the active annotation of medical texts remained a feature of monastic life in the early twelfth century. A copy of the *Passionarius* ('Book of Diseases') of Gariopontus from the monastic library (now British Library, Royal MS 12.c.xxiv) was intended as a practical manual of medicine and was annotated by subsequent users.[44]

Baldwin the builder

Abbot Baldwin was an impressive builder, and according to the Domesday Survey, by 1081 there were 342 new houses in the *banleuca* on land that had been under the plough in the time of King Edward. This suggests a rapid and planned expansion of the town, probably in a westward direction from the Abbey towards Angel Hill, Abbeygate Street and the huge open market on Cornhill. Historians are divided, however, on whether the town's celebrated 'Norman grid' plan was the work of Baldwin or his twelfth-century successor Anselm.[45] Either way, it seems likely that Anselm completed the project of improving the town that Baldwin began. In fact, the first laws and customs of the town of Bury appear in Baldwin's reign, such as a requirement for the townsmen to provide gatekeepers.[46]

Baldwin also provided the townsmen with two churches. Significantly, these were located on the west side of the Anglo-Saxon main street, which may therefore have represented the boundary of the monastic precinct. The 'grand and beautiful' church of St Denis, named after the abbey where Baldwin had first become a monk, was located under the north end of the west front of the later Abbey Church, and may have been served by a college of canons who ministered to the townsfolk.[47] There was also the chapel of St Margaret, which seems to have been a tower joined to a chapel, but it is unclear where

---

41 Banham (2014), pp. 236–8.
42 Ibid., pp. 239–41.
43 Ibid., p. 243.
44 Véronique Thouroude, 'Medicine after Baldwin: the evidence of BL, Royal 12. c. xxiv' in Licence (2014), pp. 247–57, at p. 251.
45 Gransden (1981), p. 74 considered Baldwin to be responsible; Statham (1996), p. 12 attributed the grid to Anselm.
46 Gransden (1981), pp. 68–9.
47 Bates (2014), p. 10.

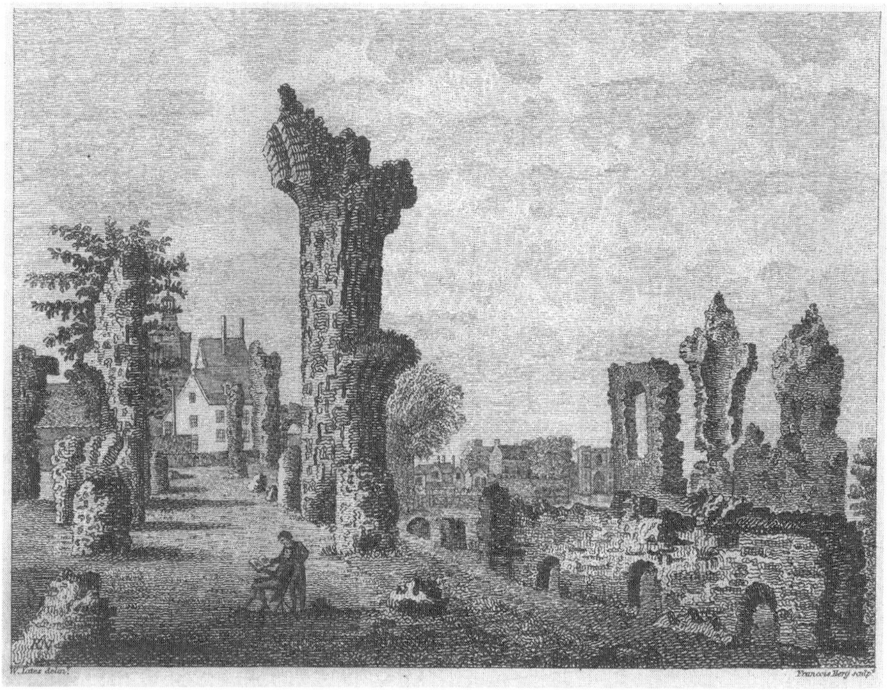

Figure 16 One of the massive crossing piers of Baldwin's church, looking west (1804). Engraving from Richard Yates, *An Illustration of the Monastic Antiquities of the Town and Abbey of St Edmund's Bury* (1843), facing p. 29.

this was located.[48] In a later era, the chapel of St Margaret was close to where the Shire Hall is today, on the south-east corner of St Mary's Churchyard. St Margaret's was constructed by the priest Ailbold to house a female recluse, Langlifa.[49]

Baldwin may have begun his new minster as early as 1081, following his final victory over Herfast at the court of King William.[50] The consecration of the crypt was celebrated in subsequent centuries on 5 November, but the year of its completion is unclear. The stone for the edifice came from Barnack in Peterborough and was conveyed to Bury by boat from Gunwade. Two stones lying in Castorfields, near Peterborough, were anciently known as 'St Edmund's stones', presumably because they had been intended for the Abbey; William instructed the abbot of Peterborough to allow Baldwin to transport the stone without hindrance.[51] Whittingham thought that the position of the church may have been determined partly by the existence of a natural spring underneath the crypt, which became a site of pilgrimage.[52]

The presbytery and choir were sufficiently complete to be consecrated on 8 April 1093,

---

48 Gem and Keen (1981), p. 2.
49 Van Houts (2014), p. 63. See also Gransden (2009), p. 117.
50 Fernie (2014), p. 77.
51 Whittingham (1952), p. 170.
52 Ibid., p. 174.

an event attended by 'almost every prelate in the land'.[53] The completion of the presbytery did not require the demolition of the old rotunda but it did necessitate the demolition of old St Mary's Church, which made way for the south transept. The open crypt of Baldwin's minster still survives among the Abbey ruins, and this would have been the first part of the building to be built, with the choir above it. The church was apsidal, like Norwich Cathedral, and the shrine of St Edmund would have stood on the floor above the crypt. The construction of an ambulatory around an apse was new to England and was a feature of the great French pilgrimage churches. With an ambulatory of seven bays, Bury had the largest and most elaborate in the world at the time, and Baldwin probably designed it in the knowledge that pilgrims would be visiting multiple shrines – those of St Botolph, St Thomas and St Jurmin as well as St Edmund.[54]

It was standard practice for the choir of a Norman church to be completed first, allowing for the celebration of mass and the divine office as soon as possible in the sanctuary. The nave and transepts, which accommodated pilgrims and additional chapels, could come later. During the building work, St Edmund continued to repose in his shrine in the old rotunda, which Baldwin incorporated into the north side of his minster. However, on 29 April 1095 the saint was translated with magnificent ceremonial into his new shrine in the choir by Bishop Walkelin of Winchester. The Feast of the Translation of St Edmund would be celebrated for centuries to come as a festival second only to St Edmund's day on 20 November.[55]

Stephen Heywood has argued that Baldwin's construction of the Abbey Church was (at least in part) an exercise in one-upmanship against Herfast's successor, Bishop Herbert de Losinga, who finally moved his see to the rapidly expanding town of Norwich in 1094 and began work on a huge cathedral minster in 1096.[56] However, Losinga faced a further humiliation when he was banned from supervising the translation of St Edmund in 1095; this was because he had been forced to go to Rome as penance for buying his bishopric.[57] Although both the Pope and King William II forgave Losinga and restored him to his see, Baldwin gained yet another victory.

In the battle between Bury and the bishop, it seems that Bury was the clear winner in more ways than one: the bishop had failed to establish his see at Bury, but he also had no spiritual jurisdiction over the town at all. Furthermore, whereas the Abbot of St Edmunds wielded spiritual and temporal power over the Liberty of St Edmund, a well-established jurisdiction, the bishops of Norwich had little temporal power at all. Add to this the fact that Norwich had no famous shrine, and it begins to be obvious why the bishops of Norwich felt threatened by the Abbots of St Edmunds, who vied with them to be the most powerful clerics in East Anglia. Baldwin had a thirty-year head start in building on the bishops, having been in post even before the Conquest, and they simply could not compete with his ruthless determination to establish the privileges of his house against all comers.

---

53   Crook (1998), p. 34.
54   R. Gilyard-Beer, 'The eastern arm of the Abbey Church at Bury St. Edmunds', *PSIAH* 31 (1969), pp. 256–62, at p. 260.
55   Gransden (1981), pp. 74–5.
56   Stephen Heywood, 'Aspects of the Romanesque Church of Bury St Edmunds Abbey in their regional context', in Gransden (1998), pp. 16–21, at pp. 19–20.
57   Fernie (2014), p. 82.

Anselm, 1121–48

Abbot Baldwin died at the end of 1097 (or possibly early in 1098), leaving the Abbey in an immensely strong position financially, politically and ecclesiastically – so much so that King William II kept the abbacy vacant for three years after Baldwin's death in order to receive the revenues of the Liberty of St Edmund and the Abbey's other possessions. Meanwhile, Herbert de Losinga busied himself in trying to undermine the Abbey's privileges. In 1098, immediately after Baldwin's death, he again petitioned the king to allow him to move his see to Bury, in spite of the fact that he had already begun a cathedral at Norwich. Only in 1101 did he confirm by charter his intention to establish Norwich as his see,[58] and even then he kept up the fight. In 1101–2 he travelled to Rome in an effort to seek the right to preach, celebrate mass and ordain clergy in the Abbey Church. He then launched a suit against the Abbey at Westminster in 1102.[59] Robert, an illegitimate son of the Norman nobleman Hugh d'Avranches, earl of Chester, was appointed Abbot in 1100, although he was only just old enough to be canonically eligible.[60] Robert d'Avranches was deposed after two years by Archbishop Anselm of Canterbury, and between 1102 and 1106 Henry I prevented the consecration of Abbot Robert II in order to appropriate the Abbey's revenues.

In 1107 Robert II was deposed by the king and there was no Abbot until 1114, when Alebold was elected.[61] Alebold had been a clerk at Bari in Italy before entering the monastic life at Bec in Normandy, subsequently serving as prior of St Nicaise at Melun.[62] He brought some measure of stability to the Abbey, but he ruled only until 1119. After a further vacancy, in 1121 St Edmunds received its second great Abbot. Like Baldwin, Anselm was a foreigner, although this time an Italian. He was the nephew of his more famous namesake, St Anselm, archbishop of Canterbury (c. 1033–1109), and began his monastic career as a monk of the abbey of St Michael at Chiusa in Piedmont. One day, while serving at the altar, the young Anselm accidentally spilled some dark communion wine on the white linen corporal. Fearful of being discovered, he prayed to the Virgin Mary and the stain miraculously disappeared. Shortly after this incident Chiusa received a visit from Anselm's uncle, and the young Anselm accompanied his uncle to France.[63] In around 1093, when the elder Anselm was appointed archbishop of Canterbury, the younger Anselm accompanied him and became a monk of Christchurch, Canterbury until 1109, when his uncle died and the younger Anselm returned to Italy. He became abbot of the monastery of Saints Alexius and Saba on the Aventine Hill in Rome.

When he was elected Abbot of St Edmunds, therefore, Anselm was eminently qualified to serve in this office, both because he had already been an abbot and because he had already spent time in England at Christchurch, Canterbury. Furthermore, in the 1080s a contingent of monks from the Abbey of Bec, where Anselm's uncle was then abbot, had visited Bury and may have brought books with them.[64] Anselm presided over the

---

58 Fernie (2014), p. 82.
59 Foot (2014), p. 49.
60 C. P. Lewis, 'Avranches, Hugh d', first earl of Chester (d. 1101)' in *ODNB*, vol. 3, pp. 1–3.
61 Thomson (1972), p. 629.
62 Gransden (2009), p. 115.
63 Gransden (2004), p. 644.
64 Thomson (1972), at p. 624.

completion of Baldwin's Abbey Church, but his first priority was the reconstruction of the ancient church of St Mary, which Anselm may have erected in its present position at the extreme south-west of the monastic precincts. Construction of the church had already begun under the sacrist Godfrey, but Anselm presided over its consecration. He also insisted that a mass in honour of the Virgin Mary should be celebrated every day, and ordered the observance of the Feast of the Annunciation on 18 December (a feast usually celebrated on 25 March).[65]

Anselm went further, and commanded the celebration of the Conception of the Virgin Mary on 8 September, a feast that had been celebrated in some pre-Conquest English religious houses (Winchester and St Augustine's and Christchurch, Canterbury) but whose theological basis was disputed by some Norman theologians. Celebration of the conception of Mary implied belief in its miraculous nature (an idea later known as the Immaculate Conception). Anselm became involved in a controversy over the celebration of the feast when he was asked by Osbert of Clare, prior of Westminster, to uphold the doctrine against the bishops of Salisbury and St Davids. In 1129 King Henry I confirmed the celebration of the Feast of the Conception, perhaps under Anselm's influence.[66] It is clear that Anselm's interest in devotion to the Virgin Mary was deeply personal, based on the miraculous experience he had in his youth, but it would have far-reaching consequences for English religious history. By putting his weight behind the campaign for Marian festivals, Anselm helped establish England as a European centre of Marian devotion, a status it retained until the Reformation.

Anselm's first monastery, Saints Alexius and Saba, was a double foundation containing both western and Greek monks, where both the Latin and Greek liturgies were celebrated, and it has been suggested that Anselm's interest in miracles of the Virgin Mary and promotion of the Feast of her Conception derived from Greek influence.[67] Anselm may have brought works of the Greek Fathers with him to Bury. The Abbey's library contained works by Origen at a very early date, and in the thirteenth century there was even a book in Greek which the monks asked Robert Grosseteste to translate for them. Anselm's 'Italo-Byzantine' background and frequent trips back to Italy also account for a number of pagan Classical texts that appeared in the monastic library at this time. These included the first known manuscript of plays by Plautus and Terence in England.[68] As might be expected, the Abbey also had an impressive collection of the works of Anselm's uncle, St Anselm of Canterbury.

In addition to promoting the cult of the Virgin Mary, Anselm also introduced the cults of St Saba and St Faith to the Abbey, and Bury was the only church in England where St Saba was venerated. However, Anselm's most lasting achievement, owing to a much later historical accident, was his foundation of the church of St James. Anselm had wanted to go on pilgrimage to Compostella but the elder monks persuaded him to found a church dedicated to St James instead, which replaced the old St Denis as a parish church for the townsfolk.[69] Rebuilt in the early sixteenth century, this church survived the dissolution

---

65 Gransden (2004), p. 646.
66 Ibid., p. 648.
67 Thomson (1972), p. 631.
68 Ibid., pp. 632–3.
69 Gransden (2009), p. 116.

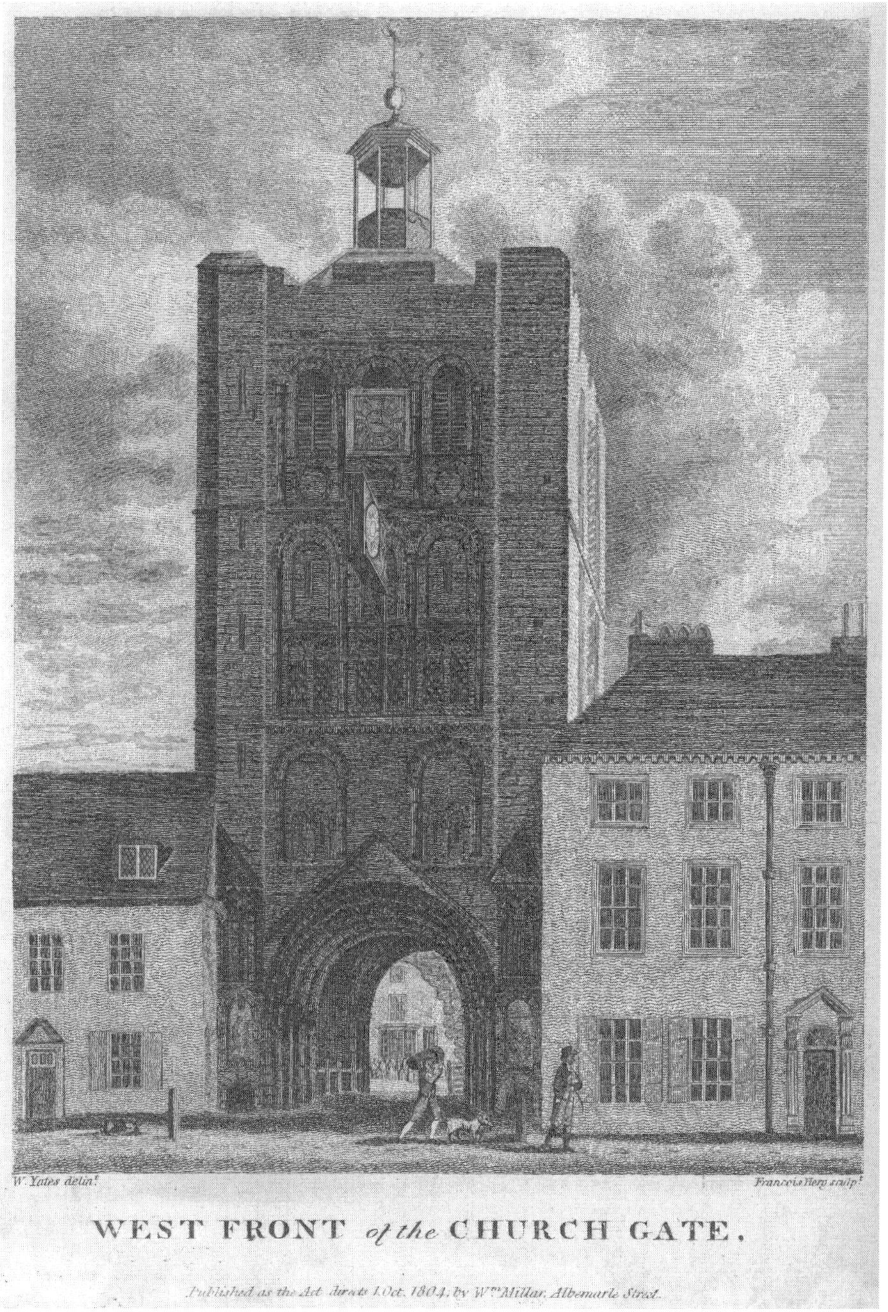

Figure 17 Abbot Anselm's Norman Tower (1804). Engraving from Richard Yates, *An Illustration of the Monastic Antiquities of the Town and Abbey of St Edmund's Bury* (1843), plate facing p. 11.

and was chosen in 1914 to become the cathedral of the new Diocese of St Edmundsbury and Ipswich.

In 1136 Anselm was nominated bishop of London in succession to Gilbert the Universal, but his election was never confirmed by the king, and although he travelled to London in expectation of taking up his see, his election was disputed by William, dean of St Paul's.[70] In Anselm's absence the prior, Ording, was elected Abbot,[71] which caused some problems on Anselm's return to Bury in 1138. Anselm was a close friend of Henry I and spent a lot of time in Normandy and Italy, as well as at the royal court and on Papal embassies as a legate. In spite of his interest in books, however, he seems to have had trouble reading and writing into his twenties and beyond.[72]

Development of the Abbey Church

At Baldwin's death in 1097, the only parts of the great Norman minster to have been completed were the crypt, choir and presbytery. Under Abbot Robert II (1102–7) Godfrey the Sacrist developed the north transept, at which time the ambulatory around the old rotunda was probably knocked down and the central part of the building incorporated as a chapel attached to the transept's east wall.[73]

Successive abbots continued the church westwards, and the nave altar was dedicated in the reign of Anselm. This implies that the nave was complete at that time, because the purpose of the nave altar was to provide a focus for masses celebrated for pilgrims, who would have gathered in the nave. A chapel at the west end of the church was dedicated by Bishop John of Rochester, who died in 1142, suggesting that the entirety of the church was completed during Anselm's reign; all that was left for Abbot Samson to do in the 1180s was to complete the towers on the west front.[74] Anselm's church:

> consisted of a five-bay east arm with an ambulatory and three radiating chapels (all, except for the western bay of the presbytery, raised on a crypt), transept arms of five bays each with an eastern aisle and apses, a nave of twelve bays, and a western massif of great breadth and complexity.[75]

In Fernie's view, the Abbey Church had a clerestory comparable with that at Ely. Indeed, the Norman portions of Ely Cathedral may offer some idea of what the church at Bury looked like. According to Hermann, the Abbey Church was covered by a *testudo* (literally 'the shell of a tortoise'), which probably means a stone vault. This was unusual at a time when wooden ceilings were more common. Fernie saw Bury as part of 'the north French great church tradition', with close parallels in the cathedrals of Winchester and Tours. The Abbey Church at Bury 'stands at the climax of a massive increase in the size of Norman

---

70 G. R. Evans, 'Anselm (*d.* 1148), abbot of Bury St Edmunds and hagiographer', in *ODNB*, vol. 2, p. 258.
71 Yates (1843), p. 211.
72 Evans (2004), p. 258.
73 Gem and Keen (1981), p. 2.
74 Fernie (2014), pp. 77–8.
75 Fernie (2014), pp. 77–8.

churches in England in the 1070s', rivalling for the first time the size of Roman and Byzantine structures.[76] Unusually for the time, Anselm built a nave that was wider than the choir, with the result that the cross-arm of the church was the largest in England at the time. The impressive Cluniac priory church of Castle Acre, which was built around the same time, would have fitted inside the transepts with room to spare.[77]

Fernie has argued that Anselm deliberately copied from Norwich the huge crossing piers that still stand as the tallest features of the ruins, in an effort to outdo Herbert de Losinga's minster.[78] He has also noted that the measurements of the Abbey Church correspond to those of Old St Peter's Basilica in Rome,[79] which Baldwin and his successors may have been trying consciously to imitate – perhaps as a statement of the Abbey's sole dependence on the Pope. Less clear is whether the establishment of a grid plan for the town preceded or followed the construction of the Abbey Church. Churchgate Street served as an impressive approach to the Abbey and was aligned with the minster, but its construction may have come later, perhaps as a consequence of Anselm's erection of the so-called 'Norman Tower'.

Fernie has drawn attention to a strong resemblance between the lowest tier of the Norman Tower and the west front of Laon Cathedral, begun in 1155, which further reinforces the connection with north French churches.[80] The tower is certainly the most impressive surviving built legacy of Abbot Anselm, although it remains unclear whether it served merely as a gate for pilgrims approaching the west front of the Abbey Church or whether it was also a bell tower for the church of St James, the role it still plays today. That the tower was originally the home of a gatekeeper is suggested by the discovery of a filled-in well underneath it and remains of meals during an excavation in 1973.[81]

Master Hugo

Master Hugo, who was active at Bury between 1130 and 1150, is the first artist in England whose name is known to history, along with specific surviving works that can be attributed to him. In spite of his association with the Abbey, it is unlikely that Hugo was himself a monk, since he is consistently referred to in contemporary documents as *magister*, a title given to travelling master craftsmen. It is by no means certain – indeed, it is rather unlikely – that Hugo was an Englishman. Medieval master craftsmen were a cosmopolitan caste who moved from country to country, but Hugo seems to have remained at Bury for a considerable time under the patronage of the community. Although it is impossible to imagine that Abbot Anselm himself did not patronise Hugo in some way, his primary patrons were two monks who were also brothers by blood, Hervey the Sacrist and Prior Talbot, who was in office between around 1125 and 1136.

Hugo was a multitalented artist of breathtaking skill, who worked in illumination,

---

76 Ibid., pp. 78–9.
77 Gilyard-Beer (1969), pp. 260–1.
78 Fernie (2014), p. 82.
79 Ibid., pp. 88–9.
80 Ibid., pp. 89–93.
81 P. L. Drewett and Ian W. Stuart, 'Excavations in the Norman Gate Tower, Bury St. Edmunds Abbey', *PSIAH* 33 (1975), pp. 241–50.

painting, metalwork and walrus ivory. His best-known work is the Bury Bible (Cambridge, Corpus Christi College MS 2, part 1), described by Christopher de Hamel as 'one of the noblest and most sublime of all English Romanesque manuscripts', and dating to the period 1130–35. The Bury Bible was the first appearance in England of huge, monumental Bibles, a trend that began in Italy, and its full-page opening illuminated initial is unique in England. No calfskin of adequate quality could be found locally to make the Bible, so parchment had to be purchased from *Scotia* (Scotland or Ireland), and unusually, the illustrations of the Bury Bible are pasted in (presumably because the imported parchment was so expensive).

The Bible was originally in two volumes, each featuring twelve illustrations, which are celebrated for Hugo's use of the 'damp-fold' technique to portray drapery. This was borrowed from Byzantine art, and together with the figures' large staring eyes, it strongly suggests that Hugo spent time in the Eastern Mediterranean. Hugo also portrays dark-skinned North Africans realistically, and De Hamel concluded that he had spent time either in Italy, Cyprus or Constantinople, and may have taken part in the English recovery of the Latin Kingdom of Jerusalem. The Bible was probably intended for the refectory of the monastery, to be read aloud there during mealtimes.[82]

Today, only the first volume of Hugo's monumental Bible survives, running from Genesis to Job, and only six of the twelve original illustrations remain. The manuscript was part of the collection of Archbishop Matthew Parker (1504–75), but it seems that bookbinders got hold of the Bible before Parker, as a small fragment of the second volume has been recovered amongst sixteenth-century bookbinder's waste from Oxford. Bookbinders regularly recycled vellum in the post-Reformation period as a cheap binding for books, without regard for the significance of the manuscripts they cut up.

It is possible that Hugo was not the first artist patronised by the Abbey; the anonymous 'Alexis Master', so called after a life of St Alexis illuminated by him, was active at St Albans and Bury St Edmunds between around 1120 and 1140, and it is even possible that the Alexis Master overlapped with, or taught, Master Hugo. At some point after 1125 the Alexis Master illuminated *The Miracles and Passion of St Edmund* (New York, Pierpont Morgan Library MS 736). One scene features the coronation of St Edmund in heaven, wearing a crown that Charles Dodwell considered more German than English, and which led him to believe that the Alexis Master came from Germany (Dodwell also thought his stay at Bury was brief).[83] Another masterpiece of illumination produced at Bury at this time was a narrative picture cycle of the ministry and passion of Christ, skilfully drawn in outline and then later coloured in by a less skilled painter (Cambridge, Pembroke College MS 120).[84]

Two of Hugo's works certainly do not survive: a great bronze bell cast for the crossing of the Abbey Church (which was probably destroyed during the great fire of 1465) and a set of bronze doors on the west front of the Abbey, which seem to have still been visible when John Leland visited in the 1530s, and were therefore in all probability melted down after the dissolution, when they became the property of the crown. Hugo may also have been

---

82 Binski and Panayatova (2005), pp. 81–3. On the Bury Bible see also T. A. Heslop, 'The production and artistry of the Bury Bible', in Gransden (1998), pp. 172–85.
83 Charles R. Dodwell, *The Pictorial Arts of the West, 800–1200* (New Haven, Conn.: Yale University Press, 1993), vol. 27, pp. 332–3.
84 Binski and Panayatova (2005), pp. 83–5.

responsible for one twelfth-century seal of an abbot, which features a figure with similar facial features and drapery to those found in the Bury Bible.[85]

In addition to the Bury Bible, two other surviving works have been attributed to Master Hugo. One is a fresco of St Paul being bitten by a viper on the island of Malta in the chapel of St Anselm in Canterbury Cathedral, although this could also have been the work of a follower of the artist.[86] More speculatively, Hugo has been identified as the creator of the 'Cloisters Cross' in the Metropolitan Museum of Art in New York, a sculpture of walrus ivory that has long been associated with Bury St Edmunds and is controversial both in its attribution and for its subject-matter. The Cloisters Cross is 23 inches high with an arm span of 14.5 inches, and is carved on all sides and even on the edges. Elizabeth Parker and Charles Little describe it thus:

> Distinctive to this double-sided Latin cross are the central medallions and the arms ending in inhabited square terminals …. On the front these elements are tied together by the representation of a tree trunk with severed branches, making the cross a Tree of Life. The terminals display scenes related to Good Friday (on the right), Easter (on the left), and the Ascension of Christ (at the top). Scrolls held by the figures in these and other scenes bear quotations from the Scriptures which serve to identify the characters and to comment on the action. Represented in the central medallion, which is supported by wingless angels, are Moses with the Brazen Serpent raised up on a forked stick before the Israelites, St Peter, St John, Isaias, and Jeremias. Above this medallion and standing over the placard, which incorporates the Hand of God in a stylized cloud, are the high priest and Pontius Pilate debating the inscription, or titulus … the cross originally possessed a corpse, which is now lost …. On either side of the shaft and on the edges are Latin couplets engraved lengthwise in majuscules. One reads: 'The earth trembles, Death defeated groans with the buried one rising. / Life has been called, Synagogue has collapsed with great foolish effort.' The other reads: 'Cham laughs when he sees the naked private parts of his parent. / The Jews laughed at the pain of God dying.' Adam and Eve appear at the foot of the cross clinging to the Tree of Life.[87]

It is clear from other figures, such as a personification of Synagogue holding a broken lance on the other side, that the iconography of the cross is consciously antisemitic. The provenance of the cross is obscure; according to one story, in the 1930s it was owned by a priest living at the Cistercian monastery of Zirc in Hungary's Bakony mountains. In the aftermath of the Second World War, the cross fell into the possession of the Yugoslavian art dealer Ante Topic Mimara, who sold it to the Metropolitan Museum of Art in the early 1960s; the British Museum refused it because Topic Mimara would provide no details of the cross's provenance.[88] The cross was always thought to be English, and it was the curator of the Cloisters, Thomas Hoving, who first suggested an association with Bury

---

85 Timothy Graham, 'Bury St Edmunds, Hugo of (*fl. c.*1130–*c.*1150)' in *ODNB*, vol. 9, pp. 71–2.
86 Ibid.
87 Elizabeth C. Parker and Charles T. Little, *The Cloisters Cross: Its Art and Meaning* (New York: Metropolitan Museum of Art, 1994), pp. 13–14.
88 Ibid., pp. 14–15.

St Edmunds, although Hoving believed that the cross dated from the early part of Abbot Samson's reign in the 1180s.

Elizabeth Parker made a convincing case for strong stylistic similarities between the Cloisters Cross and the Bury Bible of Master Hugo, pushing the creation of the cross back to Anselm's reign.[89] Although comparison of the two very different works in different media is far from conclusive, no better analogue can be found.[90] In 1973 Norman Scarfe produced a new hypothesis that the cross dated from the period 1135–54 (the reign of Abbot Ording) when Jews began to move out from London into other English towns and cities controlled by King Stephen. He drew attention to Jocelin de Brakelond's remark that during the vacancy following the death of Abbot Hugh, Jews wandered into the Abbey Church and past the altars because of the laxness of the sacrist, William Wiardel, and suggested that this may have been the norm before Samson's time – in other words, the Cloisters Cross was deliberately made by Master Hugo in Ording's time to be seen by Jews and stood on the 'small altar' of the choir.[91]

Scarfe went on to speculate in the 1980s that the cross was part of 'the treasure of our church being carried to London for the ransom of King Richard' in 1192. Samson travelled to Dürrenstein Castle on the Danube where Richard was being imprisoned, and Scarfe argued that the cross probably travelled with him.[92] It is certainly true that had the cross been in the Abbey Church at this time it might have been taken for the ransom, since its antisemitic message was no longer relevant in a Bury St Edmunds where there were no more Jews, following the expulsion of 1190 (see Chapter 3). Another approach has examined the cross in relation to liturgical practices at Bury and found suggestive echoes,[93] and yet another draws theological links with the work of Hugh of St Victor and his school.[94] The attribution of the Cloisters Cross to Master Hugo remains speculative, but Parker and Little concluded that the cross 'exhibits characteristics that can be said to assert Bury's distinguished roots in East Anglian culture':

> Compatible with both the approach and the style of Master Hugo's Bury Bible, the singular sophistication of the program of the Cloisters Cross and the quality of its execution suggest that if it were seen as the product of this abbey in mid-century, both intellectually and artistically Bury St Edmunds could certainly equal, if not surpass, the achievements of other, now better-known centers of English monasticism.[95]

The end of Abbot Anselm's reign did not mark the end of Master Hugo's career, and indeed it is quite possible that Hugo produced some of his masterpieces in the reign of

---

89 Elizabeth C. Parker, 'Master Hugo as sculptor: a source for the style of the Bury Bible', *Gesta* 20 (1981), pp. 99–109.
90 Parker and Little (1994), pp. 198–206.
91 Norman Scarfe, 'The walrus ivory cross in the Metropolitan Museum of Art: the masterpiece of Master Hugo at Bury?' in *Suffolk in the Middle Ages* (Woodbridge: Boydell, 1986), pp. 86–9 (an updated version of Scarfe's article 'The Bury St Edmunds Cross: the work of Master Hugo' in *PSIAH* 33 (1973), pp. 75–85).
92 Scarfe (1986), pp. 97–8.
93 Parker and Little (1994), pp. 206–12.
94 Ibid., pp. 222–7.
95 Ibid., p. 227.

Anselm's successor, Ording. However, the period from the election of Abbot Baldwin to the death of Anselm was formative for the development of the cult of St Edmund, the Abbey's contribution to England's cultural life, and the buildings of the Abbey. At the time of Anselm's death the Abbey Church was complete (apart from the west front), as were the Norman Tower and the churches of St James and St Mary. Between them, Baldwin and Anselm can be credited with establishing St Edmunds as England's greatest abbey and the pre-eminent shrine of the Norman era.

Chapter 3
The age of Samson and the age of Magna Carta, 1148–1229

The abbacy of Samson of Tottington between 1182 and 1211 is the best attested of any abbot of St Edmunds, or indeed of any abbot of any English house during the entire Middle Ages, owing to the remarkable *Chronicle* compiled by Jocelin de Brakelond. Although his intentions were not biographical, Jocelin has been seen as the foremost biographer of the twelfth century, and it is certainly true that the personality and character of Samson is vividly conveyed in his pages. However, Jocelin's *Chronicle* is more than just a literary production or a character sketch; it is a uniquely valuable source for the history of the Abbey, both during the abbacy of Samson's predecessor Hugh I (when Samson was subsacrist) and for much of Samson's own reign, although the narrative finishes in 1202. Samson's reign has sometimes been seen as the high point of the Abbey's history, but it was also clouded by the persecution, massacre and expulsion of Bury's Jewish community.

The reign of Samson's successor Hugh of Northwold was similarly eventful, and it is now clear that Hugh played a pivotal role in ensuring that King John signed Magna Carta. The Abbot defied the king over his disputed election, setting a precedent for the barons, who came to Bury to swear an oath to compel John to enshrine the rule of law in October 1214. At the same time as he was forced to confirm Magna Carta at Runnymede, John was also forced to back down over Hugh's election and confirm him as Abbot. St Edmund had struck another blow for English liberty, establishing the Abbey's reputation as 'the shrine of the king, the cradle of the law'.

Ording and Hugh I, 1148–80

Ording, who succeeded Anselm as Abbot, was an unlearned man – Jocelin de Brakelond described him as *illiteratus*, meaning that he could not read or write Latin. Ording continued Anselm's building programme and his patronage of Master Hugo. After a fire in 1150 which damaged some of the conventual buildings, Ording presided over the construction of a new infirmary by his sacrist, Elias, and introduced the cult of St Giles, to whom he asked the bishop of St Asaph to consecrate a chapel in the south transept.[1] The infirmary lay to the east of the cloister, and as a result of its reconstruction the tower of St Benedict's (built by Ælfric before the Conquest) and the adjacent chambers of Abbot Baldwin were pulled down,[2] although the altar in the infirmary continued to be dedicated

---
1 Gransden (2009), p. 117.
2 Ibid., p. 121.

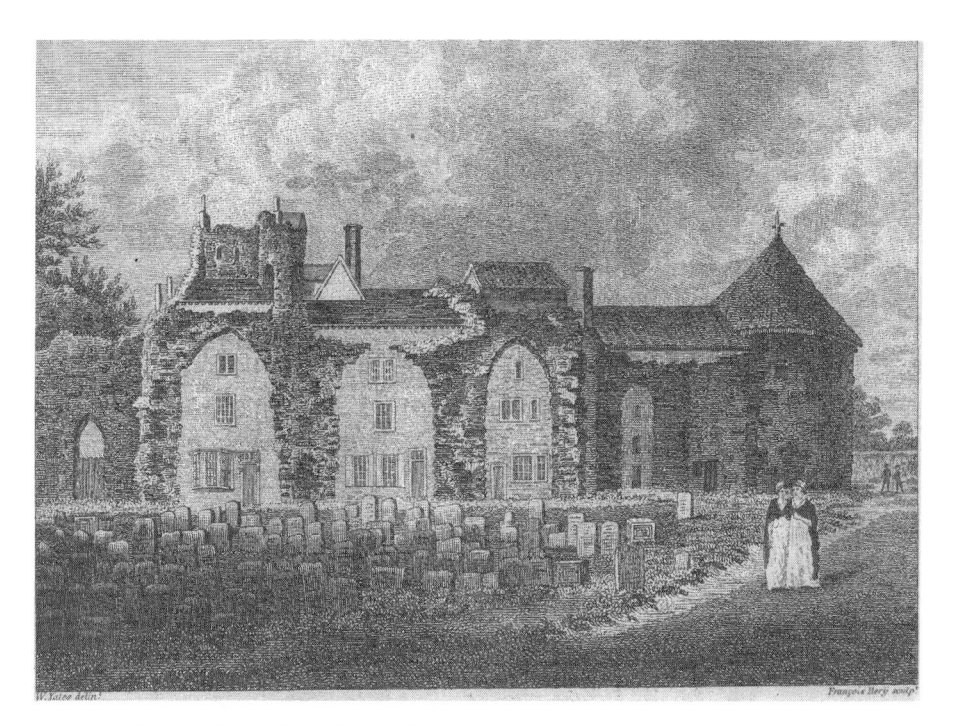

Figure 18 The west front of the Abbey Church (1804), begun by Samson as subsacrist and completed when he was Abbot. Engraving from Richard Yates, *An Illustration of the Monastic Antiquities of the Town and Abbey of St Edmund's Bury* (1843), plate facing p. 35.

to St Benedict, perpetuating the connection.[3] Elias the sacrist was also responsible for commissioning a cross with relics set in the back of it which was set up in the chapel of St Peter, otherwise known as the chapel of the Cross.[4] In 1155 Ording obtained papal confirmation from Pope Adrian IV that the town of Bury St Edmunds belonged to the sacrist and that its income was due to the Abbey.[5]

Ording may also have been responsible for the purchase or construction of a house for the Abbot in London, known as the *hospitium* – usually translated as 'inn', but in this case more like the London palaces of great ecclesiastical magnates such as the bishop of Ely's palace at Holborn. The Abbot's London palace was located at Aldgate, close to the priory of Holy Trinity, and is first mentioned in charters dating from around 1150. It was still standing in 1598 when the antiquary John Stowe described it and explained that its original name, 'Buries markes', had become corrupted to the modern name of the street where it once stood, Bevis Marks (there is also a Bury Street, presumably named after the Abbey, nearby).[6] 'Mark' in this case derives from the Old English word meaning a plot of land or territory, which implies that the *hospitium* had extensive gardens – which is

---

3   James (1895), p. 147.
4   Ibid., p. 139.
5   Gransden (2009), p. 22.
6   Gransden (2015), pp. 131–2.

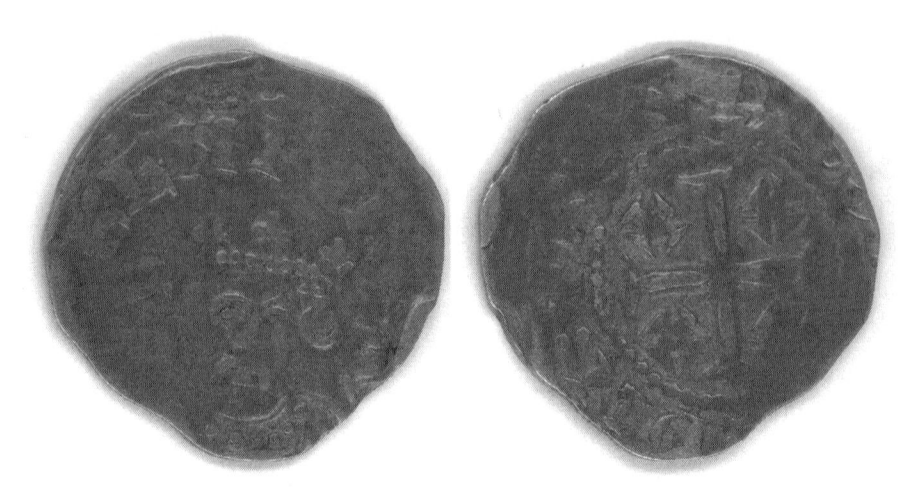

Figure 19 A 'Tealby' penny of Henry II minted at Bury during the reign of Abbot Hugh I between 1158 and 1180. Photo by the author.

confirmed by Stowe. No trace of the *hospitium* survives today, and Bevis Marks is now famous as the location of Britain's oldest synagogue, built in 1701.

During the reign of Abbot Hugh I (1157–80), Bury became involved in a dispute with St Albans Abbey about which house should take precedence as the foremost abbey in England. At the Council of Tours in 1163, Hugh was horrified to discover that the abbot of St Albans took the seat of honour among the English abbots, and as a result he occupied the seat all night to ensure that St Albans did not take it the next day.[7] In 1158 Hugh obtained papal confirmation that elections of abbots of St Edmunds would be free from external interference,[8] and in 1172 he obtained confirmation from the papacy that St Edmunds would be free of any ecclesiastical jurisdiction other than the pope's.[9] The need for a second confirmation arose in 1175 because the archbishop of Canterbury, Richard of Dover, threatened a visitation of the Abbey under his legatine powers. Hugh was forced to sell church ornaments in order to raise money to pay for a bull from Pope Alexander III, confirming that Bury was free from the jurisdiction of anyone other than a legate *a latere*. Nevertheless, Hugh did manage to erect the great rood on a beam behind the high altar.[10]

Jocelin accused Hugh of being too trusting, although he was pious and good, and noted that Hugh ran up enormous debts with Jewish moneylenders,[11] especially Benedict of Blakeham, the brother of the prominent Jew Jurnet of Norwich, who lent a considerable sum towards the repair of the monastic great hall.[12] Although the first Jews arrived in

---

7   Yates (1843), p. 212.
8   Gransden (2009), p. 153.
9   Ibid., p. 21.
10   Ibid., p. 109.
11   Ibid., p. 23.
12   V. D. Lipman, *The Jews of Medieval Norwich* (London: Jewish Historical Society of England, 1967), pp. 101–2.

England shortly after the Norman Conquest, it is likely that they arrived in Bury only in the 1130s, during the reign of Anselm. The oldest surviving secular stone building in the town, Moyse's Hall on Cornhill, dating from around 1180, has persistently been associated with the Jewish community, but the attribution is disputed. Certainly it seems most unlikely that the building was ever a synagogue as traditionally claimed, and the name Moyse is common in Suffolk and need not have any Jewish association. The story that the building was a synagogue seems to appear no earlier than the seventeenth century.[13] Overall, it is more likely that Moyse's Hall was built as accommodation for pilgrims who could not be given lodgings in in the Abbey's guesthouse.[14]

The Jews of Bury were neither 'men of St Edmunds' nor Christians bound by canon law, so were free to practise usury. Jews were under the special protection of the crown, and for this reason the monks resented their appearance in the *banleuca* because they had no kind of feudal dependence on the Abbey. The antisemitic message underlying the Cloisters Cross may have emerged during this period, and in April or June 1181, during the vacancy that followed the death of Abbot Hugh, a young boy named Robert was found murdered in the town. The circumstances of the murder seem to have resembled those that attended the murder of William, son of the priest Wenstun, who in 1144 had been found buried in a shallow grave in Thorpe Wood, just outside Norwich, with signs of torture on his body.

A Norwich Jew had confessed to the murder of William, and thereafter he was venerated as 'Little St William of Norwich' in the cathedral. The murder of 'Little St Robert' was, therefore, an opportunity for the Abbey both to draw pilgrims away from Norwich and to undermine the Jewish community. Robert was entombed in the Abbey Church with great honour, and the cult of 'Little St Robert' sprang up in the crypt; the altar of his chapel still survives.[15] Part of the martyrdom narratives of William and Robert included the idea that the boys were ritually murdered at Passover by Jews wishing to re-enact the murder of Christ and drink the boy's blood. This was the origin of the infamous 'blood libel' that lies at the root of much subsequent antisemitism,[16] which was undoubtedly East Anglia's least glorious contribution to European culture.

There is no evidence that any Jews were found guilty of or punished for Robert's death, but resentment simmered, stimulated by crusading zeal. In his brief record of the events of 1190, John de Taxster made clear the connection: 'Many going to Jerusalem killed Jews – at Norwich – at Stamford – at York – at Bury St Edmunds, where the Jews were killed on 19 March, that is to say on Palm Sunday. Those who remained, when Abbot Samson was in charge, were ejected from the aforesaid town.'[17] The men going to Jerusalem were

---

13 Ibid., p. 22.
14 Julie Kerr, *Monastic Hospitality: The Benedictines in England, c. 1070–c. 1250* (Woodbridge: Boydell, 2007), p. 148. On Moyse's Hall see Margaret E. Wood, 'Moyse's Hall: a description of the building', *Archaeological Journal* 108 (1952), pp. 165–7; E. R. Samuel, 'Was Moyse's Hall, Bury St Edmunds, a Jew's house?', *Transactions of the Jewish Historical Society of England* 25 (1977), pp. 43–7; Robert Halliday, 'Moyse's Hall, Bury St Edmunds', *Suffolk Review* 25 (1995), pp. 27–44.
15 On the cult of 'Little St Robert' see H. Copinger Hill, 'S. Robert of Bury St. Edmunds' in *PSIAH* 21 (1932), pp. 98–107.
16 Gransden (2009), pp. 117–19.
17 Quoted in Copinger Hill (1932), p. 102: *Multi jerosolimam tendentes judaeos occiderunt – apud Norvic – apud Stamford – apud Eboracum – apud Sanctum Edmundum occiduntur Judaei xv Kal.*

crusaders, vowed to slaughter the infidel – and the Jews were the infidels in their midst. Just a few days after the infamous massacre of Jews in York Castle, the people of Bury St Edmunds murdered fifty-seven Jews, probably in Hatter (anciently 'Heathenman') Street, which was the Jewish quarter of the town.[18]

Lisa Lampert has argued that it is significant that the murder of 'Little St Robert' took place during the vacancy following the death of Abbot Hugh. Jocelin de Brakelond described another candidate, William the Sacrist, as the 'father of the Jews', and in Lampert's view, Samson (then subsacrist) aligned himself with a popular antisemitic movement as part of his bid to take power in the monastery.[19] Jocelin certainly regarded the expulsion of the Jews from Bury later in 1190 as one of Samson's three greatest achievements, but for the modern observer the taint of antisemitism indelibly marks Samson's abbacy, and makes it difficult to make a thoroughly positive evaluation of his legacy.

Earlier in Hugh's reign, in 1173, the Abbey had been directly threatened by the outbreak of civil war, as Henry II's eldest son 'Henry the Young King' and Queen Eleanor of Aquitaine mounted a rebellion against him. One of Henry the Young King's supporters, Robert de Beaumont, third earl of Leicester, invaded East Anglia with an army of Flemish mercenaries, intending to link up his forces with those of another rebel, Hugh Bigod, earl of Norfolk. Leicester's army sacked Norwich and attacked Dunwich (which was then a large and flourishing coastal port) before marching back to Leicester, via Bury:

> Trusting in the number and valour of his allies – for he had about eighty picked horsemen and four or five thousand valiant infantry – and reckoning also that no-one would oppose him on the way, because he had many friends among those who appeared to favour the king's side, [Leicester] set out boldly with all his forces, taking with him his wife and a certain French noble called Hugh 'de Châteauneuf'. But the barons of the royal party were at Bury St Edmunds watching his movements with a considerable force, and when they had come up with him, they led forward their army drawn up in battle order against his troops. The latter, unable to wheel either to the right or to the left, made a virtue of necessity and boldly pushed on with all speed using their cavalry as a screen. And so began a desperate battle, the king's troops fighting for glory and the rebels for safety; but victory fell to the royal army.[20]

The battle took place on 17 October 1173 at Fornham St Genevieve, at a site which may have been within sight of the great Abbey Church. The royal army was led by Roger Bigod, later created earl of Norfolk in 1189, who rode out from Bury at the head of the Knights of St Edmund, carrying St Edmund's banner and with Abbot Hugh's banner.[21]

Aprilis, scilicet in die Palmarum: qui vero remanserunt procurante Abbate Sampsone, de predicta villa perpetuo sunt ejecti.

18 Gransden (2009), p. 29.
19 Lisa Lampert, 'The once and future Jew: the Croxton "Play of the Sacrament", Little Robert of Bury and historical memory', *Jewish History* 15 (2001), pp. 235–55, at p. 238.
20 William of Newburgh, 'The history of England', in David C. Douglas and George W. Greenaway (eds), *English Historical Documents, 1042–1189*, 2nd edn (London: Routledge, 1981), pp. 347–403, at p. 375.
21 Gransden (2009), p. 58.

Abbot Hugh and the monks must have greeted the victory with considerable relief, since if Leicester had won it is highly likely that the Abbey would have been plundered by rebel troops.

Samson of Tottington, 1182–1211

Samson of Tottington, who was born in the Norfolk village of Tottington in 1135, had an early connection with the Abbey of St Edmund; as a child of nine he dreamed he was standing in front of the cemetery gate of the Abbey when the devil tried to seize hold of him, but St Edmund saved him and held him in his arms. Samson's mother therefore took him to the Abbey, and a further connection was furnished by the fact that the son of Samson's teacher, Master William of Diss, was a monk of the Abbey. Samson studied at the University of Paris, gaining degrees in both arts and medicine, and became a schoolmaster in Norfolk.

In 1159–60 the Abbey employed Samson, then still a lay clerk, to go to Rome in order to protest about the alienation of a pension from Woolpit church from the Abbey by the crown. Samson was robbed on the way back from Rome and, although he managed to hold on to his letter from the pope, his journey was slowed down by the fact that he had to beg all the way. He arrived in Bury too late – a royal clerk had already been presented to the living of Woolpit, against the Abbot's wishes, and Abbot Hugh was so angry with Samson that the young man hid under the shrine of St Edmund for protection. He was exiled, in fetters, to Castle Acre in Norfolk, but eventually Abbot Hugh seems to have forgiven Samson, since he was professed as a monk of St Edmunds in 1165 or 1166.

Samson's first appointment was as novice-master, where he first encountered a young Jocelin de Brakelond, his future chaplain and biographer. Samson progressed quickly through the offices of the monastery, serving successively as guest master, pittancer, third prior and subsacrist; Jocelin claimed that his rapid movement from one office to another was because he was frequently accused of misconduct. The most prominent characteristic of Samson's character seems to have been obstinacy, and he was plainly unsuited to the life of obedience enjoined by the Rule of St Benedict. Abbot Hugh died on 14 November 1180, and a vacancy of fifteen months followed, during which Samson, as subsacrist, embarked on a building programme. He began a new infirmary and a new chapel of St Andrew in the cemetery, to replace an earlier one built next to the sacristy by Abbot Anselm.[22] Samson also created the choir screen and, most ambitiously of all, began building the west tower of the Abbey Church. He was accused of misappropriating alms, and eventually King Henry II forbade building works during the vacancy.[23]

In theory, the Abbot of St Edmunds was elected – and could only be elected – by the monks, but in practice, because the king had the power to withhold the Abbot's barony (and therefore his temporal power), royal confirmation of an election was necessary. An election initially took place in the Chapter House, and then a second election before the king in the royal chapel at Westminster. Augustine, bishop of Nidaros in Norway, who was then in exile at Bury St Edmunds, interceded with the king in favour of a free election, and Samson was duly elected Abbot in spite of his lack of high birth and connections.[24]

---

22 Ibid., pp. 12–14.
23 Ibid., pp. 15–16.
24 Ibid., pp. 18–20.

Samson was blessed at Marwell on 28 February 1182 by Richard, bishop of Winchester, who invested him with a mitre and abbatial ring.[25] Samson was the first mitred abbot of Bury St Edmunds, and he assumed the mitre without express papal sanction, much as he also chose to interpret a papal bull of 1187 granting him the right to administer solemn episcopal benediction in the *banleuca* as giving him the right to do it anywhere.[26]

Samson immediately set about the reform of the Abbey's property and finances, and in April 1182 he began a tour of all the Abbey's manors. He dispossessed the tenants and brought most of the manors back under the Abbey's direct control, and by means of skilled management was able to pay off the debts run up during Hugh's reign.[27] One of Samson's early achievements, in 1189, was the recovery of the manor of Mildenhall, an ancient property of the Abbey granted by Edward the Confessor but which had fallen into the possession of the Crown. Samson managed to raise the money to buy Mildenhall back from King Richard I, although the exercise proved costly and he was even forced to sell treasures of the church in order to pay the 1,000 marks required by the king.[28]

In 1190 Samson expelled all Jews from Bury St Edmunds – those who had survived the Palm Sunday massacre – on the grounds that Jews were under the special protection of the crown and therefore their presence in the *banleuca* undermined the Abbot's right to exclude royal officials.[29] His expulsion of the Jews from Bury anticipated by a century Edward I's expulsion of all Jews from the kingdom, and in Samson's case there may have been other factors at play as well as the Abbey's traditional liberties. Thanks to the cult of 'Little St Robert', which was fostered by Jocelin de Brakelond's account of the boy's 'martyrdom' (now lost), Bury had become a centre of antisemitism, and the expulsion of the Jews also drew a line under the bad old days of Abbot Hugh in which the Abbey was in debt to Jewish moneylenders to the tune of hundreds of pounds.

During Samson's reign the division between the rights of the Abbot and the rights of the Convent (the rest of the monks) came into sharp relief. Under normal circumstances, monks could appeal against an abbot's abuse of power to the local bishop or, failing that, the archbishop of Canterbury or a papal legate. However, Samson exercised the powers of a bishop and was subject to no one other than the pope himself. At the start of his reign, he confiscated all private seals owned by individual monks, other than the prior and sacrist, and ordered houses in the cemetery erected by the sacrist, William Wiardel, to be pulled down on the grounds that they were used for 'frequent wine-bibbings'.[30] Shortly thereafter, Samson deposed Wiardel and replaced him with Samson the precentor.[31]

Samson's relations with the Convent's other obedientary, the cellarer, were equally poor, and he regularly accused the cellarer of overspending, eventually deposing him and replacing him with his own personal appointee in 1197. The cellarer was in charge of obtaining food and drink for the monks and guests. Opposition from the monks was

---

25 Ibid., p. 20.
26 Ibid., p. 79.
27 Ibid., pp. 24–6.
28 Ibid., pp. 27–8.
29 Lampert (2001), p. 237.
30 Gransden (2009), pp. 32–3.
31 Ibid., p. 88.

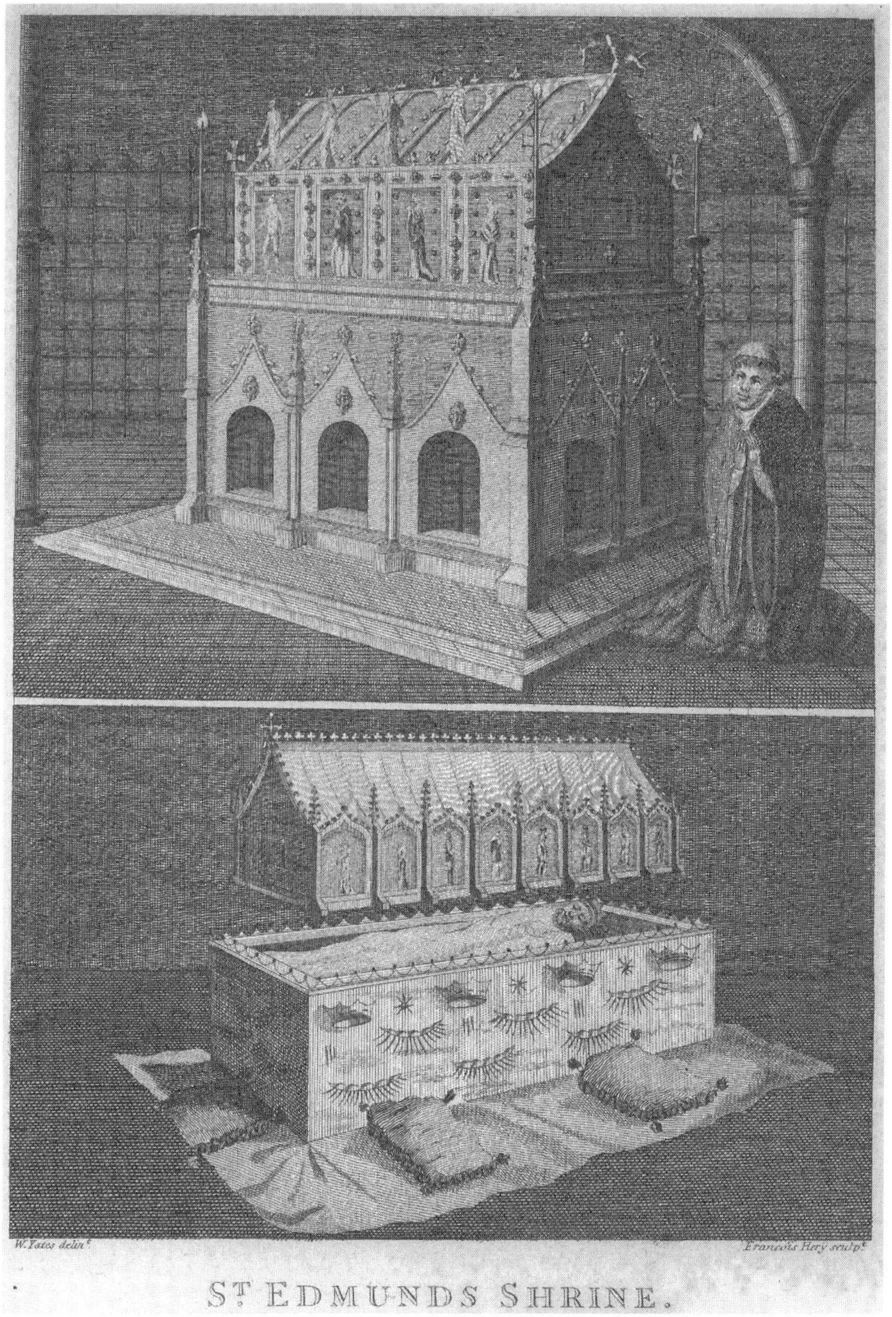

ST EDMUNDS SHRINE.

Figure 20 The shrine and feretory of St Edmund. Engraving from Richard Yates, *An Illustration of the Monastic Antiquities of the Town and Abbey of St Edmund's Bury* (1843), plate facing p. 39.

so strong, however, that Samson was eventually forced to restore the cellarer.[32] The next cellarer, Jocellus,[33] who was appointed in 1198, fell out with Samson over the case of Ralph the gatekeeper, who was accused by the monks of launching hostile suits against them and was therefore deprived of some of his income. Ralph appealed to Samson, who took his side and ordered Jocellus to restore the money. Jocellus, supported by half of the monks, refused; Samson ordered that the cellarer should eat and drink nothing until he obeyed the Abbot, and then left the Abbey for eight days. During the interval, a group of older monks persuaded Jocellus's party to yield to the Abbot, and on his return Samson excommunicated the leaders of the dispute on both sides.[34]

Samson faced one of the greatest challenges, but also one of the greatest opportunities of his abbacy when, on the night of 22 June 1198, a wooden structure for candles behind the high altar caught fire. This was apparently caused by the carelessness of the shrine keepers who, to save money, stacked used candles on top of one another to make new makeshift candles. One of these candles toppled over and set light to a cloth on top of the wooden structure and then to the wood itself, which was surrounded by iron grilles. By the time the fire was discovered at matins the feretory of the martyr itself was alight, and the monks were forced to use their cowls to try to put out the flames. When water was poured on the still-smouldering feretory it cracked the gems, and the silver plates fell off onto the floor, although the gold image of Christ in majesty attached to the shrine was apparently undamaged.

Fortunately, the rood beam above the shrine had been removed for redecoration so the *camisia* (shirt) of St Edmund and other relics were saved. The monks saw that the box containing the cup of St Edmund had been completely burned, but the fire had not consumed the cup itself, which was still inside wrapped in its half-burned linen cloth. The monks did their best to cover up the damage to the feretory, but it was obvious to pilgrims that something was amiss and rumours began to circulate that the body of the martyr had been damaged. When Samson returned to the monastery he declared his intention to adorn the feretory in gold and raise it on a new foundation of marble. On 23 November the feretory was placed on the high altar while Samson proclaimed a three-day fast for the inhabitants of the *banleuca* in preparation for the translation.[35]

The coffin of St Edmund remained in its original position on the foundation of the old shrine, and after lauds Samson and a small number of other monks unwrapped the coffin (or *loculus*) from its silk and linen coverings. Jocelin described what he saw on the outside of the coffin:

> Over the breast of the martyr there lay, fixed to the surface of the coffin, a golden angel about the length of a human foot, holding in the one hand a golden sword, and in the other a banner; under this there was a hole in the lid of the coffin, on which the ancient servants of the martyr had been wont to lay their hands for touching the sacred body.

---

32   Ibid., pp. 34–5.
33   Gransden (2009), pp. 9–10 dismisses the idea that Jocelin de Brakelond and Jocellus were one and the same person, advocated by Norman Scarfe (see Norman Scarfe, 'Chronicles of Bury Abbey', in *Suffolk in the Middle Ages* (Woodbridge: Boydell, 1986), pp. 99–121; Norman Scarfe, 'Jocelin of Brakelond's identity: a review of the evidence', *PSIAH* 39 (1997), pp. 1–5).
34   Gransden (2009), p. 38.
35   Ibid., pp. 95–8.

And over the figure of the angel was this verse inscribed: Behold the image of Michael guards the body of the martyr.[36]

The coffin was then taken to the high altar and placed in the feretory. However, on the night of 25 November Samson summoned Hugh the sacrist, Walter the physician and ten other monks to open the coffin. Once the lid of the coffin was removed, only Hugh and Walter were allowed to witness the unwrapping of the body. Samson did not dare to unwrap the body completely, but he held the martyr's head and declared, 'Glorious martyr, St Edmund, blessed be the hour when you were born! Glorious martyr, do not cast me, a miserable sinner, into perdition for presuming to touch you: you know my devotion, you know my intent.'[37]

The martyr was reverently wrapped up again and the coffin sealed, and in the morning Samson announced to the convent what he had done and the monks sang a tearful *Te Deum*. Although the fire might have been disastrous for the Abbey, by not only translating the body of St Edmund but also providing a new witness testimony to the incorruptibility of the martyr, Samson had immeasurably increased the renown of the shrine. Translations of relics were often followed by stories of new miracles, as the power of the saint was rediscovered, and Samson's inspection of the holy body must have been widely publicised at the time by the monks, and no doubt resulted in a renewed influx of pilgrims. However, Gransden's hypothesis that Samson committed a 'pious fraud' by substituting a recently dead body for the inspection is implausible,[38] and hardly consonant with the genuine devotion to St Edmund which Jocelin, a man who knew him well, discerned in Samson.

In Gransden's view, Samson adopted an enlightened attitude to the Abbey's relations with the townsfolk, and 'He was the last Abbot of St Edmunds to ward off conflict between the burgesses and convent by making concessions to them.'[39] In around 1185 he also founded a hospital specifically for the 'infirm and poor' townsfolk, St Saviour's Hospital at Babwell outside the town's North Gate, which enjoyed papal protection (secured in 1186) as well as healthy revenues from the manor of Icklingham. Samson's foundation of a free school for poor boys within the monastic precincts was far-sighted. He also bought houses in the town to provide free lodgings for forty poor scholars, who were to include two clerks and an usher. In the first instance these were to be relatives of Bury monks, but thereafter they were chosen by the schoolmaster.[40] Samson's was one of the earliest endowments of free education, and the school at Bury, refounded after the Reformation as the Bury Grammar School by King Edward VI, would go on to be one of the most illustrious schools in East Anglia.[41] Perhaps Samson's own low birth, combined

---

36 Jocelin de Brakelond, *Chronica Jocelini de Brakelond*, ed. J. Gage Rokewode (London: Camden Society, 1840), pp. 82–3: *Jacuit super pectus martiris affixus loculo exterius angelus aureus ad longitudinem pedis humani, habens ensem aureum in una manu, et vexillum in altera; et subtus erat foramen in operculo, ubi antiqui custodes martiris solebant manus imponere ad tangendum sanctum corpus. Et erat versus superscriptus imagini: Martiris ecce zoma servat Michaelis agalma.*
37 Gransden (2009), pp. 99–100.
38 Ibid., pp. 102–4.
39 Ibid., p. 47.
40 Ibid., pp. 49–51.
41 On the foundation of the Grammar School see R. W. Elliott, *The Story of King Edward VI*

with the fact that he had once been a schoolmaster, made him sympathetic to poor scholars.

Samson showed no lack of personal courage, and in 1193 he donned armour and rode at the head of the Knights of St Edmund, under the banner of St Edmund, to the siege of Windsor Castle. John, count of Mortain (the future King John) was in rebellion during his brother King Richard's captivity in Germany. Jocelin was impressed, but worried that this would set a dangerous precedent for the Abbot leading military expeditions abroad.[42] In theory, canon law prohibited clerics from bearing arms and shedding blood, but it did not specifically ban them from wearing armour and leading armies, and some clerics notoriously carried heavy clubs covered in velvet into battle, so that any blow they inflicted was unlikely to draw blood. In the reality of twelfth-century England, the Abbot was expected to defend his temporal possessions just as any secular lord would have been.

The Knights of St Edmund, who had originally been enfeoffed on the lands of the Abbey by King William I, ended up causing some problems for Samson. There were officially forty knights but twelve more had become enfeoffed, contrary to the Abbey's arrangement with the crown, during the reigns of Ording and Hugh. Samson insisted that he only owed service of forty knights and no more, but he encountered a further problem when King Richard asked Samson to send the Knights of St Edmund to France. The Knights had never fought abroad and did not consider this part of their 'scutage' (knights' service), and Samson was forced to placate Richard by buying some mercenaries for his army.[43]

During the 1190s and 1200s Samson was regularly commissioned to act as a papal judge delegate – so much so that he had little time to take care of the Abbey. But as Gransden has pointed out, the Abbey depended on the papacy for its privileges so Samson had little choice but to serve.[44] In 1195 the same problem arose as had faced Abbot Hugh in 1175, when the Pope gave legatine powers of visitation to Archbishop Hubert of Canterbury. Samson initially invited Hubert to St Edmunds as a guest, in an effort to pre-empt a visitation, but then offended the archbishop by obtaining a letter from the pope to Hubert warning him against attempting a visitation in 1196. The next year, the two ecclesiastics eventually met on the road between Waltham and London and had a heated argument.[45] Samson managed to obtain a number of other special powers and privileges from Rome, such as the right of the Abbot to wear episcopal vestments (a dalmatic under a chasuble),[46] the right to determine matrimonial causes, usually reserved to bishops, and the right to tonsure clerics and admit them to minor orders below subdeacon.[47] In effect, Samson could do everything a bishop could do other than ordain clergy to the major orders and consecrate altars and churches.

    School Bury St. Edmunds (Bury St Edmunds: Foundation Governors of the School, 1963), pp. 7–10.
42 Gransden (2009), p. 58.
43 Ibid., pp. 56–9.
44 Ibid,. pp. 68–78.
45 Ibid., p. 79.
46 The only differences between the vestments of a mitred abbot and those of a bishop were that the abbot's mitre could not feature precious stones and he held the crozier in his right hand rather than his left (Yates (1843), p. 184).
47 Gransden (2009), p. 81.

Samson established strong personal relationships with Henry II and Richard I. Henry came to the shrine in 1188 to pray before setting out on crusade, as he had done in 1177, and at some point he donated a golden chalice worth 100 marks. Richard stayed at the Abbey for at least a week over the Feast of St Edmund in the year of his accession, 1189, on one of his rare visits to England. Richard dedicated his crusading fleet to the protection of St Edmund, St Thomas and St Nicholas, and in 1191 he sent the Abbey the banner of the defeated ruler of Cyprus, Isaac Comnenus. Samson's visit to the captive Richard in Germany was mentioned in the previous chapter, and a degree of personal friendship between the two men is suggested by the fact that Richard spent around two weeks at the Abbey in March 1194 on his return from captivity.[48] Richard regarded St Edmund as a perfect warrior-king, but King John's devotion to the martyr was more lukewarm. On his first visit his only offering was a silk cloth that he had borrowed from the sacrist anyway, and on another occasion he gave only thirteen shillings as an offering at mass.

In 1207 the bedroom of Samson's manor house of Stapleford Abbotts was the scene of an important meeting between John and his ally Otto, King of the Romans to discuss how to proceed against Phillip Augustus of France.[49] This would suggest that Samson was held in high regard by John. However, on 24 March 1208, in retaliation against the papal interdict against England, John confiscated all of the Abbey's property, although St Edmunds was not special in this regard. However, as an exempt abbey under the sole authority of the pope, John may have seen an attack on Bury as a way of annoying the papacy. Three weeks later John relented 'on account of reverence for St Edmund' and restored the Abbey's privileges, but Gransden thought that Samson would have had to pay a great price for the concession, and the cellarer later calculated the losses incurred during this period at 4000 marks.[50]

A further disaster occurred in 1210 when the central spire of the Abbey Church collapsed. It tottered menacingly in the direction of the presbytery, choir and chapel of St Mary. In the end, however, it fell to the north and did little damage, although 'the posts of the campanile ... fell about in all directions'. The spire could not be rebuilt during the Interdict and it was probably not restored until the 1230s, under the sacrist Nicholas of Warwick.[51] However, Bury continued to enjoy one privilege during the dark time of the Interdict, which was the right to celebrate mass on the porphyry altar supposedly brought back from Rome by Abbot Baldwin, and which was exempt from any interdict imposed on the kingdom.[52]

The library and scriptorium

Although the earliest evidence for books at Bury St Edmunds is the list compiled by Leofstan in the eleventh century, the first library catalogue dates from shortly after 1150, and on the basis of this and a number of surviving books bearing the 'Bury press-mark', 110 books have been identified that survive from the Abbey's twelfth-century library.[53]

---

48   Ibid., pp. 63–4.
49   Ibid., p. 65.
50   Ibid., pp. 66–7.
51   Whittingham (1952), p. 175.
52   Yates (1843), p. 98.
53   Thomson (1972), p. 619. See also Richard Sharpe, 'Reconstructing the medieval library of

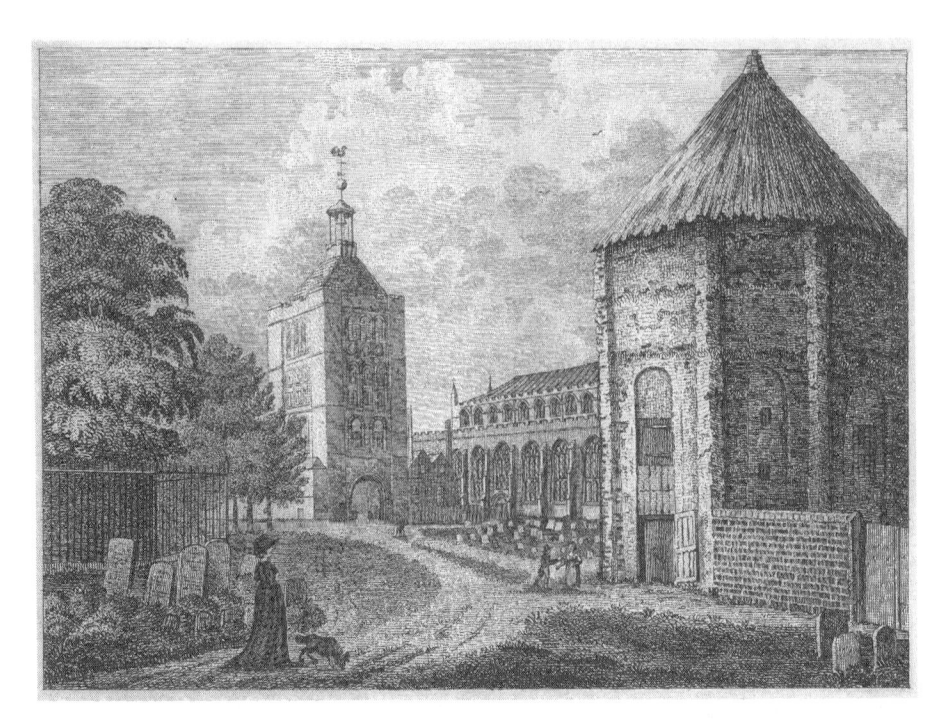

Figure 21 Samson's Tower from the south-east (1804) before Victorian 'improvements' damaged its original appearance. The tower is all that remains of the two unique octagonal towers at the ends of the western transepts. Engraving from Richard Yates, *An Illustration of the Monastic Antiquities of the Town and Abbey of St Edmund's Bury* (1843), plate facing p. 14.

Works of the Fathers predominated, as might be expected.[54] Fifteen pre-Conquest books survive with a Bury press-mark, but it is doubtful that these were all at the Abbey when they were first created, and they may have been later acquisitions. One manuscript which is likely to have been created in an eleventh-century scriptorium at Bury is the Bury St Edmunds Psalter in the Vatican Library, in which feasts specific to the Abbey are given special prominence and illuminated in gold.[55]

Rodney Thomson believed that Baldwin established a scriptorium at Bury soon after 1081, which perpetuated Anglo-Saxon writing styles rather than adopting new ones from the Continent. Thomson attributed to the scriptorium at Bury the so-called 'Bury Herbal' (Oxford, MS Bodley 130), whose contents coincide with Baldwin's medical interests. In the nineteenth century a lead book cover was discovered in the Abbey ruins, which is now in the Pitt Rivers Museum in Oxford.[56] In the early twelfth century, the Abbey's

---

Bury St Edmunds Abbey: the lost catalogue of Henry of Kirkstead', in Gransden (1998), pp. 204–18, at p. 204.
54 Thomson (1972), p. 621.
55 Ibid., pp. 622–3.
56 Ibid., p. 626.

library holdings expanded to include Latin translations of the Greek Fathers,[57] but only three books can be securely tied to the Bury scriptorium at this time, an indication of the unsettled nature of the Abbey in the early years of the century. Thomson believed that the scriptorium revived again and operated continuously under Prior Baldwin, who served under Abbot Anselm in the 1120s, and his successor Prior Talbot.[58] However, books produced during this period were 'workman-like' rather than beautiful, perhaps because Bury was racing to catch up with other Abbeys and ensure that it had all the books it needed in its library.

During Samson's reign the Abbey appears to have had close relations with the Suffolk-born Robert Grosseteste, bishop of Lincoln (although Gransden disputes the evidence for this). Grosseteste was famed for his learning, and the Abbey certainly lent him a copy of the *Hexaëmeron* in exchange for a set of commentaries on the Fathers.[59] Another important manuscript acquired by the Abbey at this time was a deluxe version of the *Canon* of Avicenna, which is evidence for a continuing interest in medicine in Bury. It may have been given by the infirmarian, Master Stephen of Caistor. Gransden has suggested that Stephen studied medicine at Bologna and brought the *Canon* to England with him; as a qualified physician as well as the monastic infirmarian, Stephen would have been able to make a considerable income from medical practice and was therefore in a position to give rich gifts to the Abbey.[60]

Gransden has suggested that a book of psalms in Hebrew Ashkenazik square script owned by the Abbey in the thirteenth century and now Oxford, Bodleian Library Hebrew MS 117 was probably in the possession of one of the Jews expelled from Bury in 1190. If so, then the influence of the Jews lingered on in the form of an interest in Hebrew studies at the Abbey, exemplified in the thirteenth century by the anonymous monk who added the Latin *incipit* (opening words) beside each psalm – a considerable feat of learning at a time when most monks were entirely ignorant of Hebrew. Furthermore, at some point in Samson's reign the Abbey acquired a Hebrew liturgy; fragments of prayers for the Day of Atonement were later reused in binding other books.[61] Perhaps the book was considered unworthy of a place in the Abbey's library, but the possibility that the libraries of learned Jews were absorbed into the Abbey's collection in 1190 is an intriguing one.

Samson the builder

When Samson succeeded as Abbot the Abbey Church as a whole had not yet been consecrated. Baldwin failed to obtain permission from King William II to have the unfinished minster consecrated, and by Samson's time the church was nearing completion. Samson managed to obtain a licence to consecrate the church from Pope Innocent III but the ceremony never took place, either because Samson would not allow the bishop of Norwich to officiate within the *banleuca* or because the king could not be present (which Samson

---

57 Ibid., p. 628.
58 Ibid., p. 630.
59 Gransden (2009), pp. 221–4.
60 Ibid., pp. 225–8.
61 Gransden (2015), p. 247.

insisted upon).[62] Instead, Samson turned his attention to completing the west front of the Abbey, following a vision in which St Edmund rose from his shrine and pointed to Samson, saying 'This is the man who will cover my feet.'[63]

The west front was a unique structure with some highly unusual features, such as a western tower and a western transept; the closest parallel to these features occurs at Ely. The distinctive construction of the west front was described by Philip McAleer:

> At the core or centre of the complex was a western transept with an axial tower rising over its intersection with the nave. This transept, a nave-like space, and a feature within this period normally found at the east end of the church, as indeed was true of Bury, was (presumably) about as wide and as tall as the nave. However, unlike a normal eastern transept, including the one at Bury, the western transept did not extend beyond the line of the aisle walls. Flanking each end wall of the transept, north and south, were two-storeyed chapel blocks which consisted of a nave and apse. And then beyond these was found at each end a large octagonal structure, most probably very like a tall chapter house in appearance.[64]

Gransden has argued that the west tower at Bury was a self-consciously Anglo-Saxon feature,[65] since Ely and Winchester had similar towers. However, the octagons at each end of the west front are harder to explain, and it is unclear how tall these originally were. They may have been intended to recall the old rotunda of St Mary and St Edmund.[66]

Samson also presided over the construction of a new infirmary and the chapel of St Andrew in the cemetery, as well as a new larder, the restoration of the Abbot's Hall and a new bath-house and guest-house.[67] Even more impressive, however, was the construction of a 2 mile long aqueduct by Samson's sacrist Walter of Banham, which may have run from the source of the River Linnet at Horringer to a cistern above the cloister range, where a system of lead water pipes and drains distributed water to different parts of the monastery.[68] The Abbey likewise constructed a large number of windmills and watermills on its manors during Samson's reign, which took advantage of the latest technology available and greatly increased the Abbey's income.[69]

Hugh of Northwold, 1215–29, and Magna Carta

When Samson died on 30 December 1211, the monastic annalist recorded that 'He had ruled the abbey successfully for thirty years (less two months), freed it from manifold

---

62 Gransden (2009), pp. 83–4.
63 Ibid., p. 85.
64 J. Philip McAleer, 'The west façade complex at the Abbey Church of Bury St Edmunds: a description of the evidence for its reconstruction', *PSIAH* 39 (1998), pp. 127–50, at p. 127.
65 Rushforth has argued, on the basis of inscriptions in the Bury St Edmunds Psalter, for an ongoing interest in the Anglo-Saxon House of Wessex and its Scottish successor, the House of Dunkeld, at St Edmunds (Rushforth (2005), pp. 255–61).
66 Gransden (2009), pp. 86–7.
67 Ibid., p. 89.
68 Ibid., pp. 90–1.
69 Ibid., pp. 288–316.

debts, enriched it with most ample privileges, liberties, possessions and buildings, and put religious observance within and without the church on a proper footing.'[70] Although Samson died during the Papal Interdict (23 March 1208–2 July 1214) when burials in consecrated ground were forbidden, even for bishops, Samson seems to have been buried in the Chapter House like his predecessors – a powerful assertion of the Abbey's exemption from an Interdict on England because it was under special papal protection.

On account of the Interdict, the abbacy remained vacant for some time after Samson's death, but in Chapter on 7 August 1213 the monks elected the subcellarer, Hugh of Northwold, as Abbot Hugh II.[71] The monks did so under the terms of the confirmation obtained by Hugh I in 1158 that elections at St Edmunds were a purely internal matter, but King John took a different view. Even though Hugh II immediately went to Corfe Castle to seek the king's confirmation, John had expected the election to take place in the royal chapel at Westminster in his presence, and refused to acknowledge Hugh II. The monks appealed to Pope Innocent III, who in October 1213 accepted that the king's assent was needed. On 21 November 1214 John issued a charter to St Edmunds confirming that he would accept any abbot whose election was canonical.[72]

Gransden has suggested that John's charter of 21 November may have been influenced by his visit to St Edmunds on 4 November, when he had demanded that Hugh II resign and Hugh refused, supported by the vast majority of the monks. Nevertheless, the convent was divided over the election, with monks associated with the cellarer supporting Hugh and those associated with the sacrist, Robert of Graveley, opposing his election. Violence erupted in Chapter on more than one occasion, with the monk Thomas of Walsingham being pushed down by force when he tried to speak in favour of Hugh.[73]

The period of Hugh II's disputed election was recorded in detail by the monk Nicholas of Dunstable in his *Cronica de electione Hugonis abbatis postea episcopi Eliensis* ('The chronicle of the election of Abbot Hugh, afterwards Bishop of Ely'). Strangely, however, Dunstable omitted from his chronicle any mention of the most famous story concerning the Abbey during this period: the oath supposedly taken by the barons on the high altar of the Abbey Church that they would withdraw their fealty to John and make war on him if he did not confirm the laws of Edward the Confessor and the Coronation Charter of Henry I. This oath led directly to the barons compelling John to confirm Magna Carta in 1215. The story is found only in the writings of Roger of Wendover, who does not specify when the meeting took place other than late 1214. The most likely date was traditionally considered to be 20 November 1214, when a large gathering of barons could have descended on Bury under the cover of a pilgrimage for St Edmund's day. J. C. Holt cast doubt on the authenticity of the story, based on John's known movements and other evidence.[74]

---

70 Antonia Gransden, 'Samson (1135–1211), abbot of Bury St Edmunds' in *ODNB*, vol. 48, pp. 809–11.
71 Gransden (2009), p. 151.
72 Ibid., pp. 153–4.
73 Ibid., pp. 156–8.
74 J. C. Holt, *Magna Carta*, 3rd edn (Cambridge: Cambridge University Press, 2015), pp. 335–9. For an alternative view see Gransden (1974), p. 359n.; Antonia Gransden (ed.), *The Customary of the Benedictine Abbey of Bury St Edmunds in Suffolk* (London: Henry Bradshaw Society, 1973), p. xxv, n. 5.

Holt's sceptical view of the barons' meeting was not held by Gransden, however, and recently David Carpenter has argued convincingly that the meeting did indeed take place – and, just as importantly for the history of the Abbey, that Hugh of Northwold was probably there. In Carpenter's view there is no need to assume that the barons could only have visited St Edmunds 'for the sake of prayer' on 20 November, since pilgrims arrived throughout the year. On 13 October Abbot Hugh arrived back in England from a meeting with John at Poitou, at which he had hoped to resolve the issue of his election, and he was back in Bury on 24 October. Between 18 and 20 October John wrote to Hugh with the message that he hoped for a quick resolution of the disputed election. However, on 28 October he accused Hugh of fomenting war (*bellum*) against him. Carpenter argues that this dramatic change of tone in John's dealings with Hugh can only be explained by the fact that he had learned of the barons' meeting, which probably took place after 24 October when Hugh was back in Bury.[75]

The veracity of Roger's account is further confirmed by the 'dramatic dash' that John made for Bury on 1 or 2 November, arriving on 4 November, when he entered the Chapter House followed by the earls of Winchester and Norfolk and Robert Fitzwalter and Geoffrey de Mandeville, with the sheriff of Northumberland, Philip Oldcoates, holding a drawn sword before him. As Carpenter observes, 'Its edge was directed not just at the abbey but at those who had so recently defied the king'.[76] Who exactly the barons were who swore the oath is more difficult to establish with certainty, but they were probably from the north and were likely to have included Roger de Cressy, who held lands in East Anglia.[77] John stayed at Bury only for a day (unusual for the time), and Carpenter's explanation of John's visit as implying a threat against Hugh is surely more plausible than the idea that he came to resolve the election dispute – which remained unresolved anyway.

The oath of the barons is a narrative that has become immensely important to the identity of Bury St Edmunds. The Victorians erected a plaque on one of the surviving piers of the Abbey Church to commemorate the event in 1847, which featured in the great open-air pageants of 1907, 1959 and 1970. When Stephen Dykes-Bower's choir for St Edmundsbury Cathedral was completed it was even decorated with the painted shields of the Magna Carta barons, and the borough's motto *Sacrarium regis, cunabula legis* ('The shrine of the king, the cradle of the law') refers to the event. The idea that the barons who came to Bury were exactly the same men who compelled John to seal Magna Carta at Runnymede must be dismissed, as well as the attendance of Archbishop Stephen Langton (the 'high-soul'd priest' of the Victorian inscription). By contrast, Carpenter's interpretation puts Hugh of Northwold centre-stage in the story of Magna Carta, and the barons' decision to come to Bury was probably informed by the fact that the Abbot-elect had recently defied John, setting a precedent they wished to follow. The fact that it was in the meadow at Runnymede that John finally gave his formal consent to Hugh's election, on 10 June 1215, adds further weight to the idea that the election of Hugh of Northwold was intimately tied up with this great event in English history.[78] 'The high soul'd priest' was Hugh, not Langton.

John did not of course honour Magna Carta, and on the outbreak of the First Barons'

---

75 David Carpenter (ed.), *Magna Carta* (London: Penguin Classics, 2015), p. 292.
76 Ibid., pp. 293–4.
77 Ibid., p. 295.
78 Gransden (2009), p. 156.

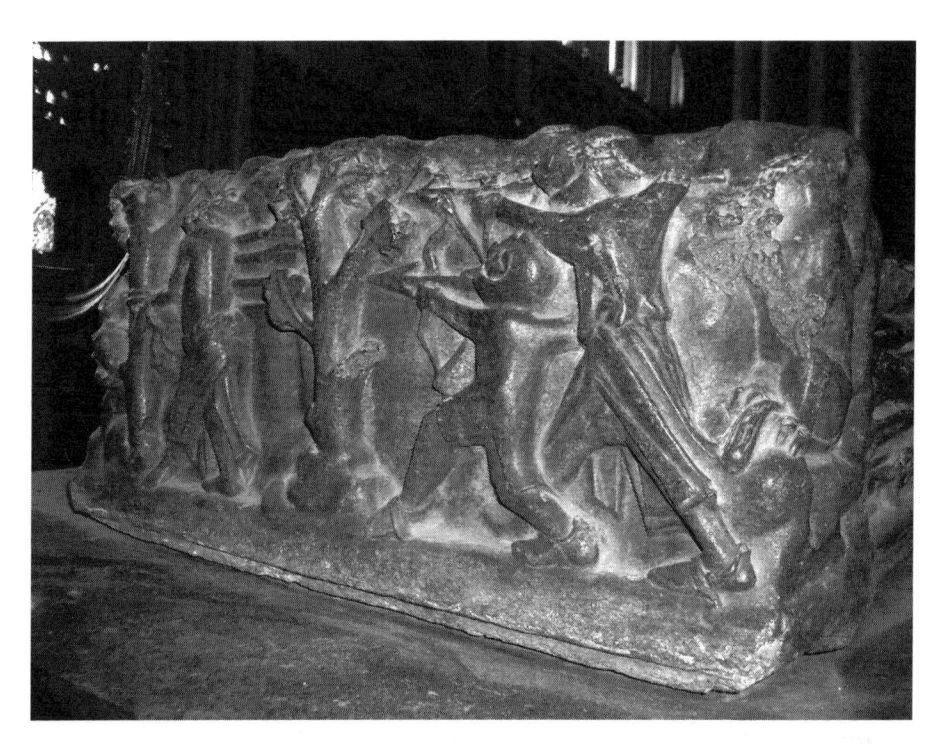

Figure 22 The martyrdom of St Edmund, depicted at the foot of the tomb of Abbot Hugh of Northwold in Ely Cathedral (1229). Photograph by the author.

War disorder and violence once more threatened Suffolk. On 21 May 1216 the dauphin of France, Louis (the future Louis VIII), landed in Kent, and after being proclaimed king in London, he made his way through Essex to East Anglia. Here, according to Roger of Wendover, he 'miserably despoiled' (*miserabiliter spoliavit*) the region.[79] This single phrase later gave rise to a speculation, otherwise entirely unsupported by evidence, that Louis took the body of St Edmund, and that at the siege of Toulouse a few years later, he gave it to the basilica of St Sernin in that city. This was supposed to explain how it was that Toulouse claimed to be in possession of the body of St Edmund from the 1440s onwards, although the story connecting the supposed relics to Louis appeared only in the work of a seventeenth-century lawyer, Pierre de Caseneuve, in 1644.[80] The idea that St Edmund's body was abducted in 1216 has been dismissed by all serious scholars. As Thomas Arnold observed:

> Had the entire relics of St. Edmund been removed at this time by Frenchmen into France, it is scarcely credible that no triumphant mention of any such thing would exist in any French source … Is it conceivable that the cry of rage and consternation which would in that case have arisen from all of Suffolk, would have left absolutely no trace

---

79 Arnold (1890–96), vol. 3, pp. xl–xli.
80 On the cult of St Edmund at Toulouse see Young (2014), pp. 22–32.

in the voluminous county records, both monastic and secular, that have come down to us from this period?[81]

In reality, there is absolutely no evidence that St Edmunds was threatened or plundered in 1216, and certainly no evidence that the body of the saint was taken away.

In comparison with the reign of Samson and the election of Hugh of Northwold as Abbot, Hugh's reign at Bury is sparsely documented. Between 1220 and around 1234 the sacrist, Richard of Newport, embarked on a new building programme, demolishing the Chapter House and rebuilding it from the foundations (leaving the tombs of Ording, Hugh I and Samson in their places). He also completed the great bell called 'Newport' for the central bell tower, and built a new hall and solar at the Abbey's manor of Manhall, near Saffron Walden.[82] Hugh set an important precedent concerning the primacy of the Abbots of St Edmunds by presiding, with the Abbot of St Albans, over the first General Chapter of the English Benedictines in the Province of Canterbury in 1218–19. Like his predecessors, Hugh was involved in the great affairs of state, and in 1225 he was a witness to the reissued Magna Carta and Charter of the Forest.[83] However, in 1229 Hugh was elected bishop of Ely – the only Abbot of St Edmunds ever to be elevated to a bishopric.

It is on account of this historical accident that Hugh of Northwold's is the only tomb of an Abbot of St Edmunds to have survived the Reformation, as it is located on the north side of the presbytery of Ely Cathedral (which Hugh himself had constructed). The tomb consists of a magnificent effigy of Hugh in Purbeck marble, holding a crozier in his left hand and lifting his right hand in blessing. It is evident that Hugh never lost his devotion to St Edmund, since at the foot of the effigy are small embossed figures depicting the martyrdom of St Edmund.[84] At the east end of the tomb is a stone panel once belonging to a throne, featuring the wolf holding St Edmund's head. This may have been part of Hugh's throne as bishop of Ely, or even his throne as Abbot of St Edmunds, transported to Ely on his election to that see in 1229.

---

81 Arnold (1890–96), vol. 3, p. xli.
82 On Richard of Newport's building projects see Gransden (2009), pp. 229–35.
83 Gransden (2009), p. 172.
84 Ibid., p. 176.

Chapter 4
A century of troubles, 1229–1329

The period following the death of Hugh of Northwold saw the Abbey become embroiled in a series of disputes over papal visitations, royal taxation and the arrival of the Franciscan friars, who were potential rivals for the spiritual dominance of Bury St Edmunds. In the 1260s, the Barons' War led to heightened tension between the Abbey and townsfolk, and relations with the town would become the Abbey's greatest challenge. Eventually, the suppressed aspirations of the townsfolk resulted in an explosion of deadly and destructive violence against the Abbey in 1327 which threatened the very survival of St Edmunds.

Richard of the Isle to Edmund of Walpole, 1229–56

Richard of the Isle, who probably took his name from the Isle of Ely,[1] was prior of St Edmunds for much of Hugh II's reign until he was elected abbot of Burton, Staffordshire, in 1222. He had belonged to the party which opposed Hugh's election in 1214, but on 5 June 1229 he was elected Abbot of St Edmunds in Chapter, and after receiving royal and papal confirmation he was enthroned on St Edmund's day. In 1231, Richard set another important precedent for the privileges of the Abbots of St Edmunds by administering the episcopal blessing in the presence of the bishop of Norwich.[2] However, in 1232 Pope Gregory IX appointed two special visitors for exempt abbeys, the Cistercian abbot of Boxley and the Premonstratensian abbot of Bayham. Exactly what the new visitors did at Bury we do not know, but Richard was concerned enough to travel to Rome in 1233 in order to complain directly to the Pope and ask for new visitors. Unfortunately Richard never reached Rome and died at Pontigny in Normandy on 29 August 1233.[3]

On 27 September the Chapter elected Henry Wodard, alias Rushbrook, as Richard of the Isle's successor. Henry had served as chaplain to Hugh II and subsequently as cellarer and prior.[4] The first challenge confronting Henry was the legatine visitation threatened by Gregory IX. Partly as a result of the efforts of Richard of the Isle, Gregory replaced the abbots of Boxley and Bayham with the Benedictine abbot of Waltham, the Gilbertine prior of Sempringham and the Augustinian prior of Holy Trinity, London. The visitation took place on 10 June 1234, and the visitation articles primarily concerned food and drink. The eating of meat and drinking of beer and wine were restricted, and the monks

---

1 Gransden (2009), p. 167.
2 Ibid., pp. 177–8.
3 Ibid., pp. 178–9.
4 Ibid., p. 180.

were strictly forbidden to take food away from the refectory. In Gransden's view, 'the visitors wished to respect the abbey's ancient, though unwritten, customs', even when these did not always coincide with the letter of the Rule of St Benedict.[5]

Another significant challenge faced by Henry of Rushbrook was the arrival of the Franciscan and Dominican friars. The friars were a new kind of religious order, professed religious not attached to a specific house as monks were, but authorised to beg for alms while preaching and serving the people. In December 1233, probably in response to a request from Henry as Abbot-elect, Gregory IX issued a bull reinforcing the fact that no chapel or oratory could be erected in the *banleuca* without the Abbot's consent. The probable purpose of the bull was to exclude the friars from Bury. In 1238 the Franciscans returned, this time supported by the Dominicans, but the papal legate Otho ruled that they had no authority to set up a friary within the town.[6] This was to be just the first of several skirmishes between the Abbey and the friars.

On 7 July 1248 Edmund of Walpole, a junior monk of less than two years' standing in the monastery, was elected Abbot in succession to Henry and enthroned by the former Abbot, Bishop Hugh of Ely. In the intervening interregnum, even though it lasted only three months, Henry III managed to extract 1,200 marks from the Liberty, which put the Abbey in a difficult financial position.[7] Two monks travelled to Rome to seek confirmation of Edmund's election from Innocent IV, where they were treated with derision and their candidate rejected. However, Innocent then called the monks back and confirmed Edmund as Abbot in exchange for 800 marks. The monks were apparently so upset by their treatment that they died on the return journey.[8]

The chronicler Matthew Paris was critical of Edmund's reign, accusing him of weakness. In 1250 he took the cross, meaning that he committed himself to go on crusade, which Matthew believed set a bad example to other monks and was done simply to ingratiate himself with Henry III. On another occasion Edmund failed to give sanctuary to William Lupus, archdeacon of Lincoln, who was embroiled in a dispute with his bishop. On the other hand, Edmund defended the Abbey's interests against Richard de Clare, earl of Gloucester, who in 1251 claimed Mildenhall and Icklingham. This resulted in a two-year trial in London, in which the Abbey's attorneys (Simon of Luton and Robert Russel) were forced to produce Edward the Confessor's charter and Hermann the Archdeacon's *De miraculis*.[9]

Gransden has argued that during Edmund's reign King Henry III increasingly imposed heavy financial burdens on the English church. In 1255 King Henry pledged 700 marks in security from St Edmunds against the expedition to recover the Kingdom of Sicily for his son Edmund. Abbot Edmund partly made up for such losses by seizing the goods of felons within the Liberty – a right that the Abbots possessed but had never before exercised.[10] During Edmund's reign the Hospital of St John (otherwise known as Domus Dei) was

---

5   Ibid., pp. 203–5.
6   Ibid., pp. 183–4.
7   Ibid., p. 191.
8   Ibid., pp. 185–6.
9   Ibid., pp. 188–90. On the resolution of this dispute by Simon of Luton see Gransden (2015), pp. 22–5.
10   Gransden (2009), pp. 191–2.

founded in Southgate Street, the first hospital to be dedicated entirely to the care of the poor and relief of beggars.[11]

Simon of Luton, 1257–79

Simon of Luton served as prior of the monastery under Abbot Edmund, having been elected in Chapter rather than simply appointed by the Abbot.[12] This was unusual, and Gransden has argued that it is evidence for a 'democratic movement' among the monks at this time, who insisted that they should have a say in who assumed high office within the Convent.[13] The monks obtained a royal licence to elect a new Abbot in January 1257, and on the next day Simon was elected. Robert Russel was sent to Italy to obtain confirmation of the election from Pope Alexander IV. However, while Russel was in Italy, Alexander issued a letter from Viterbo on 3 August insisting that abbots-elect of all exempt monasteries had to come to be blessed personally by the pope in order to validate their election. Accordingly, Simon left for Rome and was blessed on 22 October, the first Abbot of St Edmunds to be installed directly by the pope. This was in some ways beneficial to the Abbey, since it was a direct demonstration of the fact that the Abbot was under the pope's sole authority. On the other hand it was also an extremely costly exercise, and set the Abbey back 2,000 marks.[14]

The first challenge faced by Abbot Simon was the intrusion of Franciscan friars into the *banleuca*, which had occurred during the long vacancy when, on 17 February 1257, the friars had obtained a licence from Pope Alexander for an oratory in the town.[15] The friars had previously tried (unsuccessfully) to set up a chapel in the town in 1233 and 1238. Their interest in Bury St Edmunds was part of a wider strategy targeting large urban centres for preaching and mission, but it was also an indication that the Abbey's exemptions of the tenth and eleventh centuries were being sorely tested by the changed economic and social conditions of the thirteenth century. Baldwin successfully neutralised the threat from the bishops of Norwich, while Samson expelled 'the King's Jews' as intruders in the Liberty in 1190, but in both cases the Abbot seems to have had the support of the townsfolk. The Franciscan friars, whose vowed poverty stood in stark contrast to the conspicuous wealth of the Abbey, presented a more profound existential challenge to the monks because they had the potential to draw the loyalty of the town away from St Edmunds.

On 22 June 1257 the friars were admitted to the town by Sir Roger of Harbridge, and they celebrated mass in his house on the east side of Northgate Street. While Sir Roger and the friars were at dinner, officials of the Abbey smashed the makeshift chapel and then ejected the Franciscans. When the friars appealed to Rome the pope excommunicated some of the monks and reprimanded the rest, as well as appointing the archbishop of Canterbury, Boniface, and the dean of Lincoln, Richard of Gravesend, as papal judges

---

11   J. Brian Milner, *Six Hospitals and a Chapel: The story of the medieval hospitals of Bury St Edmunds, Suffolk* (Bury St Edmunds: St Nicholas Hospice/Suffolk Institute of Archaeology and History, 2013), pp. 39–40.
12   Gransden (2009), p. 194.
13   See Antonia Gransden, 'A democratic movement in the Abbey of Bury St Edmunds in the late twelfth and early thirteenth centuries', *Journal of Ecclesiastical History* 26 (1975), pp. 25–39.
14   Gransden (2015), pp. 3–7.
15   Ibid., p. 17.

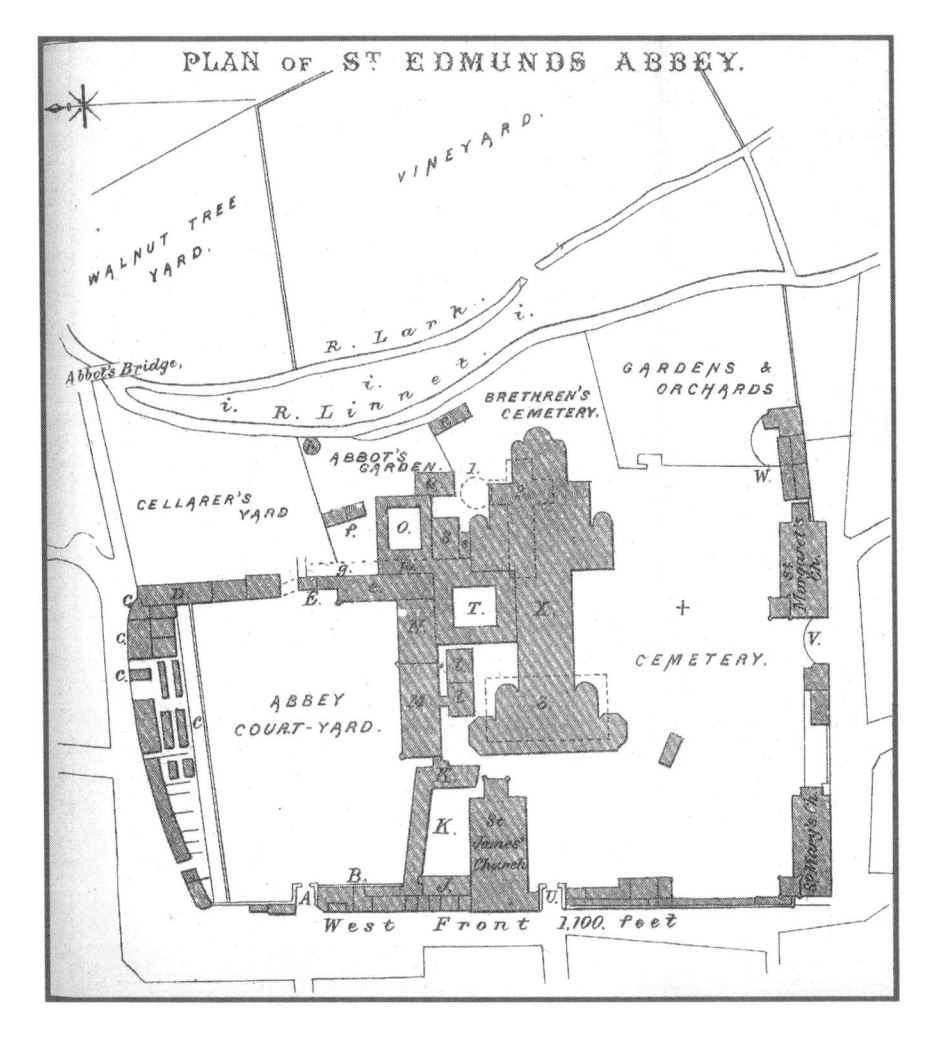

Figure 23 Plan of the Abbey precincts. From J. B. Mackinlay, *Saint Edmund King and Martyr* (1893), facing p. 352.

---

delegate sitting in St Mary's Church. The judges ruled in favour of the friars, who were then given a site on the western side of the *banleuca* which belonged to the king, which made the Abbey's position even more difficult. The Abbey could prevent its vassal Sir Roger transferring property to the friars but it could not prevent the king from so doing.[16]

The Abbey expelled the friars anyway, and then appealed to Magna Carta to justify its

---

16   Ibid., pp. 17–18. The exact site on the western side of Bury has never been identified.

References.

A Abbey Gate.
B Guest-house, Almonry and St. Laurence's Chapel.
C Stables, Offices &c., for strangers.
ccc North Gate, Prison, House of Pleas.
D Cellarer's Offices — Beodric's Messuage.
E Abbot's Palace.
e Abbot's Dining-hall.
f Abbot's Yard and Garners
g Supposed open Ambulatory.
h Dovecote.
iii Crankles or Fish-ponds.
J The Mint.
KK The Lesser Monastery.
ll Kitchens.
M The Great Refectory surmounted by the Dormitory.
N Scriptorium, Infirmary and Infirmary Chapel.
O Infirmary Cloisters.
p Supposed site of Lavatory.
Q Prior's House.
R The Bath.
S Chapter-house, surmounted by the Library.
s The Vestiary.
T The Monastery Cloisters.
U Norman Gateway, called the Great Gate of the Church of St. Edmund.
V St. Margaret's Gate.
W Abbot Samson's Schools.
X Great Church of St. Edmund.
1 Site of ancient round Chapel, where St. Edmund's Body rested till 1095.
2 Site of the Church of St. Sigebert, Bishop Theodred I. and King Canute.
3 Probable site of Ailwin's and previous Monasteries.

position. Furthermore, the monks drew up a set of propositions to be sent to Rome, appealing to Pope Gregory IX's letters of 1233 and 1238 and citing the fact that papal legates had decided in favour of the Abbey on both previous occasions. The monks claimed that the friars had acted dishonestly, not mentioning the Abbey's privileges in their letter to Pope Alexander and proceeding during a vacancy, when the Abbey was at its most vulnerable. They also dismissed the friars' claim that the people of Bury were not being instructed in the Christian faith. On 1 November 1257 Alexander IV confirmed the Abbey's privileges, but the friars ignored this change of heart by the papacy and appealed directly to King Henry III. Gottfried argued that Henry was influenced by Queen Eleanor, a supporter of the friars, to intervene in their favour.[17] He instructed one of his justices, Gilbert of Preston, to seize the site on the west side of the town and put the friars in possession. Accordingly, in the worst instance of a violation of the *banleuca* since the Norman Conquest, Gilbert rode into Bury with an escort of armed men on 25 April 1258 and forcibly established the friars.[18]

The friars remained in possession for the next five years and even started building a 'sumptuous' church, but in 1261 Urban IV, who was less favourably disposed towards the friars, was elected pope, and in 1263 he ordered the Franciscan Provincial in England to withdraw the friars from Bury and to pull down the church already built. On the Vigil of the Feast of St Edmund, 19 November 1263, the friars finally left. According to one account, the friars humbly submitted themselves to Abbot Simon in Chapter, but Gransden argues that such a harmonious end to the bitter dispute was unlikely, and it seems that the friars carried on building works after they left Bury. Presumably they retained hope that they might be able to return to their convent buildings at a more favourable time. However, Abbot Roger of St Augustine's, Canterbury, who had been deputed to enforce Pope Urban's will, had to order the alderman and bailiffs of Bury to demolish the buildings by force on 26 November. As a concession to the friars, Simon

---

17 Gottfried (1982), p. 221.
18 Gransden (2015), pp. 18–20.

then granted them a site at Babwell, outside the town's North Gate between Bury and Fornham St Genevieve (the present Priory Hotel). The dispute was over, but the financial cost of repeated appeals to the Roman Curia and the royal court had been immense.[19]

Trouble was brewing from another quarter, however, and on 4 May 1264 the young people of Bury St Edmunds rebelled against the alderman and bailiffs, as well as the Abbey's obedientaries, by forming the 'Guild of Youth' and refusing to recognise the authority of other officials. The context for the rebellion was the Barons' War, a confrontation between Henry III and his barons which culminated in the battle of Evesham in 1265, at which the barons' leader, Simon de Montfort, was defeated by the king. One of the leaders of the barons came to Bury to mediate between the Guild of Youth, the alderman and bailiffs, and the Abbey, but Abbot Simon appealed to the king who sent Gilbert of Preston back to Bury, this time to conduct an investigation into offences against the Abbey committed by the Guild of Youth. The townsfolk submitted to the Abbot in October.[20]

Simon was evidently trusted by Henry III, and in 1259 he was sent to negotiate a treaty with the French king. In 1260 Simon and the abbot of Glastonbury were the only two abbots to turn up in London after Henry summoned those barons loyal to him, and in 1267 Simon led the Knights of St Edmund to Stratford Langthorn in Essex with the intention of helping Henry besiege London.[21] The monks, on the other hand, seem to have admired Simon de Montfort. The Bury chronicler John de Taxster made a comment (later expunged from one copy of the chronicle) that stories of miracles circulated around Simon's body after death, and a motet in honour of de Montfort was composed at the Abbey.[22] Furthermore, the Steward of the Liberty of St Edmund, Henry of Hastings, was a determined supporter of the rebellion.[23] Gransden attributed the monks' enthusiasm for de Montfort to the influence of the friars, but it could also be seen in the context of the Abbey's earlier opposition to King John and St Edmund's reputation as defender of the English people – one of the major grievances of the barons and their supporters against Henry III was his willingness to put 'aliens' in possession of lands in England.

In spite of his loyalty to Henry, Abbot Simon was financially and politically penalised because he had obeyed an injunction of the baronial government in 1264 ordering the defence of the East Anglian coast, to prevent Queen Eleanor landing a French army to defeat the barons. Henry confiscated the Abbot's temporalities in 1265 and again in 1266 – for brief periods each time, but even in a short while the king would have been able to drain considerable resources from the Abbey's possessions. In 1265 Simon was fined 800 marks and 400 marks in 1266, and on 27 May 1266 a party of armed men led by John de Warenne and William de Valence arrived in Bury to seek out disinherited rebel barons who were hiding out in the town, perhaps believing that they would be safe from the king within the four crosses of the *banleuca*. Warenne and Valence accused the Abbot of favouring the rebels, but Simon successfully pinned the accusation on the townsfolk instead and even made them pay a fine to the Abbey.

However, rebel barons had followed the example of Hereward the Wake two centuries

---

19 Ibid., pp. 21–2.
20 Ibid., p. 28. On this incident see also Gottfried (1982), pp. 218–19.
21 Gransden (2015), p. 29.
22 Ibid., pp. 26–7.
23 Ibid., pp. 29–30.

earlier and holed themselves up in the Isle of Ely; Henry arrived in Bury on 6 February 1267 and summoned an army to besiege Ely. Accompanying the king was the papal legate Ottobuono, who held a council in Bury that excommunicated the disinherited rebel barons (only a legate *a latere* had the power to do this within the *banleuca*). Henry left on 22 February for Cambridge, where he began preparations for the siege.[24]

The rest of Simon's reign was comparatively peaceful but dogged by financial difficulties created by the vacancy, the dispute with the Franciscans and the depredations of the Barons' War. Simon seems to have made it his priority to rebuild and restore the Abbey's fortunes, but in the first instance he was forced to borrow from Italian moneylenders.[25] In order to repay these loans the Abbot ensured better management of the Abbey's estates and obtained a licence to live abroad with a small household between June and December 1268 in order to cut the costs of his household at Bury. He granted a life-lease of his London palace to Sir Philip Basset in 1271, no doubt for a handsome fee.[26] Leases of rich manors owned by the Abbey added further to the cashflow without alienating any land from the Abbey's possession.[27] However, the Abbey was also forced to defend itself against Edward I's campaign to force liberties to produce evidence of their freedom from royal interference (the so-called *Quo Warranto* ('by what warrant?') campaign), which resulted in extensive research into the Abbey's history and the copying of ancient charters.[28]

Pilgrimage was another source of revenue, and in 1261 Simon obtained indulgences for pilgrims venerating the 'black cross' at the foot of St Edmund's shrine, as well as for visitors to the chapel of St Mary and St Edmund, where the bier of St Edmund was venerated.[29] This chapel was the remains of the old rotunda consecrated in 1032, which was probably attached to the east wall of the north aisle of Baldwin and Anselm's Abbey Church, but which had long since lost its original ambulatory. However, in 1275 Simon embarked on his most ambitious building project: the construction of a splendid Lady Chapel in the position of the old rotunda. The ancient chapel was accordingly knocked down, and the monks discovered the remains of the ambulatory. Prior Russel laid the foundation stone of the new Lady Chapel on 1 July 1275. It was meant to replace the original chapel of St Mary, which was probably the easternmost of the apsidal chapels of Baldwin's ambulatory. Unlike previous building works, the new chapel was paid for entirely by Abbot Simon's relatives and friends, so its construction did not have an adverse effect on the Abbey's finances. The bier of St Edmund was moved to a new chapel in the cemetery, dedicated to St Edmund and St Stephen, on 28 December 1275.[30] This became a very important site because it was where pilgrims left their offerings.

The construction of a lavish Lady Chapel was appropriate given Bury's significant role in the development of the cult of the Virgin Mary in the reign of Abbot Anselm, but it also reflected the fashion of the period for large, semi-separate Lady chapels in which Lady masses could be celebrated for pilgrims, often to the accompaniment of elaborate

---

24 Ibid., pp. 30–1.
25 On Simon's debts see ibid., pp. 119–29.
26 Ibid., pp. 130–1.
27 Ibid., pp. 132–5.
28 Ibid., p. 54.
29 Ibid., pp. 208–9.
30 Ibid., pp. 209–10.

polyphony. The popularity of Lady masses was due partly to the sumptuous ritual that surrounded the cult of the Virgin, but also to the fact that no rood screen or pulpitum separated the faithful from the altar in Lady chapels.[31] Although it is several decades younger than the chapel at Bury, the Lady Chapel of Ely Cathedral is roughly the same size and shape as Abbot Simon's chapel, and gives some sense of the distinctness of the cult of the Virgin Mary as an adjunct of the main church. The chapel at Ely is also in roughly the same location in relation to the main church as Simon's chapel. Gransden has suggested that the construction of Abbot Simon's Lady Chapel coincided with a flowering of Marian poetry in Anglo-Norman French at St Edmunds, notably by the monk Everard of Gateley.[32]

In addition to building the new Lady Chapel, Simon of Luton was also responsible for relocating Abbot Edmund's hospital for the poor, God's House or Domus Dei, to a better site outside the South Gate and for providing the hospital with an altar and chaplain. He also founded a college dedicated to St John the Baptist at Palgrave.[33] Gransden's assessment of Simon's reign was positive:

> The abbey's quarrels with the Friars Minor and with Richard de Clare, earl of Gloucester, were settled, the abbey's troubles during the Barons' War overcome, and various measures taken which seem to have alleviated the abbey's financial problems. Positive achievements under Simon were the building of the splendid new Lady Chapel and the notable improvement in the abbey's provisions for poor relief. At the same time, there was an advance in the care of the convent's archives, and a revival of its historiographical tradition.[34]

John of Northwold, 1279–1301

Gransden suggests that John of Northwold was probably related to Abbot Hugh of Northwold, and there seems no reason to doubt this. Simon of Luton died on 9 April 1279 and John of Berwick was appointed keeper of the Abbey during the vacancy. In spite of its short duration (the Abbot's temporalities were restored on 5 November) Edward I took advantage of the vacancy to despoil the Abbey's possessions. John of Northwold, who was then interior guestmaster (the official in charge of guests staying in the convent itself rather than dignitaries visiting the Abbey) was elected Abbot in Chapter on 5 May. Like his predecessor Simon, John went personally to Rome and was blessed by the pope at Viterbo. He did not get back to Bury until 28 December 1279.[35]

Gransden has argued that John may have made a bargain with the monks, in exchange for his election, to correct abuses of the Convent's rights committed in Simon's reign, although direct evidence for this claim is lacking.[36] What is certain is that John set about clarifying the distinction between the property of the Abbot and the property of the

---

31 Eamon Duffy, 'Devotion to the Mother of God in the Medieval English cathedral', lecture delivered at Ely Cathedral, 1 September 2014.
32 Gransden (2015), pp. 212–13.
33 Ibid., pp. 213–17.
34 Ibid., p. 287.
35 Ibid., pp. 7–11.
36 Ibid., pp. 47–8.

Convent. Clarity on this matter was extremely important because on an Abbot's death his property reverted to the Crown for the duration of the vacancy that followed, but any manors belonging to the Convent could not be touched. Although a practical distinction had existed between the Abbot and Convent since Abbot Baldwin's time, it had never been codified in law.[37] Two vexed questions were whether the king had the right to take over administration of the town of Bury St Edmunds during a vacancy, and whether he had the right to take over the mint. Both of these were not under the direct jurisdiction of the Abbot but under the sacrist, who was of course a member of the Convent.

The separation of portions was physically represented by the division of the Abbey precincts into sacred and secular zones. The sacred zone centred upon the Abbey Church and the secular focused on the Abbot's Palace. This building was complete by around 1281, and was an extension of a structure originally known as Samson's Larder. The Abbot's Palace was a long range of buildings running north to south between the Abbey Gate and the River Lark, with a garden towards the river which is still marked by a surviving octagonal dovecote. The main part of the Palace consisted of the Queen's Chamber over Samson's Larder and the Abbot's Wardrobe, which was raided by rebels in 1327. The Queen's Chamber was probably so called because it was used by Queen Eleanor when she visited. In Whittingham's view, John of Northwold would have waited until he had received confirmation of the separation of portions between Abbot and Convent before he started building the Palace.[38] In the event, the Palace was one of the last of the monastic buildings to disappear, and was not demolished until 1720.

On 16 December 1280 a writ of Edward I confirmed that the town and mint would remain under the sacrist's jurisdiction during vacancies. Gransden attributes the success of the Abbey in obtaining this concession to the efforts of William of Hoo, who became sacrist in the spring of 1280.[39] William, who may have been a relative of Abbot Simon, was an extremely able administrator who was also employed as an attorney by the Abbey in its negotiations with the Exchequer and by the papal nuncio Geoffrey of Vezano, charged with collecting taxes due to the papacy.[40] As sacrist, William had responsibility for ensuring that the bailiffs administered justice in criminal matters in the Abbot's court,[41] but he was also archdeacon within the Liberty of St Edmund, meaning that he presided over a church court (consistory) that had the power to impose penances for ecclesiastical offences, such as adultery. As archdeacon, Hoo also had direct jurisdiction over anyone who could be considered a cleric.[42]

As both governor of the town and ecclesiastical commissary, the sacrist had almost complete control over every aspect of the lives of Bury's citizens – except that the alderman and bailiffs made obeisance to the Abbot rather than to the sacrist. The sacrist was also charged with maintaining the privileges of the two schools in the town – the grammar

---

37 On the division of portions between Abbot and Convent see Antonia Gransden, 'The separation of portions between Abbot and Convent at Bury St Edmunds: the decisive years, 1278–1281', *English Historical Review* 119 (2004), pp. 373–406.
38 Whittingham (1952), pp. 183–4.
39 Gransden (2015), p. 102.
40 Ibid., p. 104.
41 Ibid., pp. 109–10.
42 Ibid., pp. 111–13.

school and song school founded by Abbot Samson – and regularly prohibited the establishment of illegal 'adulterine' schools. However, William's dealings with the grammar school were made more complicated by the fact that its master was one of the few men outside his jurisdiction, since it was a condition of Abbot Samson's endowment that the master should be appointed directly by the Abbot and enjoy a handsome salary of three marks a year. Hoo was unsuccessful in his attempt to try a case of defamation against a scholar in his consistory court, as the master was able to appeal to the Abbot that he had the right to try the case himself.[43]

On 24 February 1285 Edward I visited Bury, bringing with him his clerk of the market, Ralph of Middlington, who inspected the weights and measures in use in the town in the tollhouse. The monks protested to the king that this represented an infringement of the privileges of the *banleuca*, but Edward replied that Ralph claimed to have inspected weights and measures during Henry III's visit as well. Edward appointed auditors to hear the case, who were unable to reach a verdict, as the Abbot and Convent refused an inquest. Edward decided that, when the royal court was at Bury, royal officials should inspect weights and measures and receive the revenues from this, but he later conceded that the Abbey would retain the proceeds.[44]

In spite of Simon of Luton's efforts to defend the Abbey, Edward I continued to press *Quo Warranto* claims against it, examining the authenticity and completeness of the Abbey's claims to be exempt from royal jurisdiction. At Ipswich on 3 November 1286 the king's justice, Solomon of Rochester, began hearing the Abbey's case in defence of the Liberty of St Edmund. Jurors accordingly testified that the Abbot had the right to appoint his own justices and that all writs concerning matters in the Liberty were passed to him. However, in 1291 judges ruled, paradoxically, that the Abbot's rights to administer justice in the eight and a half hundreds did not extend to the *banleuca* itself (Bury was not itself part of any one of the hundreds that composed the Liberty of St Edmund).[45] The importance of the Abbot's right was not just jurisdictional but also financial, as it gave the Abbot the right to confiscate the goods of felons convicted in the Liberty.

In spring 1290 Abbot John petitioned Edward for the restoration of his right to the proceeds of convictions, and some of the Abbey's ancient charters were read out in Parliament. John was the leader of a group of abbots seeking concessions from Edward. According to a story later recorded (around 1370), John declared to the king, 'I am broken by age and exhausted by my labours to recover these [privileges]; I can do no more, but I commit the case between the martyred Edmund and his church, and you, my earthly Lord, to the Supreme Judge.' That night Edward awoke in terror, saying that he had seen a vision in which St Edmund threatened to punish him as a second Sweyn. It is certainly true that Edward had a change of heart, and in May 1290 he restored all privileges of the Liberties as they had been in the year 1234.[46]

John of Northwold also continued to face trouble from the townsfolk. In 1290 they attacked a new dam erected by the cellarer on Tay Fen, and the violence resulted in a royal inquest which lasted until 1293. In 1297 the alderman, Peter of Ellingham, and a former

---

43   Ibid., pp. 113–15.
44   Ibid., pp. 54–5.
45   Ibid., pp. 55–6.
46   Ibid., pp. 58–60.

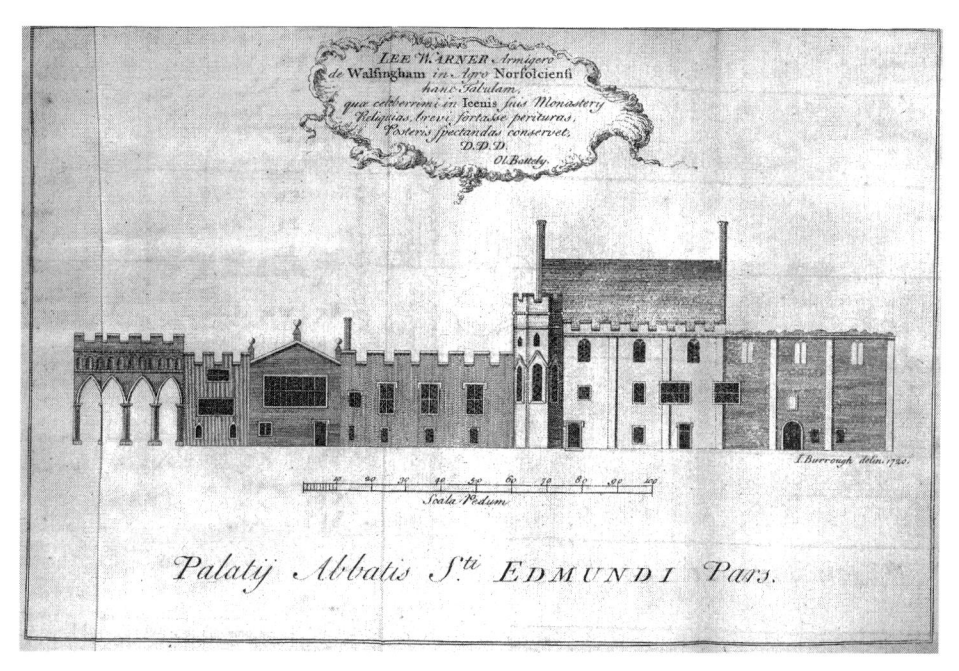

Figure 24 The Abbot's Palace, drawn by Sir James Burrough in 1720. Engraving from John Battely, *Antiquitates Sancti Edmundi* (1745), endpapers.

bailiff, Stephen son of Benedict, had charters to the Abbey confirming the liberties of the town read in the tollhouse without the Abbot's knowledge. John was outraged that the townsfolk should even have copies of these charters, and the men were arrested and the copies confiscated. They were brought before the Chapter and fined 320 marks for their presumption.[47]

Edward I was a frequent visitor to St Edmunds, which was a conveniently located staging-post between London and Scotland, where Edward was engaged in warfare for much of the 1290s. He stayed at the Abbey and at the manor of Culford between 28 April and 8 May 1292, arriving in time for the Feast of the Translation of St Edmund, and again between 16 and 20 January 1296 and 8 and 11 November the same year. He was at St Edmunds again between 8 and 11 May 1300. Gransden has speculated that Edward may have used a Bury monk, John of Shottisham, as an expert to prepare his case for overlordship of Scotland in the trial held at Norham in 1291–2. Shottisham was pardoned for stealing venison from the king's forest in 1292 and was later appointed precentor of the Abbey, and Gransden argued that Bury documents from this period contain extremely detailed information about the trial at Norham. This suggests the involvement of a Bury monk in the proceedings.[48]

On 20 November 1296 Edward summoned a parliament at Bury, and at high mass in the presence of the archbishop of Canterbury, the bishop of Durham and the counts

---

47   Ibid., pp. 76–7.
48   Ibid., pp. 80–1.

of Holland and Flanders, the Welsh prince Rhys ap Rhys bowed his head and submitted to the king. This marked the end of Edward's long campaign to subdue the Welsh, and the monks attributed it to the intercession of St Edmund, the protector of England.[49] Indeed, Edward's own devotion to St Edmund was predicated on his belief that Edmund would give him victory in battle, and in 1300 he gave specific instructions that none of the Abbey's liberties should be harmed, 'for I have no doubt that [St Edmund] will be in Scotland to protect me and mine, and to conquer the enemy; he will come brandishing his weapons, ready for battle'.[50]

John of Northwold was responsible for only one major addition to the Abbey buildings, which was the Chapel of the Charnel in the churchyard. This building is still partially standing today, in the middle of the 'Great Churchyard' between St Edmundsbury Cathedral and St Mary's Church. According to the official story, Abbot John was concerned that overcrowding of burials in the churchyard was resulting in the violation of graves (perhaps by animals), which were too close to the surface – although Gransden suggests that it may have been a petition from the townsfolk rather than the Abbot's own concern which brought about the change. The purpose of the Chapel of the Charnel was to provide a consecrated space to which bones from pre-existing graves could be moved in order to allow space for new burials. The foundation charter of the chapel, dedicated to God, the Blessed Virgin Mary, St Edmund and All Saints, was issued on 11 September 1300. Although the Charnel Chapel may not appear a very impressive ruin today (after the Reformation it served successively as an alehouse, a smithy and a private mausoleum), what survives is just the remains of the lower vault which was intended to house the bones. Above this there would have been an upper chapel in which mass was celebrated for the souls of those whose remains reposed within.[51]

Although on a larger scale, the chapel may have somewhat resembled Prior Crauden's Chapel in Ely, which likewise consists of a lower vault and a richly decorated upper chapel. The construction of the Chapel of the Charnel was accompanied by the endowment of a second chantry within the Abbey Church itself, which was a sign of the growing popularity of masses for the dead and the tendency to commemorate all of the faithful departed on one day in the calendar – All Souls' Day on 2 November. This feast was late to get off the ground in England, but Gransden speculates that the monks may have preferred it because the traditional Benedictine practice of individually commemorating dead monks was becoming time-consuming after so many centuries, and some of their predecessors' names were hard to pronounce and remember.[52]

The same concern to increase the number of masses for the dead seems to have motivated Abbot John's reform of St Saviour's Hospital, originally founded by Abbot Samson. On 12 March 1294 he issued a new charter, bemoaning the fact that the wardens of the hospital had been admitting people for money. Henceforth, he ordained that no women should be admitted to the hospital and that it should primarily be for needy members of the clergy. He also ordained that seven chaplains were to say mass daily for him, Abbot

---

49 Ibid., p. 83.
50 Ibid., pp. 84–5.
51 Ibid., pp. 221–3.
52 Ibid., pp. 224–6.

John, a practice presumably intended to continue after the Abbot's death.[53] John died on 29 October 1301, and the kitchener's register remembered him for commissioning paintings in the choir by John Wodecroft, building the Chapel of the Charnel, and building the chapel of St Botolph.[54]

Thomas of Tottington, 1302–12

Thomas of Tottington was elected Abbot in Chapter on 3 January 1302.[55] Thomas was evidently a native of the same Norfolk village as Abbot Samson, and before his election he had been a *socius* (assistant) of the cellarer and then sub-prior from around 1280.[56] Little is known of Thomas's reign. The register named after him, the *Registrum Thome* (British Library MS Harley 230), contains many blank pages that were evidently supposed to be filled with a record of his deeds, but the compiler never did this.[57] However, Thomas's reign saw the revival of discord between the town and the Abbey, and the appearance of a new phenomenon: armed conflict between the townsfolk and the Abbey.

In 1305 three royal justices, William de Bereford, William Howard and William de Carletone, held an inquisition at Bury into charges brought against the alderman and burgesses by the Abbot. They had withheld tolls and fines, resisted officers of the Abbey and thrown stones at the roof of the Abbey Church, thereby damaging it. The townsfolk had even prevented the bailiff of the Abbey from performing his duties, threatening him with swords, bows and arrows.[58] The justices ruled in the Abbey's favour, and the burgesses were compelled to pledge 500 marks and fifty barrels of wine if they should ever rebel again.[59] As Gottfried observed, fourteenth-century England was an extremely violent place, where the bearing of arms – and frequent resort to them – was all too common. Between 1272 and 1420 at least fifty-four murders took place in Bury, a town that rarely exceeded around 4,000 inhabitants.

The uprising of 1327–29

Richard of Draughton, who was then third prior, was elected Abbot in succession to Thomas of Tottington in 1312.[60] Richard's reign is not known for any of his achievements, but rather for the crisis that beset the Abbey between 1327 and 1329. During these years the town of Bury St Edmunds was effectively in a state of civil war between the townsfolk and the Abbey and its servants. The term sometimes used to describe this period, 'riots', hardly does justice to the attacks by armed assailants on the Abbey. The long-term cause

---

53 Ibid., p. 232.
54 Ibid., pp. 289–91.
55 Ibid., p. 290.
56 Thomson (1982), p. 94.
57 Liz Herbert McAvoy, *Medieval Anchoritisms: Gender, Space and the Solitary Life* (Woodbridge: D. S. Brewer, 2011), pp. 47–9.
58 Yates (1843), p. 128. Similar accusations were levelled against the townsfolk again in 1314 (Gottfried (1982), p. 220).
59 Mary D. Lobel, 'A detailed account of the 1327 rising at Bury St. Edmund's and the subsequent trial', *PSIA* 21 (1933), pp. 215–31, at p. 217.
60 Thomson (1982), p. 94.

of the uprising was the failure of successive Abbots to accommodate the aspirations of the burgesses of Bury St Edmunds, and the 1327 riots were anticipated by the disturbances in 1296 and 1305. The proximate cause of the uprising seems to have been the Abbey's failure to honour a debt to the burgesses of £2,000,[61] but the rebellion should also be seen in the wider context of the civil disorder that accompanied the deposition of Edward II in 1326. On 24 September of that year Queen Isabella landed with her allies at Orwell, and by 29 September the Queen's army was in Bury, where Isabella helped herself to £800 deposited at the Abbey for safekeeping by the king's justice Hervey de Stanton.[62]

Robert Gottfried attributed Bury's civil disorder to the rigidity of the Abbey in the face of the restiveness of the townsfolk,[63] but Mark Bailey has argued that the townsfolk enjoyed more concessions from the Abbey than they might otherwise have received. The townsfolk were allowed a guild which could elect an alderman. However, the alderman had no formal role in the governance of the borough, which remained under the control of the sacrist, and he was more like a representative or ambassador of the townsfolk than a mayor. The fact that an increasing number of wealthy burgesses had settled in Bury meant that the townsfolk harboured ideas of independence that exceeded what the Abbey would allow.[64] Both sides were surely at fault in a situation in which the burgesses were guilty of overreaching themselves, and the Abbey failed to recognise the legitimate aspirations of the people living in its curtilage.

Disturbances began on 13 January 1327, when John Frauceys met with a group of men at a tavern in the town, including some from London who encouraged the Bury men to rebel. Frauceys and his friends, including some of the minor burgesses, converged on the Guildhall at noon and summoned the greater burgesses, who agreed to take an oath against the Abbot. The rebels then seem to have gone into the countryside gathering support, and the next day an army of 3,000 forced its way through the gateway into the great court of the Abbey in front of the Abbot's Palace.[65] They were armed with swords, bows and arrows, halberds, spears and bill-hooks. The attackers beat the monks and their servants and broke the gates and windows.[66] Although many of the rioters undoubtedly had it in mind to loot the treasures of the Abbey – and the Treasury and Sacristy were indeed plundered – the main aim of the rioters seems to have been to destroy the written word that secured the Abbey's supremacy over the townsfolk. More damaging in the long term than the theft of gold and silver was the removal of charters from Cnut, Harthacnut and Edward the Confessor.[67]

The rioters deliberately looted and destroyed legal documents and registers, to the extent that the Abbot had to plead with the king to postpone legal proceedings he was involved in. Most tellingly of all, the rioters smashed forty 'carrels' (the wooden desks at which the monks read and wrote) in the cloister, and broke open chests and presses containing

---

61 Lobel (1933), pp. 220–1.
62 Gransden (2015), p. 96.
63 Gottfried (1982), p. 215.
64 Mark Bailey, *Medieval Suffolk: An Economic and Social History, 1200–1500* (Boydell: Woodbridge, 2007), pp. 137–9.
65 Lobel (1933), p. 216.
66 Yates (1843), p. 129.
67 Ibid., pp. 130–1.

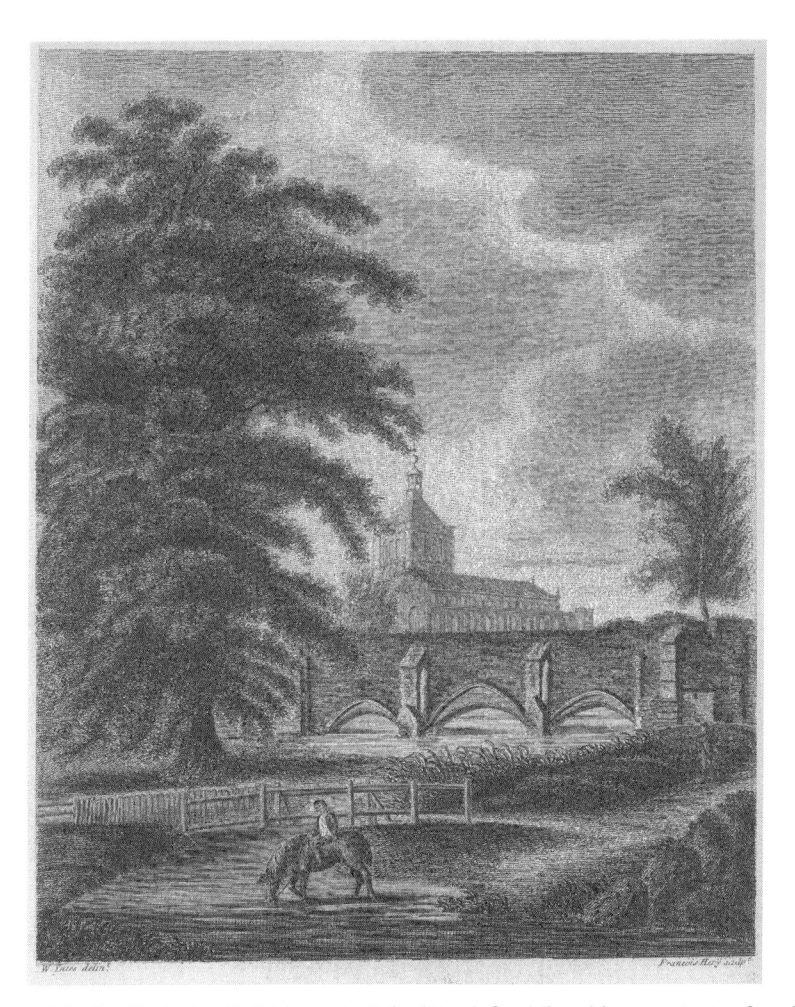

Figure 25 The fortified Abbot's Bridge (1804), built to defend the Abbey precincts after the rebellion of 1327. Engraving from Richard Yates, *An Illustration of the Monastic Antiquities of the Town and Abbey of St Edmund's Bury* (1843), plate facing p. 45.

books.[68] Because of their proximity to the Abbey Church these chests contained service books – twenty missals, twenty-four portiforia, twelve bibles, twenty psalters and ten diurnalia. They also contained books of canon law, which seem to have been a specific target of the rioters, and they carried off seven copies of Gratian's *Decretals* (the standard text of medieval canon law).[69] It is unclear whether the rioters plundered the Abbey's main library (we do not know where this was located at the time), but it seems unlikely, given the completeness of the Abbey's library in the fifteenth century. This first attack on the Abbey cannot be dismissed as mindless vandalism, therefore; it was primarily directed

---

68   James (1895), p. 146.
69   Ibid., p. 108.

against the 'secular' side of the Abbey precinct and was not an attack on the Abbey Church itself, but it did target the monks' wealth and the source of their power: the written word.

Abbot Richard was absent at the time of the attack, but the rebels captured and imprisoned the prior, Peter of Clopton, while the sacrist, Ralph Castone, only narrowly escaped to a local manor. He was then trapped as the rebels blocked every road to London. The next day nine more monks were imprisoned by the townsfolk, and the alderman, Richard of Berton, was deposed, to be replaced by his brother John, who was elected without the Abbot's approval. John of Berton appointed new gatekeepers to ensure that the town was defended by men loyal to the rebels, and on 16 January the prior and his nine fellow prisoners were brought back to the Abbey; Peter of Clopton was forced to sign the terms of the rebels, which included payment of the debt of £2,000 owed by the Abbey to the town. The burgesses then assumed the government of the town, and an axe and block were set up in the marketplace as a threat to anyone who refused to support the rebellion.

Abbot Richard arrived on 28 January to find the gates of the town barred against him. He was only admitted on condition that he sign a charter of twenty-four clauses prepared by the townsfolk which handed government of the borough to them, gave them immunity from prosecution for their rebellion and imposed a fine of £5000 on the Abbot if he failed to have the charter enrolled in the royal chancery. Gottfried argues that this charter was remarkably conservative under the circumstances; the rebels were not political revolutionaries, but 'businessmen looking for a larger personal share of the borough's wealth'.[70] However, after Richard complained to parliament that he had only signed the charter under duress, the burgesses renewed the violence on 16 February. This time they promised villeins in the Liberty of St Edmund freedom from tolls and work, and with the reinforcements of men they obtained, the townsfolk laid siege to the monastery in an attempt to prevent any provisions reaching the monks.[71] Looters brought carts to the Abbey gates, and it was during this time that Abbot Samson's remarkable aqueduct was destroyed in order to deprive the monks of a water supply.[72]

By May the king had begun to take an interest in events in Bury. A royal mandate was issued forbidding both parties from assembling, and representatives of the Abbey and townsfolk were summoned to York for arbitration. When these royal writs were ignored, the king took the Abbey under his protection on 26 May – a move that, under normal circumstances, would have provoked the indignation of the Abbot and Convent, but which in this case was welcomed, because the king's officials were given authority to arrest rebels. However, this provision came rather too late, as on 19 May the Abbey Church itself was attacked and plundered at the instigation of two clerks of the town churches of St James and St Mary. Violence was not just directed at the Abbey Church; the jewel-inlaid doors of the parish churches were ripped off and the gems distributed amongst the secular chaplains, who were asked by the burgesses to replace the monks as the custodians of St Edmund's shrine.[73]

The clerks were joined by the Franciscan friars from Babwell, who were surely seeking revenge for their ignominious expulsion from the *banleuca* in 1263, and although the

---

70 Gottfried (1982), p. 225.
71 Lobel (1933), pp. 217–18.
72 Gottfried (1982), pp. 225–6.
73 Ibid., p. 226.

burgesses refused the friars permission to settle within the town – because the chaplains saw them as rivals – the Franciscans collaborated closely with the townsfolk.[74] At around this time a number of monks took advantage of the 'confraternity' that existed between St Edmunds and the Abbey of St Bene't, at Holme in Norfolk. A confraternity was an agreement between Benedictine houses to grant rights of hospitality to brethren from another house, especially in time of need.[75] The sacrist and at least thirty-two monks, which must have been almost half the Convent, sought refuge at St Bene't's.[76]

In August Edward III wrote to inform the burgesses that he planned to proceed severely against them because they had despoiled the Abbey and its goods while it was under royal protection. On 16 October Sir John Howard became the Abbey's royal guardian, and two days later the monks attacked the burgesses while they were at prayer in the parish churches and captured some of them. When a crowd gathered outside the Abbey demanding the prisoners' release, the monks replied with 'stones and engines' (presumably stone-throwing siege machinery of some sort). This so enraged the townsfolk that they stormed the Abbey Church; the monks resisted, and the townsfolk rang the tollhouse bell and the fire bell of St James's church to summon reinforcements.[77] A group of townsfolk led by John of Berton, Robert Foxton, Richard Drayton and Alice Lickdish took an oath together, and began a four-day rampage of destruction. The group burned down the gates of the Abbey and the sacrist's offices (as well as plundering lead from the roof of the Abbey Church[78]), before turning their attention to Holderness Barns, Almoner's Barns, Haberden, Westley and other granges and manors of the Abbey, causing £1,000 worth of damage.

The next day, the townsfolk burned the Abbey's stables, malthouse, bakery and granaries on the north side of the great court, and the following day they moved further into the Abbey, destroying the guest quarters. On 21 October the cellarer's offices and the infirmary were targeted.[79] Later in the day a deputation from the townsfolk attempted to make peace with the Abbey, and asked the monks to meet them in St Mary's church. Five monks came, but the alderman demanded that the whole Convent should come. When twenty-four monks appeared, they were imprisoned.

The Abbot, who was safely in London, was so angered by this that he wrote seeking the assistance of Thomas, earl of Norfolk to raise a *posse comitatus* against the townsfolk. The alderman and burgesses backed down, and the next day soldiers entered Bury, while the townsfolk heaped the bodies of burgesses killed in the violence by the gates of the Abbey in the hope of appealing to the soldiers' sympathy.

However, the Abbot had managed to obtain from Rome the one thing the townsfolk truly feared – excommunication of the offenders. The sheriff of Norfolk took up residence in the Abbot's Palace, and the bodies of the dead were thrown into the town ditch as excommunicates, while cartloads of townsfolk (over 400 men and women) were taken to Norwich for trial. The trials lasted until May 1328.[80] However, in January 1329 the

---

74 Lobel (1933), pp. 218–19.
75 Gransden (1985), p. 23.
76 Lobel (1933), p. 220.
77 Ibid., p. 222.
78 Gottfried (1982), p. 227.
79 Yates (1843), pp. 131–2.
80 Lobel (1933), pp. 222–5.

ex-alderman John of Berton escaped from gaol and sought sanctuary with the friars at Babwell. About a month later a group of outlaws, presumably incited by John, seized control of the town gates and were welcomed by the townsfolk.[81]

Worse was to come, and on 17 October 1329 John of Berton and others launched a surprise raid on the manor of Chevington while Richard of Draughton was staying there, and kidnapped the Abbot. Stuffed into a sack, the prelate was conveyed to the house of a tanner in London and his head and eyebrows shaved in order to disguise him. A former mayor of London was then bribed to help the conspirators get the hapless Abbot out of the country to Dienst in Brabant. Both the pope and the archbishop of Canterbury excommunicated all involved, but the townsmen took advantage of the Abbot's absence and, at Christmas 1329, they forged letters from the Abbot exonerating clerks imprisoned in the town. Finally, in April 1330 the Abbot's friends discovered where he was being held and he was brought back to England. He was welcomed in Bury with a procession in his honour.[82]

The aftermath

The townsfolk were fined the vast sum of £140,000 for their rebellion, which they were unable to pay. Edward III was forced to visit Bury in person on 6 June 1331 in order to mediate, and the king arranged for the sum to be reduced. Nevertheless, the burgesses did not finally finish paying back the remaining sum until 1349.[83] The most visible legacy of the uprising today is the Abbey Gate, built between 1327 and 1346 to replace a gate damaged by the rioters.[84] The present Abbey Gate was probably built to the south of the old gate while the latter was still in use, and only when the new gate was complete was the old one pulled down. This explains why the Abbey Gate is not aligned with the main thoroughfare between the Abbey and marketplace (Abbeygate Street). The Abbey Gate contains niches for statues which would originally have concealed the defensive loopholes for archers that are now visible – a reminder of a very violent time in the town's past.

One consequence of the rebellion of 1327 was the end of the Bury mint. In January 1328 the king instructed new dies to be prepared to replace those taken by the rioters the previous year, but in 1329 a new writ noted that the Abbot had not so far exercised his right to mint coinage owing to an 'impediment' – this was, of course, his imprisonment overseas.[85] The hiatus in minting seems to have undermined Bury's status as the site of a royal mint. Nevertheless, a new moneyer, John Taloun, was appointed in May 1329, and dies were authorised for the mint in May 1340, but they were never brought into use. In Robin Eaglen's view the main cause for the demise of the mint was inflation. There was a shortage of silver and therefore it was too expensive to strike pennies, and Bury did not have permission to strike the new halfpennies and farthings. However, Abbots were under-

---

81 Ibid., p. 228.
82 Ibid., pp. 228–9.
83 Statham (1996), p. 56.
84 Whittingham (1952), p. 186. The gate can be dated from the appearance of the unquartered royal arms, used by Edward III before 1346. The upper part of the gate was not completed until after 1353 when John Lavenham became sacrist.
85 Eaglen (2014), p. 42.

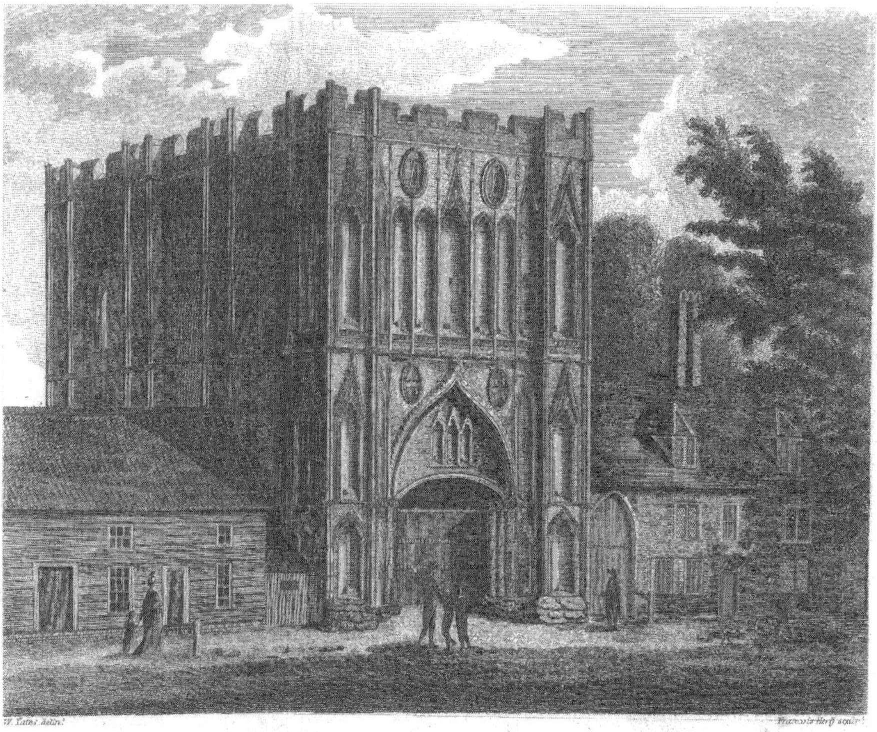

Figure 26 The west front of the Abbey Gate, rebuilt after the rebellion of 1327 (1804). Engraving from Richard Yates, *An Illustration of the Monastic Antiquities of the Town and Abbey of St Edmund's Bury* (1843), plate facing p. 3.

standably anxious not to lose the privilege of coining money even if they could not afford to do so, which is why Abbot William Bernham obtained dies that were never used.[86] Only a tiny number of coins (five) struck at Bury in the reign of Edward III have been found,[87] suggesting that the mint only operated for a short period after 1327.

Although Richard of Draughton was restored and the townsfolk were punished, it was an inescapable fact that the Abbot had been personally humiliated and the prestige of the Abbey permanently damaged. There seems little reason to suppose, as Gottfried did, that Richard was a 'competent and forceful man'.[88] Richard proved that he was incapable of dealing with outbreaks of violence without recourse to the aid of the crown and its officials, and this undermined the very essence of the Abbey's ancient liberties and privileges. Furthermore, although the rebellion resulted in the dissolution of the townsfolk's guild, this made possible the emergence of the body that would one day give rise to the modern civic identity of Bury St Edmunds: the Candlemas Guild.[89]

---

86 Ibid., p. 43.
87 Ibid., p. 203.
88 Gottfried (1982), p. 223.

Chapter 5
Plague, revolt and fire, 1329–1469

Although the Abbey survived the serious revolt against its authority in 1327–29 it was soon to face other equally serious challenges of a different kind: the Black Death of 1349 and subsequent outbreaks, a dispute over two rival claimants to the abbacy in 1379, and a further popular revolt in 1381, which resulted in the prior's head being displayed on a spike in the marketplace. Leadership of the Abbey during this period was weak and undistinguished until the election of William Cratfield in 1389, which saw a period of determined financial reconstruction followed by the election of Bury's last great Abbot, William Curteys, in 1429. Under Curteys the Abbey enjoyed a special relationship with King Henry VI, and the monk John Lydgate flourished as a literary figure of national significance. In 1447 the Abbey was once more at the centre of national events when, during a Parliament summoned by Henry VI, the king's uncle Humphrey, duke of Gloucester died while under arrest for treason. However, in 1465 the Abbey suffered a significant setback when its church was very nearly destroyed completely by a disastrous fire.

The Abbey and the Black Death, 1348–78

The hapless Abbot Richard of Draughton died in 1335 and was succeeded by William Bernham, who was then sub-prior.[1] Gottfried described Bernham as 'surely the least competent of all late medieval leaders of the abbey',[2] and during Bernham's reign the monks attracted damaging accusations of laxness in their observance of the Rule of St Benedict, as well as immoral living. A commission established by the bishop of Norwich accused the monks of living away from the monastery, wearing lay clothes and indulging in vices such as gambling and fornication.[3] In an error of judgement, Bernham decided to deny the charges to the bishop, but they were upheld.[4]

The Black Death arrived in Bury in 1349, in late winter or early spring. While the plague had been spread by rats on its initial arrival in England the previous summer, by the time it reached East Anglia it had mutated into the even more contagious form, pneumonic plague, which was spread by the sputum of coughing victims. Urban centres such as Norwich, Ipswich and Bury, where people lived close together, were the worst affected places. Owing to its proximity to the town the Abbey could not escape the general disaster, and the monks were decimated. On 19 January 1351 a bull of Pope Clement VI

---

1 Thomson (1982), p. 94.
2 Gottfried (1982), p. 232.
3 Lobel (1933), p. 220.
4 Gottfried (1982), p. 232.

granted permission for Abbot William to arrange the ordination as priests of ten monks under the canonical age of 25. Of around eighty monks, forty were dead,[5] although none of the Abbey's senior officials seems to have perished on this occasion.

Apart from the fact that it killed half of the Convent, Gottfried has portrayed the Black Death as a disaster for the Abbey. Suffolk, which had been one of the most populous areas of England before the plague arrived, was extensively depopulated for the remainder of the Middle Ages. Consequently there was insufficient labour to farm the Abbey's estates and its income fell. Although the Abbey momentarily had the advantage over the townsfolk, who were decimated while the institution of the Abbey (and its Abbot) endured, this was soon lost as the economy of the town diversified into woollen cloth by the 1370s.[6] In Gottfried's view, the Abbey's failure to adapt to new economic conditions led inexorably to its decline.

The effects on the Abbey of the second plague of 1361–62 were arguably more serious than the epidemic of 1349. The prior, Edmund Brundish, died in 1361 and the sacrist, Simon Langham, followed a few months later.[7] William Bernham also died in 1361, but the monk elected to succeed him, Henry of Hunstanton, died of the plague at Avignon on his way to receive papal confirmation before the end of the year.[8] 1361 was consequently the only year in the Abbey's history in which three Abbots ruled successively. Little is known of John Brinkley, chosen to succeed Henry of Hunstanton, and neither of the two monks had held significant office in the Abbey before their election. This is surely a mark of the devastation of the community; to have two Abbots, the prior and the sacrist die in the same year must have destabilised both Convent and town, to say nothing of the other lives lost.

The plague struck yet again in 1369, by which time the Abbey seems to have been in a state of disorder. Three of the monks, John de Norton, John de Grafton and William Blundeston, had an argument, and one night Grafton stabbed Norton to death in the monastic dormitory. The body was not found until the morning, when all the monks decided to hide the body in a shallow grave in the cemetery. By failing to inform the coroner the monks were breaking the law. Abbot John discovered the body, and Grafton and Blundeston were committed to gaol. However, a scandal erupted when Edward III pardoned both monks before they were brought to trial, on the grounds that the murder had been committed 'in hot blood'.[9] It seems astonishing that this justification for murder was applied to monks, who ought to have been held to a higher standard of behaviour than laymen, and the pardon of Grafton and Blundeston is indicative of a decline in standards of religious life at the Abbey during this traumatic period. Furthermore, it is possible that the Abbot persuaded the king to grant the pardon because there were scarcely enough monks to perform the necessary duties of the monastery, and he simply could not afford to have two of them executed – even for murder.

---

5   Ibid., p. 51.
6   Robert S. Gottfried, *The Black Death: Natural and Human Disaster in Medieval Europe* (New York: Free Press, 1983), p. 150.
7   Thomson (1982), pp. 93, 95.
8   Yates (1843), p. 218.
9   Gottfried (1982), p. 217.

Henry of Kirkstead and the monastic library

In the midst of the disorder in the religious life of the Abbey in the second half of the fourteenth century, it comes as something of a surprise to discover that a far-sighted and efficient monastic librarian was in the process of turning the Abbey's library into one of the best in England. Henry of Kirkstead was a monk of Bury between 1338 and 1378. He began his monastic career as one of the Abbot's chaplains, and was novice-master and *armarius* by 1361. In 1362 he was elected prior in succession to Edmund Brundish, who died of the plague that year, and served in this role until 1374.[10] Kirkstead devised a system according to which every volume in the library was assigned a press-mark consisting of a letter from A–Y and an Arabic numeral.[11] The letter indicated the name of the author or the main contents of the volume, while the Arabic numeral indicated 'the order of acquisition or of the natural sequence of the volume in its own class'.[12]

The binding of Bury books was also uniform, consisting in most cases of 'white skin over wooden boards: the boards and backs usually quite flat: the chain-mark almost always on the front cover at top or bottom: the commonest form of fastening is a strap with metal loop, which fits on to a pin fixed in the middle of the last cover'.[13] Kirkstead 'renewed the press marks and noted defects and also in one or two cases added notes of a literary and bibliographical sort touching the contents of a volume'.[14] As a consequence, books from the Abbey can be identified comparatively easily in modern collections. M. R. James misidentified the author of a seventeenth-century copy of Kirkstead's *Catalogus scriptorum ecclesiae* as 'Boston of Bury' (John Boston),[15] a monk active in the reign of Abbot Curteys in the fifteenth century. It is certainly true that Curteys rebuilt and reorganised the library, but R. H. Rouse and Richard Sharpe have conclusively shown that it was the fourteenth-century monk Kirkstead rather than the fifteenth-century Boston who was responsible for giving Bury books their distinctive identifying features.[16]

An anti-Abbot: Edmund Bromefield

John Brinkley died on 31 December 1378, and his death was followed by a particularly bitterly disputed election. A few years earlier, Brinkley had sent an ambitious monk, Edmund Bromefield, to Rome to act as the Abbey's representative, but Bromefield was elevated to the position of proctor in Rome for the General Chapter of the English

---

10 Thomson (1982), p. 93.
11 Press-marks are so called because they indicated which press (cupboard) the book belonged to. These presses were probably set at right angles to the wall along the length of the library, with work spaces between them in front of the windows – much like the arrangement of Duke Humphrey's Library in Oxford.
12 James (1895), p. 2.
13 Chaining of books was common at a time before printing, when manuscripts were artefacts of immense value – this was also a reason why they were the target of looters in 1327 and 1381.
14 James (1895), p. 3.
15 Ibid., p. 40. See also M. R. James, 'Bury St. Edmunds manuscripts', *English Historical Review* 41 (1926), pp. 251–60.
16 R. H. Rouse, 'Bostonus Buriensis and the authors of the *Catalogus Scriptorum Ecclesiae*', *Speculum* 41 (1966), pp. 471–99; Sharpe (1998), pp. 205–7.

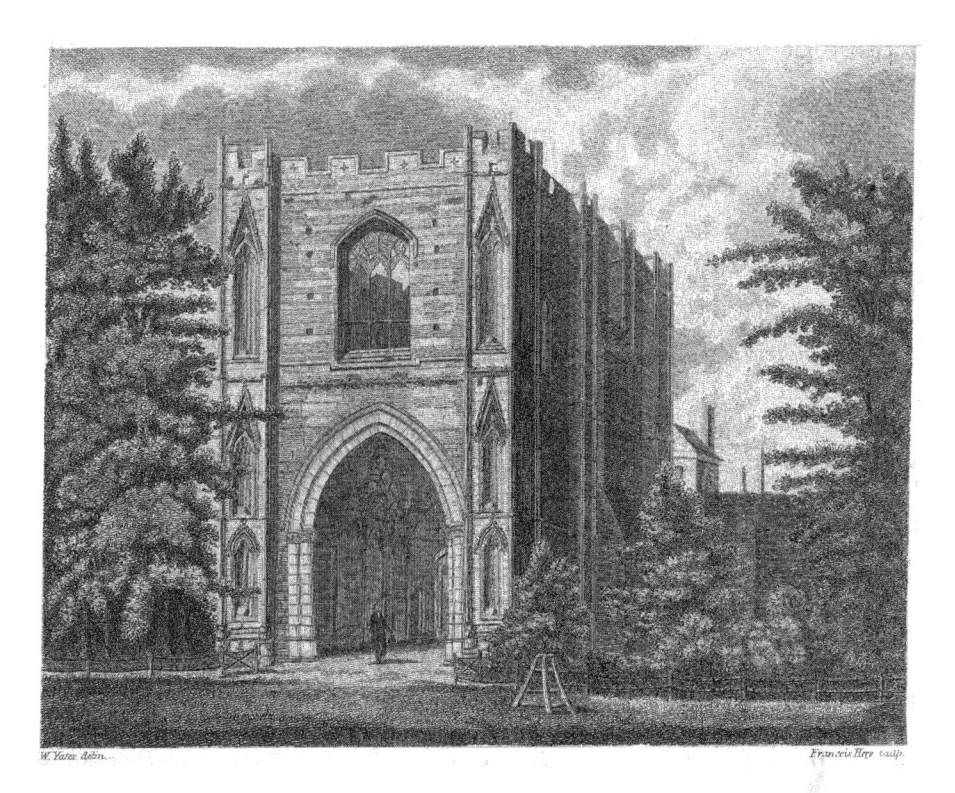

Figure 27 The Abbey Gate from the east (1804). Engraving from Richard Yates, *An Illustration of the Monastic Antiquities of the Town and Abbey of St Edmund's Bury* (1843), plate facing p. 9.

Benedictine Congregation in 1375. When he heard of Brinkley's death, Bromefield paid a Flemish lawyer in Rome, John Shipdam, to arrange for him to become Abbot of St Edmunds, or failing that, prior of Deerhurst or a bishop. Shipdam in turn bribed some of the cardinals, who persuaded the pope to appoint Bromefield to St Edmunds, claiming that the Chapter had already elected him. Accordingly, Bromefield returned to England armed with papal bulls supporting his claim.

Unaware of Bromefield's machinations, the monks had already elected the sub-prior, John Timworth, as their next Abbot. The Abbey sent two monks to Rome, armed with letters from the king and others, to persuade the pope to confirm John, but Urban VI remained committed to Bromefield. By now back in England, in October Bromefield conducted a triumphal progress around the Abbey's manors, gathering popular support. Along with the alderman Thomas Halesworth, who claimed to be Bromefield's cousin, he summoned the monks, as well as secular clergy, friars and laity, to the Chapter House where he seems to have set out a sort of manifesto for changing the relationship between the Abbey and town. Bromefield then led the people to the Abbey Church where he was invested as Abbot.[17]

---

17 Thomas of Walsingham, *The Chronica Maiora of Thomas of Walsingham, 1376–1422,* ed. David Preest and James G. Clark (Woodbridge: Boydell, 2005), pp. 94–5.

John Ridgard has noted that Edmund Bromefield was a near-contemporary of John Wyclif and, like Wyclif, an Oxford doctor of divinity. Bromefield dismissed the obedientaries and appointed new ones, although he restored the Abbot-elect, John Timworth, as sub-prior. Bromefield insisted on eating in the vestry rather than taking up residence in the Abbot's Palace. According to one account he even allowed a female lime-burner to eat from the same dish.[18] For the first time in its history, Bury St Edmunds had an Abbot and an anti-Abbot vying for recognition. Also unprecedented was Edmund Bromefield's decision to appeal to the seculars, friars and laity to support his election, and this suggests that Bromefield was a political thinker with a radical agenda rather than just another ambitious churchman. He seems to have envisaged a completely different Bury St Edmunds, in which the Abbey existed to serve the people rather than the people the Abbey, and Ridgard saw Bromefield as anticipating some of the later ideas of the Lollards.

After little more than a few days, presumably in response to the protests of John Timworth, soldiers entered the town and carried off Bromefield and eighteen monks who supported him to London. Bromefield was put on trial before the lord chancellor, who asked him why he had presumed to enter the monastery as Abbot. Bromefield replied that 'he had entered his own sheepfold as its true shepherd to bring comfort to his plague infected sheep and to provide health restoring medicines for the victims', but the lord chancellor found him guilty of treason and he was sent to the Tower of London.[19] However, Bromefield had unleashed forces of popular resentment against the Abbey that could not so easily be put down.

The revolt of 1381

The causes of the Peasants' Revolt of 1381 are notoriously diverse and difficult to pin down,[20] but East Anglia was one of the principal theatres of this episode of medieval history, and the Abbey of Bury St Edmunds was the main target of insurgents in the region.[21] On one interpretation, the attack on the Abbey was a local manifestation of a national movement against villeinage by blood and against unfair taxes, but it is impossible to read of the revolt of 1381 without considering its local historical context, most notably the earlier revolt of 1327 and popular acclamation of Edmund Bromefield as Abbot of St Edmunds in 1379. Again and again, popular aspirations had been crushed by the power of the Abbey – and even when the pope authorised the election of a sympathetic Abbot, the monks had still managed to have their own way. It is easy to imagine why the people of Bury St Edmunds and the Liberty of St Edmund were frustrated with the Abbey and its establishment.

Like the rising of 1327, the revolt of 1381 cannot simply be dismissed as an act of mass criminality and a breakdown of law and order. Rather, as Christopher Dyer argued, the

---

18   John Ridgard, 'From the rising of 1381 in Suffolk to the Lollards', in David Chadd (ed.), *Religious Dissent in East Anglia III* (Norwich: Centre of East Anglian Studies, 1996), pp. 9–28, at pp. 12–13.
19   *Chronica Maiora* (2005), p. 96.
20   See Christopher Dyer, 'The rising of 1381 in Suffolk: its origins and participants', *PSIAH* 36 (1988), pp. 274–87, at p. 274.
21   Ridgard (1996), p. 9.

rebels were interested in establishing a new law more favourable to the common people.²² In Dyer's view, the origins of the revolt can be seen brewing in the conflicts between villeins or their representatives and the Abbot over the Abbey's rights in the manor of Mildenhall, which began as early as 1321.²³ It was certainly unfortunate that on the outbreak of the revolt, the prior chose to flee to a village that the Abbey had repeatedly antagonised.

On the eve of the Feast of Corpus Christi, 12 June 1381, the rebellion was planned at Sudbury (home town of the unpopular Archbishop Simon) and the following day a party of rebels rode to Cavendish where they confiscated the goods of the chief justice of England, Sir John Cavendish. The horsemen then made a rendezvous with rebels on foot at Long Melford. After drinking a considerable quantity of Cavendish's wine the rebel army, under the command of a chaplain from Sudbury, John Wrawe, marched north, encamping outside the South Gate of Bury at nightfall. Following the Bromefield affair, John Timworth had yet to receive formal confirmation as Abbot, and the acting head of the monastery was Prior John Cambridge, in Gottfried's view 'a well-meaning but inept muddler during the best of times, and quite helpless in a crisis'.²⁴ Cambridge fled to Mildenhall, but he was apprehended by the rebels on Mildenhall Heath with 'incriminating papers' in his saddlebags and summarily executed. Ridgard interpreted these papers as referring to the disputed candidacy of Edmund Bromefield as Abbot. Along with Cambridge, the Abbey's 'baroner' (keeper and enforcer of the Abbot's baronial privileges), the monk John Lakenheath, was incompetently beheaded.²⁵

On 14 June the rebels entered Bury, and the heads of the prior and Sir John Cavendish were stuck on pikes in the market place, set up as if they were talking to each other. The rebels then offered to crown John Wrawe 'King of Suffolk' but he refused, saying that he had a hat already, and used it to crown Robert Westbrom. Westbrom had been a prominent supporter of anti-Abbot Bromefield.²⁶ As in 1327, the rebels entered the Abbey and ransacked it, beating the monks and taking the charters from the treasury and transferring them to the Guildhall. The charter extorted from the Abbey in 1327, which had been signed by the sub-prior John Timworth, was reinstated, and those monks who had supported Bromefield's candidacy assumed the governance of the Abbey.²⁷ The townsfolk also burned the Abbey's manorial rolls, symbolically rejecting its property claims over the district.²⁸ However Bromefield himself was in prison in Nottingham at the time, rendering it impossible for him to make a comeback.²⁹

The rebels' triumph in 1381 was far more short-lived than it had been in 1327, and the regime of Richard II was better equipped to suppress the revolt than that of the young Edward III. On 23 June an army led by the bishop of Norwich, Henry Despenser, arrived at the gates of the town. The burgesses gave up John Wrawe, who was hanged, disembowelled, castrated, drawn and his body hewn into quarters. The Abbey utterly revoked the

---

22 Dyer (1988), pp. 275–6.
23 Ibid., pp. 277–8.
24 Gottfried (1982), p. 233.
25 Goodwin (1931), p. 61.
26 Ridgard (1996), pp. 11–12.
27 Gottfried (1982), p. 234.
28 Dyer (1988), p. 276.
29 Ridgard (1996), p. 13.

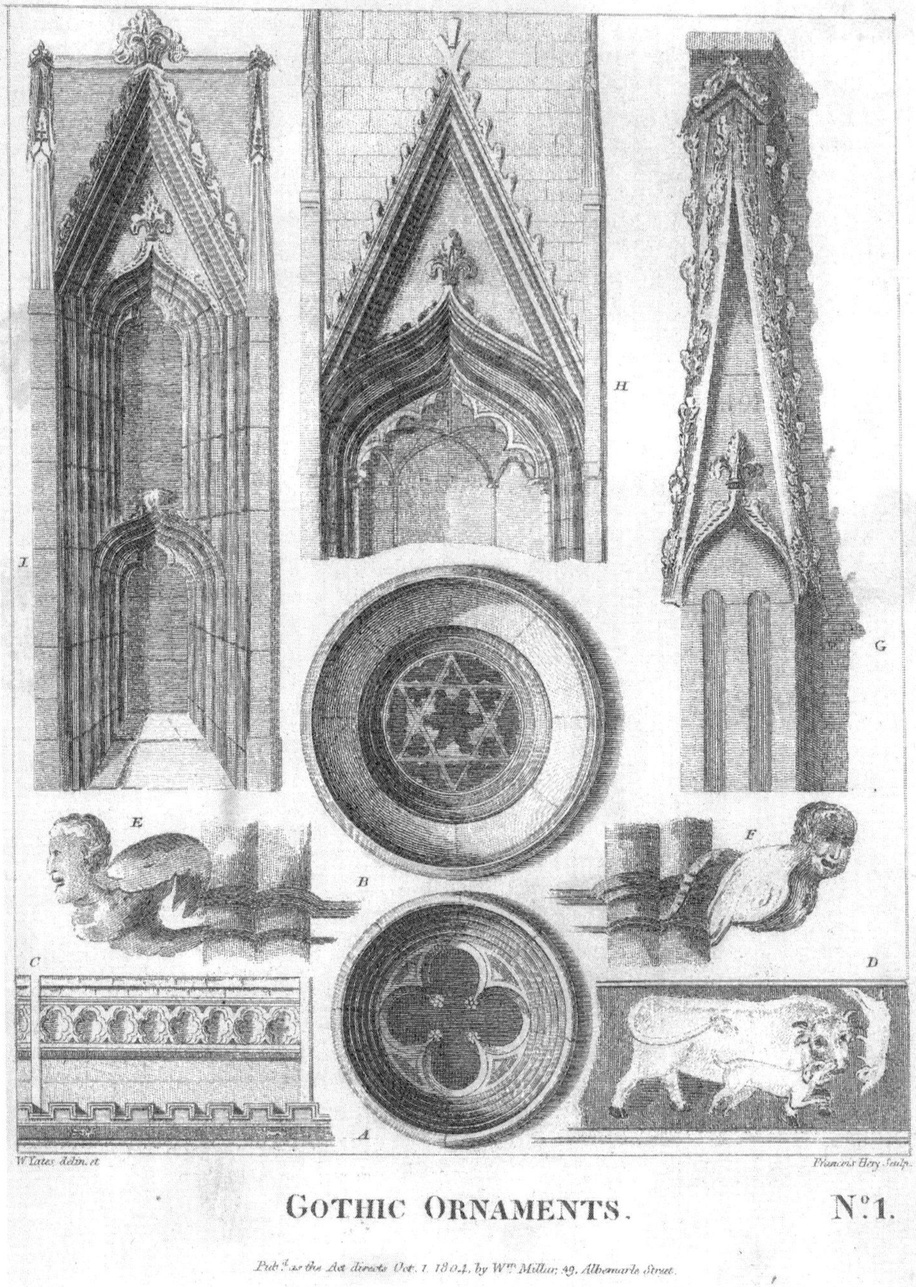

Figure 28 Decorated era sculpture from the Abbey Gate. Engraving from Richard Yates, *An Illustration of the Monastic Antiquities of the Town and Abbey of St Edmund's Bury* (1843), plate facing p. 4.

invalid charter of 1327 and imposed a fine of 2,000 marks on the townsfolk.[30] Overall, in spite of the murder of the prior, the revolt of 1381 was far less serious for the Abbey than the events of 1327. The Abbey buildings suffered no lasting damage, and owing to stronger royal authority, the rebels were not able to remain in control for more than a few days. However, the Abbey had once again been brought low and symbolically humiliated. The fact that the bishop of Norwich, under royal authority, had been forced to intervene undermined the authority and position of the Abbot, even though there was technically no Abbot in office at the time; Timworth was not officially confirmed until 1384.[31]

William Cratfield, 1389–1415

John Timworth died on 16 January 1389, leaving behind him significant debts, in spite of the fact that the townsfolk had finally paid off a fine of 2,000 marks in 1386.[32] These debts were incurred during the period between the death of John Brinkley in 1378 and John's confirmation as Abbot after the suppression of the rebellion in June 1381, when the Abbey's temporalities were in the hands of the crown and therefore systematically stripped, as was the crown's usual custom. Furthermore, Timworth had been faced with the cost of repairing the damage done to the Abbey during the rebellion itself. On 28 January 1389 the chamberlain, William Cratfield, was elected in Chapter, and the temporalities were restored on 8 October. Cratfield's register survives as British Library, Cotton MS Tiberius B.ix.

Cratfield was so concerned about the state of the Abbey's finances that he excused himself from attending the General Chapter of the English Benedictine Congregation in June 1390, and he began a concerted campaign to reduce the financial burdens on the Abbey. In August 1396 he obtained from Richard II confirmation that the monks would no longer have to pay 1,200 marks for the privilege of retaining the Convent's possessions during a vacancy (they would pay £40 a year instead). In 1398 he also obtained confirmation from Pope Boniface IX that the Abbey would no longer need to pay a tax of 1,500 florins and 500 florins for 'petty services', commuting this to an annual sum of 20 marks. Crucially for the Abbey's finances, the pope also granted permission for an Abbot-elect to choose a bishop to bless him, obviating the need for every new Abbot to undertake an expensive journey to Rome. In order to pay the £40 to the king and 20 marks to the pope, Cratfield obtained licences to appropriate two ecclesiastical livings at Harlow and Thurston.[33]

Life in the monastery during Cratfield's reign returned to normal after a long period of disruption. A surviving fourteenth-century *Rituale* (British Library, MS Harley 2977) gives some idea of the splendour of the ceremonial on major festival days in the Abbey in this era. On Christmas Day, for example, the procession consisted of a monk with an aspergilium full of holy water at the front, followed by two crucifers, two acolytes with candles and then the *feretrum* of St Edmund, the bier on which the saint was supposed to have been carried to London by Æthelwine the Sacrist in 1010. The *feretrum* was

---

30 Gottfried (1982), pp. 234–5.
31 Goodwin (1931), p. 60n.
32 Ibid., pp. 61–2.
33 Antonia Gransden, 'Cratfield, William (*d.* 1415), abbot of Bury St Edmunds' in *ODNB*, vol. 14, p. 48.

accompanied by the torn and bloody *camisia* (shirt) of St Edmund, one of the principal relics exposed to the faithful (the body of the saint itself was never shown), carried by two secular chaplains in albs and richly embroidered copes. After the bier came three sub-deacons, each carrying a 'text' (these were probably mass texts to be used by the priest on the altar), and then three deacons, the one in the centre carrying a stole and maniple for the priest, and those on the right and left bearing 'the accustomed relics'. Finally came a priest. The whole procession wound around the cloister and down into the crypt, then up into the choir and into the nave, stopping before the great rood above the nave altar.[34] Long and elaborate processions were typical of the usage of Sarum celebrated in most medieval English churches.[35]

Celebration of the Feast of St Edmund was naturally the high point of the Abbey's calendar. It began at dusk on 19 November – the Vigil of St Edmund – with the ringing, at dusk, of the holy-water bell. 'Gabriel', the cemetery or 'thunderstorm bell', then joined in, followed by the bells of St Mary's, St James's (probably in the Norman Tower) and St Margaret's. Then the younger monks, stationed in the great belfry above the Abbey Church, gave the signal for all the bells to be rung in a fourth peal, in which a *haut-et-cler* bell rose above all the others, giving this peal the nickname *le glas*, 'the clear one'.[36] In the early hours of the next morning, the monks processed into the choir for the night office, a series of twelve responsories dating back to the time of Abbot Baldwin, and possibly written by Hermann the Archdeacon.

We can imagine the air thick with the sweet smell of hot beeswax as hundreds of lights illuminated the darkness of the great church. Four great candles of 12 lb each burned at the four corners of the shrine, with twenty-four smaller candles in a circle around these; five candles burned on the high altar and a candle each in the seventeen windows of the presbytery.[37] At the climax of the solemn responsories, the monks addressed their patron directly with 'an exaggerated sense of entreaty': *O martyr invincibilis, o Eadmunde testis indomabilis* – 'O invincible martyr, O Edmund, unconquerable witness.' The liturgy collapsed the centuries that separated the monks from Edmund's martyrdom; 'commemoration blurred into re-enactment', and the monks sang of Edmund's martyrdom 'on this day'. The intensity of the ceremony was heightened by the presence of the martyr's incorrupt body; as far as the monks were concerned, Edmund their king, the true lord of the Abbey, was in their midst.[38]

Another surviving manuscript from around this time (British Library, MS Harley 3977) describes the experience of a young postulant (a man seeking admission as a monk). The postulant would be met by the novice-master in the guests' parlour before being conducted to the small parlour and then to the Chapter House, where he had to stand before the *pulpitum*. He then had to ask formally for admission to the monastery in Norman French: *Nus priuns la misericord deu e nostre dame seinte marie et nostre seignur*

---

34 James (1895), p. 183.
35 For an account of liturgy in the Abbey of Bury St Edmunds see Richard W. Pfaff, *Liturgy in Medieval England* (Cambridge: Cambridge University Press, 2009), pp. 192–9.
36 Ibid., p. 145.
37 Ibid., p. 179.
38 Henry Parkes, 'St Edmund between liturgy and hagiography', in Licence (2014), pp. 131–69, at pp. 133–4.

seint Edmun e la uostre e vous priuns par seinte charite ke vous nus grantez moniage ('We pray by the mercy of God and of Our Lady St Mary and our lord St Edmund, and yours, and we pray by holy charity that you would grant us monk-hood'). The use of Norman French was probably a relic of the twelfth century, when most of the monks would have been the sons of Norman landowners, and it may also have served to screen out men who lacked education.

The novice was then taken to the infirmary where he received the tonsure, making him a cleric. After that, he was taken to a door in the east side of the choir called the Trayle where he was warned against leaving the precincts of the monastery without permission, and then to the chapel of St Saba, where he spent a minimum of nine days learning the Rule of St Benedict and the customs of the house, including Bury's distinctive form of monastic sign language.[39] When the novice-master considered that the novice knew the Rule well enough he was sent to sit in the cloister, 'having a psalter in [his] hand and beginning to ruminate on reading', until he was called once again to the small parlour. After a year the novice was professed, taking his vows as a monk. He took off his novice's habit in the chapel of St Saba and put on a habit without a hood, entering the church carrying a hooded habit in his left hand and a breviary in his right. On the second day the profession itself took place.[40] Thereafter, if the young monk showed promise as a theologian or canon lawyer he might be sent to Gloucester Hall, Oxford, the Benedictine house of studies, in order to study for a degree.

In Goodwin's view, 'Infinite tact and a certain worldly shrewdness made Cratfield a firm but not fanatical defender of the abbey's legal and spiritual prerogatives.'[41] This tact was well illustrated when, on 1 October 1400, word reached the Chapter that the archbishop of Canterbury, Thomas Arundel, had just finished a visitation of the dioceses of Norwich and Ely and was intending to visit Bury. This implied that Arundel intended to make a visitation of St Edmunds as well – something he had no authority to do – but rather than barring the gates to the archbishop, Cratfield laid on a splendid and lavish banquet that created the impression that Arundel was an honoured guest. This headed off the possibility of a visitation, and Arundel and Cratfield parted on friendly terms.[42]

Cratfield's approach was conciliatory in other areas as well, and in 1408 he was able to bring to a satisfactory resolution a long-running dispute between the Abbey and Christchurch, Canterbury over the right of the Canterbury monks to issue writs in Monks Eleigh and Harlow. He died before he was able to resolve a similar dispute involving properties of the cathedral priory of Ely within the Liberty of St Edmund. Cratfield also adopted a new policy of admitting lay magnates to confraternity with the monks, such as John of Gaunt, duke of Lancaster and his sons the earls of Dorset and March. This was a prelude to the Abbey's identification with the Lancastrian dynasty later in the century. Cratfield was often on the move, presiding over the Benedictine General Chapter in 1408 and 1411, and in 1394 he obtained from the pope a licence to have a portable altar. He endowed chantries in the hospitals of St Nicholas and St John. During the last two years of his life he was unwell and spent most

---

39 On Bury's monastic sign-language see David Sherlock and William Zajac, 'A fourteenth-century monastic sign list from Bury St Edmunds Abbey', *PSIAH* 26 (1988), pp. 251–73.
40 James (1895), p. 178.
41 Goodwin (1931), p. 66.
42 Ibid., p. 67.

of his time on the manor of Elmswell. He died there on 18 November 1415, having done much to restore the fortunes, honour and reputation of the Abbey.[43]

John Lydgate and William Curteys, 1429–46

John Lydgate, who was born in the Suffolk village whose name he took in around 1370,[44] entered the Abbey at around the age of 15 and studied at Gloucester Hall in Oxford. Lydgate received minor orders as an acolyte on 13 March 1389, was made subdeacon on 17 November or December of the same year, and was ordained deacon on 31 May 1393. He received priest's orders on 7 April 1397. Between 1406 and 1408 Henry, prince of Wales (the future Henry V) wrote to Abbot Cratfield asking for 'our very dear in God Dom J. L., your fellow monk' to be allowed to continue his studies in theology or canon law, which was probably a reference to Lydgate.

In the early fifteenth century Lydgate began writing poetry in English, apparently inspired by the work of Geoffrey Chaucer, whom he greatly admired. His early poetry included the *Ballade of her that hath All Virtues*, *The Complaint of the Black Knight*, *The Flour of Curtesye* and the dream poem *The Temple of Glass*. Lydgate's chivalric and courtly themes, combined with the fact that he enjoyed the royal patronage of the prince of Wales, made him a popular author for commissions. Lydgate's first mature poem, *The Troy Book*, was commissioned by Prince Henry in October 1412. This work on the fall of Troy was on an epic scale, consisting of 30,000 lines of couplets in five books. Indeed, prolixity was to be a defining characteristic of Lydgate's productions.[45]

Abbot Cratfield was succeeded in 1415 by William Exeter, an obscure monk who had not previously held high office in the Convent. Exeter played a role in the global church, attending the Council of Constance (1414–18) which ended the papal schism as well as the conclave that elected Martin V in 1417, the first pope to command the loyalty of the cardinals of both Avignon and Rome. Exeter also presided over the reconstruction of the church of St Mary, and his splendid building of 1424 (which still stands today) presumably replaced Anselm's Romanesque church, which in turn replaced the oldest church in the town, to which the body of St Edmund had originally been brought.[46] Lydgate also contributed to the cult of the Virgin Mary, writing a poem on *The Life of Our Lady* in around 1421–22.

Lydgate's patron Henry V died on 31 August 1422 at Vincennes, and Lydgate may have composed a prose work warning against faction at the royal court, *The Serpent of Division*, in December of that year. However, Lydgate's star remained in the ascendant during the regency for the infant Henry VI. It may have been partly owing to the patronage of the new king's uncle, Humphrey, duke of Gloucester that Lydgate was elected prior of Hatfield Regis in Essex in 1423. Hatfield was an alien priory (a dependency

---

43 Gransden, 'Cratfield' (2004), p. 48.
44 In 2014 graffiti apparently signed by a young John Lydgate was discovered in Lidgate church; see Matthew Champion, *Medieval Graffiti: The Lost Voices of England's Churches* (London: Ebury Press, 2015), pp. 17–18.
45 Douglas Gray, 'Lydgate, John (*c.*1370–1449/50?)' in *ODNB*, vol. 34, pp. 843–8. For a longer biography of Lydgate see Walter F. Schirmer, *John Lydgate: A Study in the Culture of the XVth Century* (Berkeley, Calif.: University of California Press, 1961).
46 Goodwin (1931), p. 68.

of a foreign abbey, a type of religious house suppressed under Henry V) which became attached to St Edmunds, although Lydgate did not hold the post for long and returned to Bury in 1424. In 1426 the poet went to Paris, then under English control, where he entered the service of the earl of Warwick, acting regent of France. He composed a poem entitled *The Title and Pedigree of Henry VI* to prove Henry's right to rule France.

In 1428 the then prior, William Curteys, permitted the bishop of Norwich, William Alnwick, to carry out an investigation against Lollard heretics in Bury. Abbot Exeter died early in 1429 and was replaced by Curteys, who was elected in Chapter on 14 February 1429. The king restored the Abbot's temporalities on 18 February, and Curteys was blessed by the bishop of Ely at Blackfriars, Cambridge (the present site of Emmanuel College) on 6 March. Two days later he was enthroned at Bury. Curteys was forced to sell items belonging to the Abbot's household to pay off debts incurred by Exeter, and the fact that Curteys had allowed the bishop of Norwich to investigate heretics in the borough caused problems, because it suggested a concession with regard to the Abbey and *banleuca*'s freedom from episcopal jurisdiction. Curteys was forced to send two monks to Rome to obtain renewed papal confirmation of these exemptions, which took two years.[47] However, Curteys was no less zealous against heresy than Alnwick, and conducted his own proceedings in 1431 and 1438.[48]

In 1429 Henry VI was crowned in London as king of England and in Paris as king of France, events celebrated in verse by Lydgate, who urged the new king to suppress the Lollard heresy.[49] However, disaster struck the Abbey on 18 December 1430 when the south side of the west tower collapsed, followed by the east side on 30 December 1431. During the course of 1432 the remainder of the tower was demolished, and Curteys began to collect funds for its reconstruction through appropriations of Abbey lands as well as by obtaining a plenary indulgence of forty days for anyone who donated money or materials.[50]

On 1 November 1433, while he was at his manor of Elmswell, Curteys received the news that Henry VI intended to visit Bury. The Abbot commissioned eighty craftsmen and workmen to beautify the Abbot's Palace for the king's visit, and on Christmas Eve 1433 the 12-year-old king rode into the town with his magnates, accompanied by 500 mounted men from the borough dressed in scarlet, who had met him on Newmarket Heath. At the south gate (St Margaret's) of the Abbey, Abbot Curteys and the bishop of Norwich sprinkled holy water on the king and conducted him to the shrine of St Edmund. The king stayed for Christmas, receiving splendid gifts from the Abbot. After Epiphany on 6 January the king moved to the prior's lodgings, since they were more pleasantly situated overlooking the River Lark, and during January he went hunting in the woods on the east side of the river (the site of the present day Moreton Hall Estate). On 23 January Henry moved to Elmswell for fishing and hawking, and then back to the prior's lodgings for Lent.

---

47 Antonia Gransden, 'Babington [Babyngton], William (*d.* 1453), abbot of Bury St Edmunds', in *ODNB*, vol. 3, pp. 88–9.
48 Antonia Gransden, 'Curteys, William (*d.* 1446), abbot of Bury St Edmunds', in *ODNB*, vol. 14, pp. 760–1.
49 Pinner (2015), p. 99.
50 Goodwin (1931), p. 69.

Along with the duke of Gloucester and other members of the court he was admitted as an honorary member of the fraternity at Easter, and he finally departed on St George's Day, 23 April 1434.[51]

Henry VI's lengthy visit cemented a special relationship between the Abbey and the Lancastrian king. Both Goodwin and Pinner argue that the richly illuminated presentation copy of Lydgate's *Legend of Ss Edmund and Fremund* (now British Library, MS Harley 2278) was presented to Henry during his visit, although Gransden dissents and concludes that it was presented to Henry some years later, in 1438, to commemorate the visit.[52] However, whether presented during or after the event the manuscript constitutes a unique visual record of a royal visit, since it depicts the monks presenting the book to Henry, as well as both Henry and Lydgate kneeling at the shrine of St Edmund (a valuable record of the shrine's appearance at this date). The *Legend* itself is an epic poem of 3,693 lines in three books telling the story of St Edmund and his fictitious cousin, Fremund.[53] Its purpose was to present Edmund as an ideal model of youthful kingship, as well as to cement the king's affection for the Abbey and therefore guarantee its privileges.

Curteys was renowned for his learning, and indeed he was responsible for composing his own brief life of St Edmund, which concentrated on the implications of the martyr king's life for the privileges of the Abbey.[54] However, the most significant achievement of Curteys' reign was his construction of a new monastic library, a fact unknown until M. R. James discovered the Abbot's copy of Isidore of Seville's *Etymologies* in the Palace Green Library in Durham. This contained the words 'provided by Dom. William Curteys, Abbot of the monastery of St. Edmund at Bury ... which book he assigned and gave to the Library, constructed by himself, of the said monastery, there perpetually to remain'. James thought that the library was probably located over the cloister or the Chapter House.[55] He argued that a warning issued by Curteys to the monks to return any books they had borrowed or sold from the library or taken to university for their studies within fifteen days – on pain of suspension from divine offices – was the prelude to Curteys' better organisation of the library.[56]

Gransden has argued that the model for the new library at Bury was the library of Gloucester Hall, Oxford, the Benedictine house of studies which was heavily patronised by St Edmunds. When Curteys was prior, he had funded the construction of accommodation for Bury monks at Oxford which included a library.[57] As a result of the library, scholarship thrived at the Abbey, and in around 1435 the abbot of St Albans wrote to Curteys, asking him to send one of the Abbey's scholars to the Council of Basel to defend the privileges of the Benedictine Order. Gransden saw Curteys' reign as the culmination of archival activity at the Abbey, and the Abbot left behind the celebrated Curteys Register (British Library MSS Add. 14848 and Add. 7096) as well as other important documents produced when he was cellarer and prior. Curteys' health may have begun to fail by November 1442, when

---

51 Ibid., pp. 70–1.
52 Gransden, 'Curteys' (2004), pp. 760–1.
53 Pinner (2015), p. 89.
54 Ibid., p. 91.
55 James (1895), pp. 40–1.
56 Ibid., pp. 110–11.
57 Gransden, 'Curteys' (2004), pp. 760–1.

Pope Eugenius IV granted him permission to be admitted as a brother of St Anthony's Hospital in London. The Abbot died early in 1446. In Gransden's view, he was 'the last great ruler of that house'.[58]

Curteys was indeed a far-sighted figure. We know little of him on a personal level, but he seems to have understood that the Abbey's future was best ensured by cultivating a personal relationship with the monarch. Merely securing exemptions and privileges for the Abbey was not enough; Curteys had to show the king that he was a reliable counsellor, as well as demonstrating that he was willing to throw the weight of the church behind efforts to suppress the Lollard heresy, which was a threat to public peace as well as Catholic doctrine. Curteys was fortunate to have the services of as gifted a poet as Lydgate, and he seems to have seen the Abbey's future as a centre of learning and archival activity, an aspect of the Abbey's life sorely neglected by the fourteenth-century Abbots. By attracting such an extended royal visit Curteys may also, of course, have served to boost numbers of pilgrims. It seems very likely that the popularity of Lydgate's poem on St Edmund, which was copied numerous times, had this effect.[59]

John Lydgate did not long outlive Curteys, and probably died in 1449 or 1450. In his own time he achieved considerable fame, which continued into the sixteenth century (when his works were edited by John Stowe) and even into the eighteenth, when he attracted praise from Thomas Warton and Thomas Gray. In the nineteenth century, however, Lydgate was denounced by the critic Joseph Ritson as a 'voluminous, prosaick, and driveling monk', cementing his popular reputation as turgid and verbose.[60] However, the study of Lydgate is increasingly popular among students of medieval English literature keen to reappraise his contribution, partly because the volume of material is so great in comparison with other medieval English vernacular writers such as Chaucer and Langland.

William Babington, 1446–53

William Babington was a native of Somerset rather than Suffolk, and was still a young monk at the time he was sent to Rome by Abbot Curteys to defend the Abbey's privileges against Bishop Alnwick. Babington was a doctor of canon law at Oxford by 1442, based at Gloucester Hall, and in 1444 he became principal of the School of Canon Law. Babington's career was proof that in the fifteenth century it was possible for a monk to have a successful academic career, and Abbot Curteys would undoubtedly have encouraged Babington in this. Although Benedictine monks took a vow of stability to their house, houses of study such as Gloucester Hall were an exception, and allowed the monks to challenge the domination of the universities by Dominican and Franciscan friars.

Shortly after Curteys' death in the spring of 1446 Babington was elected Abbot in Chapter, and the Abbot's temporalities were restored on 23 May.[61] The first challenge of Babington's reign was hosting parliament, which was summoned to meet at Bury St Edmunds in February 1447. This notorious parliament, which famously features in a

---

58 Ibid.
59 Pinner (2015), p. 102.
60 Gray (2004), p. 848.
61 Gransden, 'Babington' (2004), pp. 88–9.

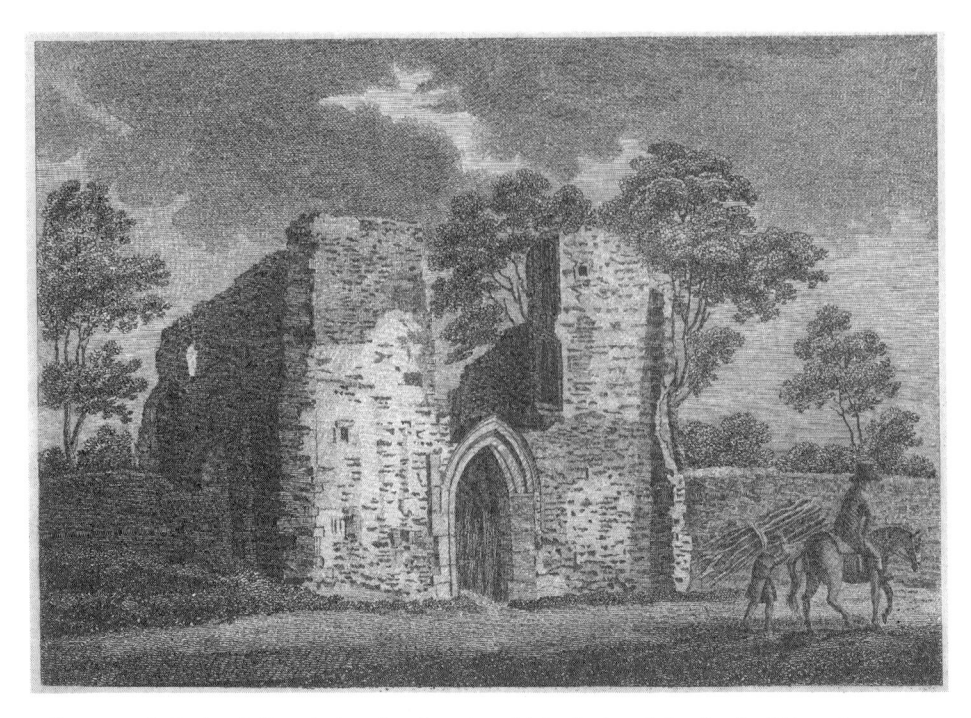

Figure 29 St Saviour's Hospital on Fornham Road (1804), site of the death of Humphrey, duke of Gloucester in 1447. Engraving from Richard Yates, *An Illustration of the Monastic Antiquities of the Town and Abbey of St Edmund's Bury* (1843), plate facing p. 48.

fictionalised form in Shakespeare's *Henry VI Part 2* (Act III, Scene 1), saw the downfall of Humphrey, duke of Gloucester. It was not unusual at this period for parliament to be summoned at a location other than the Palace of Westminster, since the peers and commons of the realm were expected to assemble around their sovereign, wherever in the country he might be, if writs were issued to that effect. William de la Pole, duke of Suffolk, managed to convince Henry that his uncle, Humphrey, duke of Gloucester was planning a popular rising to dethrone him. Armed men were stationed around the town, and Henry was heavily guarded as he processed to the monastic refectory,[62] where he opened parliament on 10 February.[63] The bill under consideration proposed to revive severe laws against the Welsh, who had recently risen up under Gruffydd ap Nicholas. Babington served as the parliament's trier of petitions, deciding which petitions should and should not appear before the king.[64]

On 18 February Gloucester, who had been in Wales putting down the rebels, rode into Bury accompanied by a small retinue (including the defeated rebel Gruffydd) and took up residence at St Saviour's Hospital on the road to Fornham All Saints, oblivious to the

---

62 Susanne Saygin, *Humphrey, Duke of Gloucester (1390–1447) and the Italian Humanists* (Leiden, Netherlands: Brill, 2002), p. 127.
63 Goodwin (1931), pp. 72–3.
64 Gransden, 'Babington' (2004), pp. 88–9.

preparations made against him by his political rival.[65] Gloucester was met by a delegation of magnates and placed under arrest on a charge of treason. Gloucester's downfall had been a long time coming, but the final act of this drama, which ultimately triggered the Wars of the Roses, took place in Bury. Meanwhile, the Welsh rebel was brought before Henry in the monastic refectory and made formal submission to the king as overlord of the Welsh – a confirmation of English dominance that was fitting for a parliament under the protection of St Edmund, the patron of the English.

After three days of confinement at St Saviour's, Gloucester fell into a coma, and shortly before 3 o'clock on 23 February he died, depriving the duke of Suffolk of the satisfaction of a trial for treason. The event is today commemorated by a large Victorian plaque on the remains of St Saviour's Hospital, now next to a Tesco supermarket. Although contemporary sources make clear that Humphrey's death was a natural one – he was emotionally overwhelmed by the experience of his own nephew turning against him – rumours immediately spread that he had been poisoned at Suffolk's instigation.[66] As a consequence of Gloucester's death, a bitter battle began for influence over Henry. A key contender was Richard, duke of York, a great-great grandson of Edward III and the head of the Yorkist dynasty, which became increasingly assertive in its claim to influence the crown owing to proximity of blood.

The duke of Gloucester had been admitted to the Chapter as a member of the confraternity in 1433, and Goodwin argued that the duke's death might have been a particular blow for the monastery. However, it was some consolation when, on 28 November of the same year, Henry VI granted a charter confirming the Abbey's privileges. Henry followed this in 1449 by exempting St Edmunds from taxation on condition of an annual payment of 40 marks.[67] At a time when taxation fluctuated wildly depending on the king's needs in peace and war, payment of a fixed subsidy to the crown was much to be preferred.

In the summer of 1450 rebellion broke out in Kent, led by a man named Jack Cade. Among other things the rioters demanded that Henry recall the duke of York from exile. Cade was defeated, but York returned in September, and in October he began a tour of East Anglia. He arrived at Bury on 16 October 1450, where he met one of his key supporters, John de Mowbray, duke of Norfolk, to discuss the candidates they would promote in elections to the forthcoming parliament. However, it is also possible that the two men discussed deposing Henry VI by force on this occasion, as Ralph Griffiths has argued. If so, Bury again played a critical role in English history as a place where royal authority was challenged in the name of the greater good of the country.[68] Eventually York challenged Henry VI for the throne in arms.

Babington's involvement in state and church affairs continued. He served once more as a trier of petitions at the parliament of 1449, and on 13 March he was appointed England's proctor to the Papal Curia. Babington set out for Rome, arriving in time for the Jubilee Year of 1450. Gransden believed that Babington asked Pope Nicholas V to place restrictions on Benedictines travelling to Rome to receive the indulgences without permis-

---

65   Ralph A. Griffiths, *King and Country: England and Wales in the Fifteenth Century* (London: Hambledon, 1991), p. 191.
66   Saygin (2002), pp. 127–8.
67   Goodwin (1931), pp. 73–4.
68   Griffiths (1991), pp. 294–5.

sion – Babington imprisoned a monk of Glastonbury, under his authority as proctor of England, for misbehaviour while he was in Rome. In effect, during this period Babington had complete authority over any English monk in the city. The pope even allowed Babington to depute priests who could grant indulgences to Benedictines throughout England and Wales who were unable to come on pilgrimage. Babington managed to continue his academic career as a canon lawyer as well; on 9 November 1450, on his way back to England along the Rhine, he was admitted to the faculty of canon law of the University of Cologne.[69]

John Bohun, 1453–69

Abbot Babington died in the autumn of 1453, and his successor John Bohun (or Boone) was elected soon after. Bohun was a safe choice, having been prior since 17 October 1437.[70] A powerful Bohun family, based at Fressingfield in northeast Suffolk, dominated county politics at this period, but Bridget Wells-Furby has rejected the idea that Abbot Bohun may have been related to this family.[71] Bohun, like his predecessors Abbots Curteys and Babington, was a committed and loyal supporter of the House of Lancaster, and in 1462 during the reign of the Yorkist Edward IV the monks foolishly pinned an inflammatory letter from the pope to the door of the Abbey Church. This granted an indulgence to supporters of Henry VI and excommunicated Edward and his followers. The king punished Bohun for the incident by demanding a fine of 500 marks.[72]

Work on the reconstruction of the great west tower, which had partially collapsed in 1430, continued in Bohun's reign. The reconstruction was supported by the townsfolk, whose relations with the Abbey were more cordial at this time than some analyses have suggested. John 'Jankyn' Smith, a powerful figure in fifteenth-century Bury who refused the position of alderman because it was controlled by the sacrist, left his 'best standing cup of silver and gilt' to the prior in his will. Another influential man, John Baret (whose remarkable chantry tomb can still be seen in St Mary's Church), left the Abbot his 'beads of white amber with the ring of silver overgilt [be]longing thereto and [a] gilt standing cup' in his will.[73]

Unfortunately, however well funded and supported it might be, the rebuilding work carried with it considerable risks. The roof of the new west tower needed to be releaded, which in turn required workmen to bring lighted braziers onto the roof, and on 20 January 1465 disaster struck. It is not possible to provide a better account of this than M. R. James's translation of a vivid contemporary description, in a manuscript he discovered at Jesus College, Oxford:[74]

> In the 1465th year of the Lord's Incarnation there took place at Bury St. Edmund's

---

69 Gransden, 'Babington' (2004), p. 89.
70 Thomson (1982), p. 93.
71 Bridget Wells-Furby (ed.), *The 'Bohun of Fressingfield' Cartulary* (Woodbridge: Suffolk Records Society, 2011), p. 3.
72 Goodwin (1931), p. 75.
73 Lobel (1935), pp. 162–3.
74 James (1895), pp. 208–12.

a dismal conflagration of the monastery of that saint on the 13th of the Kalends of February (20 January), through the negligence of some men who were repairing – or, to speak more truly, destroying – the Church with lead and fire. Now it arose this way. The sun was shining, there was neither foul weather, thunder, not high wind; all whisper of a breeze had fallen, and there was but a light air from the south, which grew strong enough, alas! afterwards. The men got ready what was necessary for their plumbing work, the fire and irons, and went up the tower. They placed their brazier in a spot exposed to the gentle draught of wind. They then set to, and worked until the dinner-hour called them away: whereupon they went down, and left the brazier very unwisely placed, between the roof and the wind. The fire was fanned by the breeze, melted the lead and penetrated into the roof, remaining unsuspected within the wooden ceiling until the whole was in flames. At last the ceiling caught, and instantly great tongues of flames shot forth into the Church. As soon as they were seen, the bells clashed out in harsh discord, and the people rushed in from all quarters, eager to help. But by this time the fire had gained such power that no one dared cope with it, partly because of the great height above the floor, and partly because of the dropping of molten lead, which it was impossible to face.

It was now midday, and the whole roof of the Church, from the west end almost up to the bell-tower (central tower) was falling in. The crowd left the Church in a panic, and prayed on their bended knees to God and St Edmund. Meanwhile some of the utensils of divine service were torn down and carried off to a place of safety: some of them were removed by unprincipled persons, never to return; and others, of the most precious kind, perished in the sudden conflagration. There was a great cry made, and great was the noise of men going and coming; sorrow and fear were on every face. Not only, moreover, were the ornaments of the Church plundered, but in other buildings and chambers every secret recess was explored, and all that could be found was removed: for destruction threatened the whole establishment. Some did this work with good intent, to save the articles from the fire, but others of malice aforethought.

The western portion of the Church was now a dismal ruin; but many thought that the flames would at any rate stop at the central tower. Yet their fury did not slacken; they made their way through openings on this side and on that, broke into the Church, and consumed the lateral parts of it [the transepts, probably] with irresistible force. Yea, and the presbytery itself, wherein the body of the Lord is kept, and where the shrine of the holy martyr Edmund in all its beauty has often stirred the heart of the devout believer to praise, was invaded by the fearful violence of the fire. The sacrament of our redemption had, however, been already removed by the Sacrist, and placed reverently in the vestry, with a lighted candle before it; for he feared to tempt the Lord his God [by forcing him to a display of miraculous power]. The whole house of God now tottered to its fall; the flames, raging high and low, caught upon the lantern that tops the spire, and is the ornament of the whole fane. This grieved and terrified the spectators more than all: all hope died when that graceful spire was seen to be in flames. By this time 'a great wind was sounding through the air', and carrying large burning sparks to a great distance: nay, what is more surprising, I saw numbers of small pieces of lead cast to a considerable distance by the combined force of wind and fire. Our groans now redoubled, and many a deep sigh was drawn. The poor monks knew not which way to turn, nor what to do, and their pitiable complaints might not inaptly have recalled Virgil's lines on Troy. 'To us too had the last day, the inevitable moment, come: we *were* monks, the glory and honour of Eastern England *was*, but the fierce fire is seizing it all, and mastering the holy temple.' Moreover, the feeling was not now chiefly of concern for the burning of the spire, but of fear for its fall; for it threatened totally to destroy the Church, and, besides, to make an end of the whole monastery. The onlookers therefore retired to a distance, some 'beholding it afar off,' others unable to bear the sorrow of seeing its fall. However, the special mercy of God, which never fails to succour His servants, did not suffer the great and noble sanctuary of His soldier to be wholly destroyed. The fire consumed the timbers which supported the steeple; and it sank, wonderfully to say, perpendicularly into the tower below, without bending to right or left. What a fiery furnace was there! What clouds of smoke, think you, what blazing heat! That exquisite choir, that left not its match in all the kingdom, – the graceful spire of the Church, – the nine bells, the great candlestick, wrought with such art and skill, were all blazing up together in one heap! What more? This enormous pyre now directed all its flames and all its force against the shrine of the martyr. Hither and thither it darted, licking up the presses and seats, the projecting images of the angels, and the huge hanging crucifix that almost touched the holy martyr, and reduced them all to glowing embers. The wooden cover of the shrine, when the rope that held it up was burnt through, fell down upon the shrine, in flames: so that the martyr, though walled about on every side with fire, as in an oven, remained scatheless. O precious boon of God! O wonderful chance, worthy to be preferred to any miracle, that all these millions of flames should have been foiled by one martyr! At this point some daring souls made a rush for the Church, broke through the windows, cast water upon the flames, and seeing that the shrine was intact, raised a cry of joy to those without; whereupon all gave thanks to God and to the holy martyr.

Another incident was very surprising, and deserves to be recorded, concerning Egelwyn, the former servant and charioteer of the martyr, and others whose bones were kept in a wooden chest, high up, near the king's tomb. Some men had employed great force in trying to move them, inasmuch as the heat had already got to them; but though the chest could ordinarily be lifted with one hand, they were now unable to stir it. Was not this truly a faithful servant, who refused to forsake his king? And, though thus overcome by the martyr, the miserable disaster did not come to an end forthwith; but redoubling its strength, breathed all its heat against the Chapel of the Blessed Virgin [that is, on the north side of the Choir, as I suppose]. The Refectory had been already consumed [perhaps only the roof: it was on the side of the Cloister furthest from the Church], and the fire had caught upon the roof of the Palace. But by great exertions it was subdued there, and now raged only in the Chapel: nor did it cease, though copiously drenched with wine and water, until it had laid it even with the ground. In the Infirmary, which was completely exposed to the danger, no damage was done, for God preserved it. The care and anxiety of all was now centred on the Vestry, where, as I have said, the body of the Lord had been placed, and where the whole treasure of the Church now lay shut up. It had been in no slight degree affected by the flames, as is witnessed to this day by the scorched walls, and the stones and timbers from which the heat has sucked out the hardness. The door opening out of the Choir into the Vestry did not escape damage, but by God's help everything that was inside remained safe. For the Lord of all, like a good Vestiary, fulfilled his office faithfully, preserving all His possessions unharmed. We owe, therefore, and we would pay, hearty thanks to God who vouchsafed to deliver Himself and His soldier Edmund out of this great fire, and who now assures us, though we were well-nigh comfortless, of the solace of so great a protector: to the praise and glory of His name; to whom is honour everlasting. Amen.

The fire left the Abbey Church gutted and its ornaments and furnishings destroyed, while the shrine of St Edmund itself only just escaped destruction. The wooden spire had also been completely consumed, and all that remained was the shell of Baldwin and Anselm's Abbey Church. The chronicler vividly conveys the monks' despair, but it ought to be borne in mind that much of the Abbey remained untouched. The roof of the Abbot's Palace had briefly caught fire, but the prior's lodgings, infirmary and refectory were unaffected, as were the secular buildings on the north side of the complex. Furthermore, it seems likely that the cloister and library were not burned as there is no evidence in surviving books from Bury of fire damage. For the remainder of his reign Abbot Bohun was faced with the considerable task of beginning the reconstruction of his church after the most damaging fire in its history.

Chapter 6
The final years, 1469–1539

The use of teleological reasoning in history – the assumption that because something happened it was always going to happen, whatever the details of events – is a grave temptation, and it has been a particularly strong one for monastic historians. The fact of the dissolution of the monasteries is etched into the British landscape, naturally giving rise to interesting counterfactual questions about whether the religious houses could have survived if a change in central policy had not determined their end. Questions about what did *not* happen are, strictly speaking, unanswerable for the historian, but it is certainly possible to challenge faulty interpretations of what did occur. In 1931, Albert Goodwin pronounced a damning historical verdict on the Abbey of Bury St Edmunds:

> Power, prestige and privilege had … proved the monks' undoing. For centuries they had lived for little else than the acquisition of papal grants or royal endowments. Increasing secularisation, set off by their inflexible and hidebound conservatism, had gradually alienated every class of the community. Their tardy attempts at reform were undoubtedly genuine but their social exclusiveness and the utter uselessness of their existence had, by the end of the fifteenth century, undermined their whole position … the very *raison d'etre* of the system of which they were the representatives had disappeared … the dissolution was neither a grave social nor a serious economic calamity. It was both just and necessary.[1]

Goodwin made his judgement on the assumption that the tide of history had turned against the Abbey; it could not resist the advance of modernity and secularisation, of which Henry VIII's suppression was just one manifestation. Yet 'modern' and 'secular' are abstract concepts constructed by later historians, and neither Henry VIII nor any other inhabitant of sixteenth-century England was aware of them. To argue that the end of the Abbey was inevitable is quite simply bad history (as indeed is virtually every appeal to the idea of the inevitability of historical events). Historians of monasticism have long since moved beyond Goodwin's dismissive attitude, and the consensus since the work of David Knowles holds that the monasteries had much still going for them at the time of the dissolution.

This is especially true of St Edmunds. In addition to the house's vast wealth, there is much evidence that the monks of fifteenth- and sixteenth-century Bury had a rich literary and academic life and were interested in beautifying and repairing their Abbey Church, a project in which the townsfolk also willingly shared. Profound conservatism with regard

---

1   Goodwin (1931), p. 73.

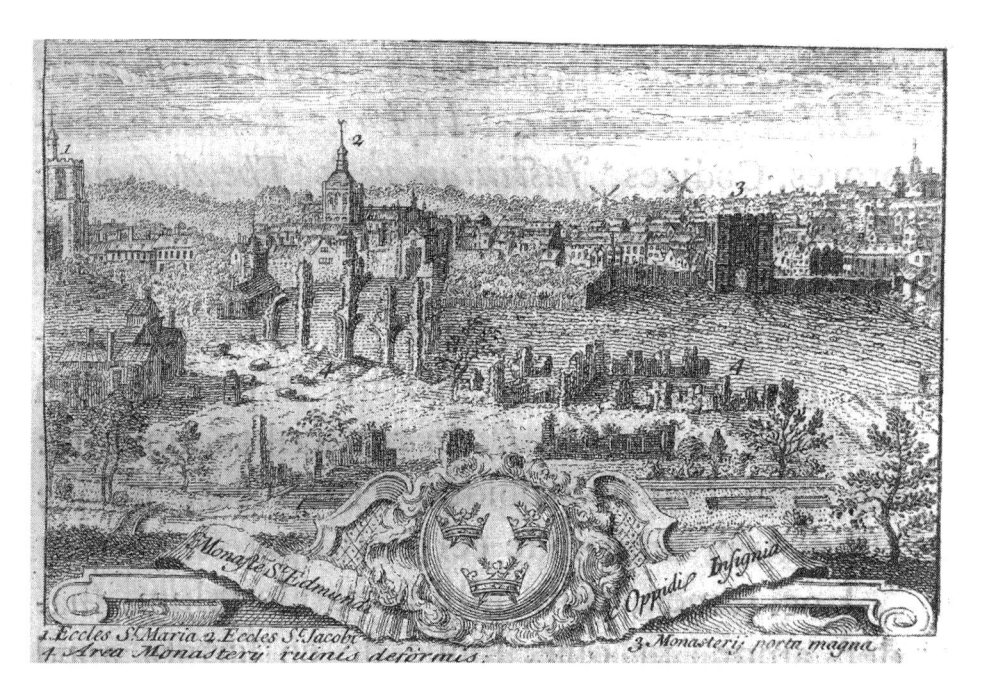

Figure 30 The outcome of dissolution: a view of the Abbey in 1745. From John Battely, *Antiquitates Sancti Edmundi* (1745), p. 1.

to authority and privilege was a feature of early sixteenth-century English society, from the king himself to the humblest subject, so it seems unfair to criticise the monks for this. The men who dissolved the Abbey were at least as interested in religion as the monks themselves, rendering suspect the idea that 'secularisation' lay behind the dissolution. Likewise, Goodwin's suggestion that the monks were 'useless' ignores the possibility that they sincerely believed in the value of their spiritual tasks, and there are good reasons to believe that the dissolution was indeed a social and economic calamity.

Late medieval Abbots

Little is known about the four Abbots who preceded John Reeve. John Bohun was succeeded, on 20 September 1469, by Robert Coote (alias Ixworth), who according to Yates was the son of Sir John Coote of Norfolk.[2] This seems unlikely, as monks took toponymic names and Ixworth is not in Norfolk. What we do know is that Robert Ixworth was prior and sacrist concurrently in late 1468.[3] Ixworth continued to face challenges from the townsfolk, and on 10 September 1471 alderman Robert Gardiner drew up a new assertion of the borough's privileges.[4] Ixworth's reign was a short one, however,

---

2   Yates (1843), p. 220.
3   Thomson (1982), pp. 93, 95.
4   Norman M. Trenholme, *The English Monastic Boroughs: A Study in Medieval History* (Columbia, Mo.: University of Missouri Press, 1927), pp. 98–102.

and he was succeeded by Richard Ingham (or Hengham) in the year of his death, 1474. In 1479 Ingham presided over a dispute with the townsfolk, when the burgesses advanced a claim that the alderman could appoint constables and keepers of the market as well as the traditional watchmen and gatekeepers. The Abbot took the matter before the king's council, which decided in favour of the Abbot, ruling that 'the abbot was lord of the whole town with power of appointing and removing aldermen and all other officials'.[5]

Ingham died later the same year and was succeeded by Thomas Rattlesden, who had briefly served as sacrist between the election of Abbot Ixworth on 20 September 1469 and 2 September 1470.[6] It was under Abbot Rattlesden that John Wastell became master mason to the Abbey in around 1486, in succession to Simon Clerk (d. 1489).[7] Rattlesden ruled until 1497, witnessing the restoration of the Lancastrian claimant Henry Tudor, and it is unsurprising that Henry VII confirmed the loyal Abbey's privileges by charter on 1 December 1488.[8] The king also visited the Abbey in 1486,[9] the final visit of a reigning monarch to the Abbey.

Abbot Rattlesden was succeeded by the cellarer, William Bunting (otherwise known as Coddenham, presumably from the village of his birth), who received the degree of doctor of divinity at Cambridge in 1501.[10] In 1506 Bunting presented a rising star in the clerical firmament from Ipswich, Thomas Wolsey, to the living of Redgrave.[11] However, Abbot Bunting's most lasting achievement was undoubtedly his decision to rebuild St James's Church from 1503 onwards, under the Abbey's stonemason John Wastell. Wastell's distinctive string-coursing along the west front of the church, featuring the scallop shell and pilgrim's pack of St James, is comparable with his more famous work at King's College, Cambridge, Canterbury Cathedral and Peterborough Abbey. Indeed, it is no accident that the central tower of the Cathedral of St James and St Edmund, completed in 2005, bears a striking resemblance to Wastell's great tower at Canterbury.

The last Abbot: John Reeve, 1513–39

Abbot Bunting died in 1513 and his successor, John Reeve alias Melford, was elected later the same year. Reeve emerged from the prosperous clothier dynasties of south Suffolk and was related to Thomas Smith of Long Melford, one of the wealthiest men in Suffolk in 1524.[12] J. R. Thompson thought that Reeve may have been related to the Reeves of Harleston on the basis of the similarity between their coat of arms and those of the last Abbot.[13] His election proved that 'new money' could successfully dominate senior ecclesiastical offices in the county. Reeve is not recorded as having held high office in the

---

5 Goodwin (1931), p. 76.
6 Thomson (1982), p. 95.
7 Francis Woodman, 'Wastell, John (d. c.1518)' in *ODNB*, vol. 57, pp. 542–3.
8 Lobel (1935), p. 163.
9 Alfred W. Morant, 'On the Abbey of Bury St. Edmunds', *PSIA* 4 (1872), pp. 376–404, at p. 384.
10 Thomson (1982), p. 97; Yates (1843), p. 220. Yates erroneously thought that Abbots Bunting and Coddenham were two different men.
11 Yates (1843), p. 220.
12 MacCulloch (1986), p. 136.
13 J. R. Thompson, *Records of Saint Edmund of East Anglia King and Martyr* (Bury St Edmunds: F. T. Groom, 1890), pp. 165–6.

monastery before his election. This fact, and his comparatively long reign of twenty-six years, suggest that he was quite young – perhaps in his early thirties – when he succeeded as Abbot. Reeve continued the Abbey's patronage of John Wastell until the stonemason's death in 1518, when he was buried in St Mary's Church.[14]

Early in his reign, in November 1515, Reeve became embroiled in a series of incidents that foreshadowed some of the later controversies of the English Reformation. Jane Wentworth, the 12-year-old daughter of Sir Roger Wentworth of Gosfield, Essex, suffered from violent fits until Lady Day (25 March) 1516, when she claimed to have received relief from a vision of Our Lady of Grace at Ipswich. Jane then demanded that she be taken to the popular shrine, where she was met by a crowd of a thousand people and Abbot Reeve, who insisted on walking the thirty miles from Bury to Ipswich on foot as a pilgrimage to Our Lady of Grace. Reeve vowed to repeat his pilgrimage every year if Our Lady of Grace effected a cure of Jane's fits.

Jane claimed deliverance but returned to Ipswich shortly after Whitsun, when she addressed a crowd of 4,000 who had come to see her. She then called the senior clergy and laity to her lodgings in the middle of the night before haranguing them for two hours. After this, her sisters and brother fell into fits and she successfully 'cured' them. The 'miracle' was documented by Robert, Lord Curzon and later by Sir Thomas More, who cited it as one of the best examples of a modern English miracle.[15] The incident certainly shows that there was an abiding thirst for the miraculous amongst the people of Suffolk a few decades before the Reformation, and Jane Wentworth's disorderly speech under supposed divine influence foreshadowed the use of the 'Holy Maid of Kent' by opponents of the religious changes of Henry VIII in the 1530s.

It seems only reasonable to attribute Reeve's involvement to personal piety, but it is also possible that the Abbot was trying to buy in to the fashionable religious trends of the day, which tended to be associated with miracles performed at or by holy images rather than the shrines of incorrupt Anglo-Saxon royal saints. The faithful wanted holy things that could be seen and even touched, while the body of St Edmund was never seen. Reeve completed a pilgrimage to the miraculous 'Good Rood' of Dovercourt in Essex after witnessing the 'miracle' of Jane Wentworth's deliverance,[16] but he was soon faced with more mundane and familiar concerns when the townsfolk of Bury launched yet another challenge against the Abbey's privileges. In around 1515 representatives of the town appeared before the Court of Star Chamber and claimed:

> that the more part of the said town is held by Katherine now queen of England by suit to her court there called the court of honour and certain rent as part and parcel of the portion to her assigned by the king's grace and the which town is and of old time hath been parcel of the earldom of the monarch and the said abbot intending to disherit the king then defraud the Queen thereof faineth all the said town to be holden of him and would cause the said inhabitants to pay him yearly XIII pence for their freeholds whereas they of right ought to pay him no penny thereof.

---

14 Woodman (2004), pp. 542–3; MacCulloch (1986), p. 136.
15 MacCulloch (1986), pp. 143–5; Richard Rex, 'Wentworth, Jane [Anne; called the Maid of Ipswich] (c.1503–1572?)' in *ODNB*, vol. 58, pp. 127–8.
16 MacCulloch (1986), p. 155.

The townsfolk went on to claim that since the death of Richard, duke of York the Abbots had 'kept no court … and do claim the lands there which appertain to the Earldom to be their proper land and thereof have made leases under their convent seal to disinherit the said king and queen'. The alderman, John Smith, demanded that the sacrist, John Eye, yield the quit rents due to him for repairing the Guildhall and other works, and complained that he was not allowed to carry out the duties of his office: surveying streets, determining weights and measures, and the assay of bread and wine. The sacrist, Smith complained, was now appointing the gatekeepers instead of the burgesses, 'against their ancient privileges', and extortionate tolls were being charged, even on inhabitants of the town who had previously been allowed to go into and out of it without charge.

Furthermore, the sacrist was exempting men from 'watch and ward' in the summer time on the grounds that they were servants of the Abbot, 'which makes the burden lie heavy upon the rest'. The Abbot was releasing men imprisoned by the alderman without payment of bail, and imprisoning townsmen without a writ from the king; Smith claimed that, by ancient custom, no townsman could be imprisoned without a writ except for treason and felony, but 'The said custom is newly broken and divers persons imprisoned.' The bailiffs and clerks of the Abbot were also accused of rigging juries and letting off bakers and brewers of substandard bread and beer. Smith also claimed that the Abbot's 'cope' of 100 marks – the town's customary payment to a newly elected Abbot – was 'an intolerable charge'.[17] It is unclear how the alderman and burgesses had got the idea that Henry VIII had granted the *banleuca* of Bury St Edmunds to Katherine of Aragon – no other record of such a grant survives.

Star Chamber rejected the townsfolk's suit, but they sent two burgesses, William Adams and John Hawkyns, to appeal directly to the king.[18] Henry appointed Humphrey Wyngfield and Francis Mountford to hear the case, but the townsfolk claimed that the Abbot would not appear before the court and 'by his cunning, craft and subtle demeanour' was delaying any action until Cardinal Wolsey conducted a visitation of the Abbey as papal legate *a latere*. Adams and Hawkyns were subsequently arrested by a sergeant at arms and brought before the Abbot. In Reeve's presence they were forced to disclose the names of the other burgesses who had financed the suit against the Abbey.[19]

The bishop of Norwich, Richard Nix, then began an investigation of other townsfolk, with the result that on 17 September 1517 most of the leading burgesses were arrested and bound over to pay £100 each. Adams and Hawkyns were sent to the Fleet prison and another of the defendants, John Pope, was committed to Ipswich gaol. For his part, Abbot Reeve claimed that Star Chamber had always dismissed the charges against him, but malicious individuals kept bringing the suit. The matter was settled when, on his way to the shrine of Our Lady of Walsingham on pilgrimage in September 1517, Wolsey stopped at Bury. The Abbot insisted to Wolsey that the charges 'grew upon none good nor substantial true matter, but only of malice without reasonable cause by them borne unto [him]'. He denied that he had persuaded the cardinal to arrest Adams and Hawkyns, and

---

17   British Library MS Add. 17391, reprinted in Trenholme (1927), pp. 102–4. On this dispute see also Lobel (1935), pp. 163–4.
18   Lobel (1935), p. 164.
19   Ibid., p. 165.

claimed he had only commissioned the bishop of Norwich to investigate because Wolsey did not have time to consider all the evidence.[20]

In Lobel's view, 'The abbot was uncompromising and probably had friends at court, with the result that the suit [in Star Chamber] dragged endlessly on.'[21] What is most interesting about this case, however, is Reeve's reliance on Bishop Nix and Cardinal Wolsey to aid and abet him in his struggle against the townsfolk. Reeve was clearly determined to criminalise dissent against the Abbey rather than answering the townsfolk on their own terms, by giving them their day in court. Yet unlike previous Abbots, who had jealously guarded their privileges against other ecclesiastics, Reeve's behaviour suggests that he saw Wolsey and Nix as allies against a common enemy – the burgesses – and he was prepared to take advantage of Wolsey's visitatorial jurisdiction rather than perceiving it as a threat.

In the 1520s, having proved himself in the dispute in Star Chamber, Reeve began taking a greater part in national and local affairs. He was sworn to the Privy Council in 1520,[22] and in 1522 he sat on a commission to determine the boundaries of the town of Ipswich.[23] In exchange for the support he received from church and crown the Abbot was expected to pull his weight, and in 1523 Reeve was appointed to squeeze money in taxation from all persons in Suffolk with £40 or more for an increasingly cash-strapped government. In 1525 Henry demanded a sixth of every man's substance, however humble.

In 1528, the insupportable pressure of regressive taxation on the poorest members of society provoked the so-called 'rising of the poor men'. In Bury St Edmunds this took the form of a gathering of two or three hundred people in the town summoned by a man called Davy, who planned to march to London and petition king and cardinal. Sir Robert Drury rather than the Abbot intervened and soon dispersed the crowd, putting paid to their plans for a march on London.[24] However, although Reeve had served as a government tax collector this small-scale revolt was not directed at the Abbey, but rather at central government – an interesting sign of the times in its own right. Even the poorest people in Bury St Edmunds realised that it was now primarily Henry and Wolsey who determined their fate rather than Abbot Reeve.

Religious life continued in Bury in the 1520s much as it had always done. One practice that was still remembered long after the Reformation (in the 1630s) was the ceremony of the 'Bury Bull', which was a rite intended to ensure female fertility. A white bull was led from Haberden meadow to the town's South Gate and up Southgate Street as far as the Norman Tower, accompanied by singing monks and the woman seeking to have a child, who walked beside the bull, stroking its 'milk-white sides and hanging dewlaps'. The procession then turned west along Churchgate Street and north onto Guildhall Street, turning east again to go down the Cook Row (Abbeygate Street) towards Angel Hill. The bull was then led away and the woman went to pray at the shrine of St Edmund.[25] This practice indicates that the Abbey was attempting to respond to popular demand by promoting St Edmund as a patron of fertility and providing religious services for ordinary

---

20   Ibid., p. 166.
21   Ibid., p. 164.
22   Page (1907), p. 66.
23   Yates (1843), p. 221.
24   Lobel (1935), p. 167.
25   Young (2015), p. 164.

people. The practice is also a reminder of the important traditional connection between St Edmund and his female devotees first remarked upon by Hermann the Archdeacon.

By the second half of the fifteenth century pilgrimages to traditional monastic shrines were in decline. Relics were less popular than holy images, but they retained their relevance when used 'for specific assistance' by the laity, as in the 'Bury Bull' ritual.[26] Eamon Duffy has noted that the survival of foundations like Bury 'depended on continuing loyalty to the patron', something ensured by Abbot Curteys' patronage of John Lydgate's poetry in the fifteenth century, but it was harder to ensure in the sixteenth.[27] Hoxne Priory, the site of a rival pilgrimage to St Edmund, recorded a very modest income from pilgrims in the late fifteenth century, and this pattern may have been repeated at Bury, from which the financial records of this period do not survive.[28] The cult of St Edmund was certainly not a significant source of the Abbey's revenue by the 1520s: of 118 wills made in Bury between 1512 and 1539 only six left bequests to the Abbey.[29] By contrast, the more fashionable 'image-centred' Marian shrine controlled by the monks, Our Lady of Woolpit, received rich offerings well into the sixteenth century.[30]

Remarkably, the cult of 'Little St Robert' in the crypt of the Abbey Church retained its popularity right up to the Reformation, in spite of the absence of Jews from England for over two centuries. In 1524–25, singers were still being paid for singing in Robert's chapel on his feast day,[31] and a convincing case has been made that 'mystery plays' based on the death of St Robert were still being performed in the town at this time.[32] Perhaps the fact that 'Little St Robert' was a saint from the town, albeit venerated in the Abbey, explains some of his enduring appeal. However, the religious certainties that sustained the Abbey were increasingly subject to criticism, even within the Abbey. Early in the 1520s, the English disciple of Martin Luther, Robert Barnes, made several visits to the Abbey where he met with two of the monks, as well as two known Lollard brick-makers, Lawrence Maxwell and John Stacy. The two monks were Edward Rougham, the future sacrist who had been a fellow student with Barnes at the University of Louvain, and the Abbey's chamberlain, Richard Bayfield (alias Somersham). In around 1526 Barnes gave Bayfield several books, including Erasmus's new translation of the Greek New Testament, the same book that had begun the Reformation when it was read by Luther.[33]

After two years Reeve apparently discovered the heretical books in Bayfield's possession, and according to the Protestant martyrologist John Foxe, Bayfield was 'cast into the prison of his house, there sore whipped, with a gag in his mouth, and there stocked'.

---

26 Yates (1843), p. 424.
27 Eamon Duffy, *The Stripping of the Altars* (New Haven, Conn.: Yale University Press, 1992), p. 196.
28 Yates (1843), p. 429.
29 MacCulloch (1986), p. 135.
30 Clive Paine, 'The Chapel and Well of Our Lady of Woolpit', *PSIAH* 38 (1993), pp. 8–12, at pp. 8–9. The proceeds of the cult had been coming to the Abbey since 1211. When the Jesuits revived a local pilgrimage in the reign of James II (1685–88) they chose Woolpit rather than Bury (see Young (2006), p. 215).
31 Gransden (2009), p. 120.
32 Lampert (2001), pp. 235–55.
33 Korey D. Maas, *The Reformation and Robert Barnes: History, Theology and Polemic in Early Modern England* (Woodbridge: Boydell, 2010), p. 13.

However, in around 1528 Rougham managed to obtain Bayfield's release, and Bayfield joined Barnes in Cambridge. He was later brought before Cuthbert Tunstall, bishop of London, who ordered him to return to Bury and do penance, but Bayfield fled to the Continent where he traded in evangelical books. In 1528 he returned to England in secret, but he was betrayed and confined in Lollards' Tower. When he was brought to trial on 11 and 16 November 1531 it was noted that Bayfield was a priest and a professed monk of St Edmunds, and one of the charges brought against him was that he had failed to fulfil 'the vow of his profession'. In his reply, Bayfield acknowledged that he had been professed a monk of Bury in 1514. On 20 November the bishop of London condemned him as a relapsed heretic, and he was burned to death at Smithfield on 27 November or 4 December.[34]

The abbots of Westminster and Waltham were involved in Bayfield's trial, probably because he was a Benedictine, but although the case must have been an embarrassment to Abbot Reeve there is no evidence that he participated in the trial. However, Bayfield was not the only Bury monk to get into trouble for heretical opinions. John Salisbury (1501/2–1573), when a student at Gloucester Hall, was imprisoned on the orders of Cardinal Wolsey between 25 February 1528 and 26 March 1529. On his release Salisbury was sent back to St Edmunds, where for five years he claimed that he was 'little better than a prisoner'. However, in 1534 Salisbury became prior of St Faith's, Horsham and therefore escaped Abbot Reeve's control. Salisbury was consecrated bishop of Thetford (a suffragan of Norwich) in 1536 and oversaw the dissolution of numerous religious houses. He continued to amass benefices in plurality in the reigns of Mary and Elizabeth, including dean of Norwich Cathedral, but he remained a religious conservative. In 1570 he was appointed bishop of Sodor and Man, but never visited his diocese and died in Norwich.[35]

In 1527 a Norfolk-born Cambridge don, Thomas Bilney, began preaching Lutheran doctrines at Hadleigh, which was a peculiar of the archbishop of Canterbury, geographically within the Liberty of St Edmund but outside the Abbot's jurisdiction. Bilney attacked pilgrimages and the veneration of images, until in 1528 he was pulled from the pulpit of St George's, Ipswich and arraigned for heresy. His execution in 1531 was followed by popular attacks on religious shrines at Sudbury and Stoke-by-Nayland, although 'No one seems to have dared to tackle St Edmund in his well-defended monastery.'[36] However, most of the attacks were directed against miraculous images, which those inspired by Reformation ideas may have considered more superstitious and idolatrous than the veneration of the body of a martyr.

Following Wolsey's fall from grace in 1529, as a result of the cardinal's failure to secure an annulment of Henry VIII's marriage to Katherine of Aragon, Abbot Reeve found

---

34 On Bayfield's trial and execution see John Foxe, *The Acts and Monuments of John Foxe* (London: George Seeley, 1870), vol. 4, pp. 680–88.
35 Ian Atherton, 'Salisbury, John (1501/2–1573), bishop of Sodor and Man' in *ODNB*, vol. 48, p. 710–11. The only other Bury monk to be consecrated as a bishop in the sixteenth century was John Brainsford, appointed a suffragan bishop in the Diocese of Lincoln in 1517 (Gordon Beattie, *Gregory's Angels: A History of the Abbeys, Priories, Parishes and Schools following the Rule of Saint Benedict in Great Britain, Ireland and their Overseas Foundations* (Leominster: Gracewing, 1997), p. 48).
36 MacCulloch (1986), pp. 150, 154–5.

himself in a difficult political position on account of his closeness to Wolsey. On 11 July 1530 Reeve was indicted on a charge of *praemunire* (subverting the laws of England by upholding papal authority) along with Bishop Nix of Norwich and others, and on 17 October he appeared before the Court of King's Bench. The charge was that Reeve and Nix had aided and abetted Wolsey in exercising his powers as a papal legate *a latere*. However, Henry had grander designs against the church and decided to drop the proceedings against Reeve and Nix.[37]

Life returned to normal for the Abbot, at least for the time being, and in 1531 he was serving on the Commission of the Peace for Suffolk, the first Abbot to do so.[38] The appointment was an ironic one, since Justices of the Peace had no authority within the Abbot's own Liberty of St Edmund (west Suffolk). In 1532 Reeve presided over the funeral of a fellow abbot, John Islip of Westminster.[39] In November of the same year came the first sign of encroachment on the Abbey's possessions by the new lord privy seal, Thomas Cromwell, when Cromwell asked Reeve for a sixty-year lease on Harlowbury Farm in Essex. Cromwell presumed to ask for an answer by return, but in fact he had already agreed with the then holder of the lease to purchase the remainder, without consulting Reeve. Cromwell vowed to do whatever he could for the monastery if the Abbot granted his request.[40] It was to be a hollow promise.

The last great ceremonial and royal event in the history of the Abbey took place on 22 July 1533. It was the funeral of Mary Rose Tudor, the youngest sister of Henry VIII. Mary had the status of dowager queen of France, having briefly been married to Louis XII of France in 1514–15. She subsequently married Charles Brandon, duke of Suffolk and the couple lived at Westhorpe Hall, regularly visiting Bury Fair where they had their own pavilion. Mary died on 25 June and her body lay in state at Westhorpe while preparations were made for her funeral at the Abbey. Among other things, King Francis I of France had to send a herald to ensure that her status as queen dowager was properly honoured. A procession involving candles, torches, banners, horse-trappings and coats of arms wound its way through the Suffolk countryside from Westhorpe to Bury, and the queen's embalmed body was covered with black cloth of gold with a white cross. Over this there was a wax funeral effigy, 'an image of the Queen apparelled in her robes of estate with a crown upon her head in her hair, as appertaineth, and the sceptre in her right hand'. The body was borne on a hearse decorated with the arms of England impaled with France.

The chief mourner was Mary's daughter Frances Grey (the mother of Lady Jane Grey). Six knights held a canopy over the hearse, which was preceded by 100 poor men holding burning torches, followed by gentlemen in pairs, knights, barons, lords, the Garter and Clarencieux Kings of Arms, then Mary's chamberlain, Lord Powis. After the hearse walked four heralds bearing banners depicting the Holy Trinity, the Virgin Mary, St Elizabeth and Charlemagne, then Frances Grey and eleven female mourners. The procession reached Bury's East Gate by 2 o'clock, where it was met by Abbot Reeve at the head of a procession of monks. The knights carried the coffin into the Abbey where a requiem mass was sung by fourteen priests. During the mass, four of the principal mourners presented four yards of

---

37 Ibid., pp. 153–4.
38 Page (1907), p. 66.
39 Yates (1843), p. 220.
40 Page (1907), p. 66.

cloth of gold each at the offertory. The Abbot of St Bene't, Holme preached on Our Lady, Star of the Sea, and at the burial itself the officers of Mary's household broke their staffs of office and sorrowfully threw them into the tomb.

Leaving the heraldic banners in the Abbey, the nobles then went to dine with the Abbot while generous alms were distributed to the poor of the town at the gates of the monastery. The tomb of Mary Tudor – the only queen to be interred in the Abbey Church – bore the inscription:

> Here lieth the right noble and excellent princess Mary, French Queen, sister to the most mighty prince King Harry the VIII of that name and wife to Lewis, King of France, which all her lifetime continuing peaceable Queen Dowager of France and in high favour and estimation of both the realms was afterward married to Charles, Duke of Suffolk.[41]

Mary's funeral was the kind of grand royal ceremonial that the Abbey did best, although Henry VIII himself was not in attendance and staged a funeral of his own for Mary – complete with empty hearse – at Westminster. Yet the funeral at Bury was the last time in history that the Abbey would serve the purpose for which it existed, as a burial place of monarchs and a centre of royal pilgrimage.

Dissolution, 1535–39

The dissolution of the greater religious houses, which was completed in 1539–40, was a complex process of several stages. The dissolution was neither a result of nor the beginning of 'the English Reformation' – except perhaps in retrospect – since Henry VIII had nothing against the *religion* of the monks in itself (even if Thomas Cromwell held reformed ideas). Indeed, reform of monastic orders and dissolution of houses deemed corrupt or unnecessary was hardly unprecedented, even if it had never taken place before on such a scale, and it could as easily be defended by zealous Catholics as by those who embraced the new evangelical religious ideas. Indeed, many of those who carried out or benefited from the dissolution were conservative in their religious opinions.

A profound change in the status of the Abbey occurred in 1534, when parliament passed the Act for the Submission of the Clergy and Restraint of Appeals. This required all dues to Rome to be paid henceforth to the king, who was declared supreme head of the Church of England. The heads of the great religious houses, including Abbot Reeve, were required to swear the oath of supremacy (which Reeve seems to have done without demur). At a stroke, the Abbey was transformed from a monastery exempt from any authority other than that of a papal legate *a latere* to a religious house wholly dependent for its survival on royal favour. All of the Abbey's ecclesiastical privileges were gone, and Henry VIII henceforth had the right to appoint any visitor to the Abbey he chose.

It is ironic that by the time of the dissolution the Abbey had almost completely severed its once close ties with the papacy anyway. The crucial moment had come in 1398 when

---

41 Mary's funeral is described in Erin A. Sadlack (ed.), *The French Queen's Letters: Mary Tudor Brandon and the Politics of Marriage in Sixteenth-Century Europe* (New York: Palgrave Macmillan, 2011), pp. 154–6.

Abbot Cratfield obtained confirmation from Boniface IX that election in Chapter constituted a sufficient title for an Abbot, allowing an Abbot to choose any bishop to bless him. Furthermore, the Benedictine abbeys were all independent houses subject to no external control from overseas superiors, unlike the Cistercians, Franciscans, Dominicans and others. Understandably, the black monks of St Benedict saw no reason why the king should treat them as potentially disloyal, especially since many Benedictine monasteries were ancient royal foundations. The monks of Evesham in Worcestershire, for example, petitioned the king to preserve their house on the grounds that it was 'of the King's Grace's most noble foundation' and offered to amend their life in any way – they seem to have envisaged the possibility that Henry might choose to turn the monasteries into colleges of canons, chantries or hospitals.[42]

It seems reasonable to assume that the idea of the total destruction of his house did not enter Abbot Reeve's darkest imaginings. The thought that Henry would eliminate the shrine of the patron saint of the English people, who had aided the country in battle on so many occasions, and been venerated by his Lancastrian and Tudor predecessors Henry VI and Henry VII, would have been inconceivable. St Edmunds was a royal abbey, not to mention the fact that Henry's VIII's favourite sister had been laid to rest there just a few years earlier. For the king to turn the Abbey into a royal peculiar like Westminster would not have been surprising. Perhaps the idea that the Abbey might be secularised, as the rebels of 1327 had fantasised, also entered Reeve's mind. He may even have wondered if Henry would erect the Abbey Church as a cathedral.[43] But no Abbot, however far-sighted, could have anticipated that Henry would deliberately destroy one of the greatest churches of Christendom, the glory of England, and leave scarcely one stone on top of another.

Historians are divided on the state of the Abbey in the 1530s. Gottfried argued that behind its splendid appearance, the Abbey was in terminal decline. Bequests to the community had been falling since 1500, but the Abbot and his officers continued to maintain their high style of living.[44] Gottfried discerned in the Abbey 'A peculiar inability to adapt to the more favourable economic conditions for great landlords' in the fifteenth century; it failed to take advantage of its position at the edge of one of England's great cloth-producing regions.[45] The Abbey responded to decline by selling off its lands from the mid-fifteenth century onwards. Initially it bought new lands elsewhere to compensate, but by the 1520s even this had ceased. The Abbey 'was like a jaded dowager, a still rich but fading institution renting out everything and increasingly forced to sell parts of its patrimony in order to remain solvent'.[46] Gottfried was ultimately at a loss to explain the Abbey's decline in such favourable economic conditions.

An analysis of land ownership in the Hundred of Thingoe, a collection of twenty-three

---

42 The letter from the monks of Evesham to Henry VIII is reproduced in George May, *A Descriptive History of the Town of Evesham* (Evesham: George May, 1845), pp. 430–32.
43 This was the fate of the abbey churches of Gloucester, Bristol and Peterborough. A local Bury tradition has it that Henry considered making the Abbey a cathedral, but this seems to be unsubstantiated by evidence and may have been inspired by the belief that the king spared Peterborough on account of the tomb of Katherine of Aragon.
44 MacCulloch (1986), p. 135.
45 Gottfried (1982), pp. 237–40.
46 Ibid., p. 244.

manors, would seem to lend some support to Gottfried's case. In 1539 the Abbey held only ten of these manors, less than half of the total: Sextens (Westley), Fresels (Westley), Great Saxham, Fornham All Saints, Chevington, Hargrave, Whepstead, Hardwick, Nowton and Great Horringer.[47] Nevertheless it remained the largest single landowner in the area, followed by John Lucas and William Drury with three manors each. Lucas held the manors of Little Saxham, Leo's Hall (Westley) and Little Horringer,[48] in addition to the manors of Lackford, Flempton and West Stow in the neighbouring Hundred of Lackford,[49] while Drury held Hawstead, Brockley and Rede.[50] Two of the remaining manors were held by absentee landlords – Barrow by Thomas, Lord Wentworth and Southwood by the duke of Suffolk, who sold it to Thomas Audley in March 1539.[51] Five manors were held singly by local families: Risby by the Jermyns, Pembroke Hall (Westley) by the Markants, Hengrave by Sir Thomas Kytson the Elder, Ickworth by Sir Nicholas Hervey and Manston (Whepstead) by the Sturgeons.[52]

Even before the dissolution, therefore, eleven manors were held by local gentry and a pattern of gentry dominance of the area was beginning to emerge. The dissolution arguably accelerated a process of economic transformation in the county that was already under way. To a certain extent the Abbey acknowledged the growing power of the gentry, granting many of them honorary membership of the Chapter as early as the fifteenth century, including members of the Drury and Paston families.[53] However, other members of the gentry lived as if the Abbey did not exist at all. It is hard to believe that Sir Thomas Kytson the elder's splendid crenellated Hengrave Hall, built between 1525 and 1538 and the ultimate expression of early modern mercantile self-confidence, was completed before the Abbey's fall, yet the building was planned even before the dissolution of the lesser religious houses in 1536.[54]

Diarmaid MacCulloch, by contrast, argued that Gottfried was relying on unreliable sources for his conclusions, and concluded that 'there is no good evidence that the Abbey's last half century was anything but a time of continued prosperity and success'.[55] Abbot Reeve was a successful administrator who forged important links with the local gentry. His will revealed his close relationships with local gentry families, notably the Heighams, Drurys and Jermyns. He was the victor in disputes with the townsfolk, like his predecessors, and a complainant remembered eighty years later that Reeve declared 'he was lord and kinge within the said town',[56] a confident reiteration of the Abbot's medieval privileges that still obtained in the first quarter of the sixteenth century. Whatever its financial woes, the income of St Edmunds Abbey in 1535, at £1,659, still vastly exceeded that of

---

47 John Gage, *The History and Antiquities of Suffolk: Thingoe Hundred* (London, 1838), pp. 87, 92, 102, 243, 325, 338, 389, 475, 489, 505.
48 Ibid., pp. 133, 92, 519.
49 Ibid., p. 50.
50 Ibid., pp. 434, 357, 374.
51 Ibid., pp. 8, 343.
52 Ibid., pp. 75, 89, 180, 293, 384.
53 Yates (1843), pp. 155–7.
54 On Hengrave Hall see Francis Young, *The Gages of Hengrave and Suffolk Catholicism, 1640–1767* (Woodbridge: Catholic Record Society, 2015a), pp. xxiii–v.
55 MacCulloch (1986), p. 136.
56 Ibid., pp. 136–7.

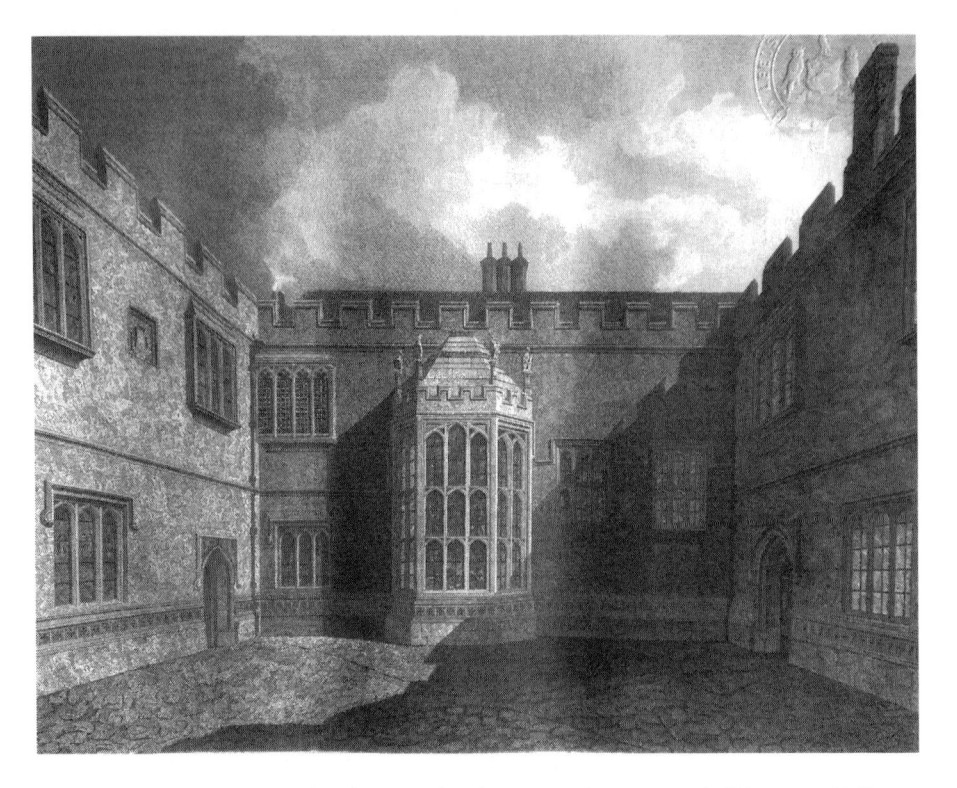

Figure 31 Gentry imitation of ecclesiastical architecture: the courtyard of Hengrave Hall (1525–38). From John Gage, *The History and Antiquities of Hengrave* (1822).

any other religious house in Suffolk.[57] By 1539 the Abbey was in possession of estates scattered from Lincolnshire to London.[58]

However, although the Abbey remained West Suffolk's largest landowner in the 1530s, it is undeniable that others were rapidly catching up. It is possible that the overall size of the Abbey's land-holdings may have masked financial decline. The Abbey's diffuse land-holdings, which were increasingly no longer concentrated in one area, may have weakened its hold on local politics, and its institutional complexity meant that it did not behave like other landlords by responding quickly and intuitively to changing circumstances. Lobel thought that high rents imposed by the Abbey meant that 400 tenements in the town had been allowed to fall into disrepair.[59] However, even if the Abbey was in decline, this was hardly an unprecedented state of affairs – the Abbey was on its uppers for much of the fourteenth century – and there was no reason why its financial woes would have resulted in its fall had Henry VIII not intervened.

Martin Heale has argued that in the new political environment of the 1530s, the Abbey's

---

57 Gordon Blackwood, *Tudor and Stuart Suffolk* (Carnegie: Lancaster, 2001), p. 309. For a different estimate of the wealth of the Abbey in the 1530s see Gottfried (1982), pp. 241–2.
58 Ibid., p. 76.
59 Lobel (1935), pp. 163–4.

great wealth was ironically its greatest weakness, since great wealth made the monasteries easy targets of criticism and rich prizes for the royal treasury.[60] However, Heale maintained that a major reason for the suppression of the monasteries was religious, since they were supposed to offer support to popular superstition. Duffy has noted that even so orthodox a prelate as John Fisher, the bishop of Rochester executed in 1535 for his opposition to the royal supremacy, encouraged benefactions to new, humanist Cambridge colleges rather than 'slack, easy-going and over-funded monastic houses'.[61] By 1538 Henry VIII, inspired by Erasmus, was engaged in a pious quest to stamp out false relics, and 'superstition' was one of the abuses that the commissioners were sent to seek out.[62]

It also seems that in spite of Abbot Reeve's pilgrimage on foot to visit the holy maid of Ipswich, spiritual life in the Abbey was less than intense. MacCulloch described Suffolk's religious houses at the eve of the dissolution as 'conscientious but not inspired'.[63] The monks of Bury mounted no acts of resistance against the Act of Supremacy like their confreres at Glastonbury, and went quietly. In 1534 Henry delegated visitatorial jurisdiction over all the religious houses of England to Cromwell, who in turn delegated the visitations to his own officials, who began compiling the *Valor Ecclesiasticus* – a complete survey of the value of church lands throughout England.

On 4 November 1535 the Abbey received a visit from two of the commissioners, Sir John Legh and John ap Rice. The following day ap Rice reported the state of the monastery in a letter to Cromwell:

> Please it your mastership, forasmuch as I suppose you shall have suit made unto you touching Bury ere we return, I thought convenient to advertise you of our proceedings there, and also of the parts of the same. As for the abbot, we found nothing suspect as touching his living, but it was detected that he lay much forth in his granges, that he delighted much in playing at dice and cards, and therein spent much money, and in building for his pleasure. He did not preach openly. Also that he converted divers farms into copyholds, whereof poor men do complain. Also he seemeth to be addicted to the maintaining of such superstitious ceremonies as hath been used heretofore.
>
> As touching the convent, we could get little or no reports among them, although we did use much diligence in our examination, and thereby, with some other arguments gathered of their examinations, I firmly believe and suppose that they had confedered and compacted before our coming that they should disclose nothing. And yet it is confessed and proved that there was here such frequency of women coming and resorting to this monastery as to no place more. Amongst the relics we found much vanity and superstition, as the coals that St Laurence was toasted withal, the paring of St Edmund's nails, St Thomas of Canterbury's penknife and his boots, and divers skulls for the headache; pieces of the holy cross able to make a whole cross of; other relics for rain and certain other superstitious usages, for avoiding of weeds growing in corn, with

---

60 Martin Heale, 'Training in superstition? Monasteries and popular religion in late Medieval and Reformation England', *Journal of Ecclesiastical History* 58 (2007), pp. 417–39, at p. 419.
61 Eamon Duffy, *Saints, Sacrilege and Sedition: Religion and Conflict in the Tudor Reformations* (London: Bloomsbury, 2012), pp. 135–6.
62 Heale (2007), pp. 420–2.
63 MacCulloch (1986), p. 133.

such other. Here depart of them that be under age upon an eight, and of them that be above age upon a five would depart if they might, and they be of the best sort in the house, and of best learning and judgement. The whole number of the convent before we came was 40 saving one, beside 3 that were at Oxford.[64]

In James's view, 'the Commissioners had ferreted about in any and every direction for scandalous tales against the abbot and the monks: and the abbey of Bury compared most favourably in respect of decent religious life with some of its smaller neighbours'. He also noted that ap Rice did not specify whether the women mentioned resorted to the church or the domestic buildings.

The conditions put in place after Legh and ap Rice's visitation made it clear that the Abbey's days were numbered. All monks under the age of 24, as well as those who had taken vows under the age of 20, were dismissed. This led to the departure of eight monks and cut off the monastery's future life. Needless to say, the Abbey was permitted to admit no new monks, and the entire community was confined to the precinct. This was especially inconvenient for the Abbot as a peer of the realm with many responsibilities, and on 6 November Reeve wrote to Cromwell begging a licence to travel abroad 'with a chaplain or two' on the business of the monastery.[65] In August 1536 the Abbot successfully obtained a licence from the king for any of his servants to shoot with a crossbow at deer and fowl in his parks and grounds. Under normal circumstances only the nobility were permitted to shoot at game, even on their own property, and the reason for the licence may have been that Reeve, confined to the precincts of the Abbey, could not obtain game because he could not shoot it himself.

As a last desperate measure, Reeve seems to have resorted to bribery of the lord privy seal. In Chapter on 26 November 1536 the Abbot and Convent granted Cromwell and his son Gregory a pension of £10 per annum from the manor of Harlow, where Cromwell already held the lease. Astonishingly, in December Cromwell's servant Sir Thomas Russhe called on the Abbot asking him to confer a larger sum. Reeve promised to do so.[66] Reeve had rightly judged Cromwell to be driven by greed, but he had not reckoned on the fact that Cromwell was also ideologically motivated. The dissolution had now been set in train and it was too late to stop it. By the end of 1536 all of the lesser religious houses in Suffolk had been dissolved, leaving the Abbey in splendid isolation.

Following the visitation of 1535 the monks began systematically disposing of books from the Abbey's great library, which MacCulloch thought was 'second only to that of Oxford University'.[67] Ironically, it was this pre-emptive dispersal which has probably led to more books surviving from Bury than from many other monastic houses. Had Reeve preserved the library until the very end, it is likely that it would have been sold off wholesale as scrap material for bookbinders. As it was, interested individuals were given the chance to acquire books they genuinely valued. One of these was William Smart, 'portman' or alderman of Ipswich. On his death in 1599, persuaded by a fellow, Richard Buckenham, Smart bequeathed his library of around 100 volumes to Pembroke College,

---

64 Quoted in James (1895), pp. 169–70 (spelling modernised).
65 Page (1907), p. 66.
66 Ibid., p. 67.
67 MacCulloch (1986), p. 136.

Cambridge, which in consequence had the largest collection of former Bury books when M. R. James investigated it.[68]

It was at around this time that John Leland made his first visit to Bury, making a list of twenty-two books he found there. In James's view, most of these were then probably absorbed by the royal library but a few later ended up in the hands of Archbishop Matthew Parker and the antiquary Sir Robert Cotton.[69] That other local people acquired significant numbers of books is attested by a bequest of Bury books to St John's College, Cambridge by Jeremiah Holt, rector of Stonham Aspal, in 1634. In the seventeenth century books from Bury were also owned by the Corporation of Wisbech.[70]

Early in 1538 John ap Rice, John Williams, Richard Pollard, Phillip Parys and John Smyth paid a second visit to the Abbey, this time to gather any precious metals and treasures they could for the royal treasury. Dissolution was now only a matter of time; the Abbey belonged to the king, who was plundering it as he pleased. The commissioners wrote to Cromwell, complaining of the effort required to destroy the shrine:

> Pleaseth your lordship to be advertised that we have been at St Edmund's Bury, where we found a rich shrine which was very cumbrous to deface. We have taken in the said monastery in gold and silver 4000 marks and above, over and besides a well and rich cross with emeralds, as also divers and sundry stones of great value, and yet we have left the church, abbot and convent very well furnished with plate of silver necessary for the same ... And this present day we depart from Bury towards Ely, and we assure your lordship the abbot and convent be very well contented with everything we have done there, as knoweth God, who preserve your lordship.[71]

The monks were now left with only the bare essentials necessary to conduct divine service. James thought that 'the defacing of the shrine need not have extended further than stripping it of the metal plating. It was very likely not opened.' Rebecca Pinner has recently identified some of the plating from the shrine as having survived, reused as a funeral brass at Frenze in Norfolk. In 1987 the brass of George Duke (d. 1551) was turned over, and on the reverse was discovered:

> an image of a king seated in bed beneath a crown-shaped canopy. The bed rests on a tiled floor raised above the grass in the foreground by a low plinth with three triangular projections. The king is pierced with a spear, from the shaft of which is suspended a drawstring bag. The king's soul, a naked infant with a grotesque face, is seized by a hirsute demon.

Pinner argues convincingly that the scene depicted is the death of Sweyn, of which there

---

68   James (1895), p. 4. For the most up-to-date treatment of surviving manuscripts from Bury, see Antonia Gransden, 'Some manuscripts in Cambridge from Bury St Edmunds Abbey: Exhibition Catalogue', in Antonia Gransden (ed.), *Bury St Edmunds: Medieval Art, Architecture and Economy* (London: British Archaeological Association, 1998), pp. 228–85.
69   Ibid., pp. 10–11.
70   Ibid., p. 22.
71   Ibid., pp. 170–1 (spelling modernised).

were several depictions in the vicinity of St Edmund's shrine. The style of the brass is consistent with the late fifteenth century, and traces of gilding found on it would suggest that it was intended to look like gold. After the fire of 1465, the addition of gilded brass plates would have been a cost-effective way of restoring St Edmund's shrine to a semblance of its original splendour, and Pinner argues that the surviving brass was one of sixteen that depicted scenes from the life and miracles of the saint.[72]

One of the great unanswered questions attendant upon the visit of the commissioners in 1538 is what happened to the body of St Edmund. The issue has been much debated, and I have treated it in a separate book. The theory that St Edmund's body was not in the shrine because it had been taken to Toulouse by Louis the Dauphin in 1217 can be dismissed as groundless.[73] Sir Ernest Clarke's theory that St Edmund's body was consumed in the fire of 1465 is likewise problematic, as the source describing the fire notes that the interior of the shrine was protected by the collapse of the canopy above it. There seems no good reason to suppose that a body was not in the shrine in 1538, and in 2013 I uncovered the first positive evidence to suggest that the saint was deliberately hidden. In the late seventeenth century the aged prior of the Benedictine Priory of St Edmund in Paris (see Chapter 7), William Hitchcock (1618–1711), told another monk that his grandfather or great-grandfather 'had seen [St Edmund's] Body put into an Iron Chest at the fall of Religion [i.e. monasticism] in England & knew w[her]e it was put'.

In 1710 Hitchcock's story reached the chronicler of St Edmund's, Ralph Bene't Weldon, who tried to get another monk to confirm it by speaking to Hitchcock, but the former prior was by then too senile to remember what he had said. Since Hitchcock took the alias Needham on his ordination as a Catholic priest, it is possible that his grandfather or great-grandfather was the Bury monk Robert Nedeham, alias Brunning, who was a schoolmaster in Lavenham in 1577 and may therefore have married and had children.[74] If true, Hitchcock's story (an oral tradition far removed from events) might suggest that St Edmund's body was concealed before, or more likely shortly after, the visit of the commissioners in 1538, when it was absolutely certain that the Abbey was doomed. The story is by no means implausible: the commissioners did not deliberately destroy the bodies of saints, especially royal ones. Edward the Confessor was allowed to remain in his shrine at Westminster undisturbed and St Cuthbert was relocated at Durham.

Stripped of its treasures, the Abbey lingered between life and death. It is possible that the Abbot's time was taken up during this period with negotiating pensions for himself and the other monks. Then on 4 November 1539, the vigil of the feast of the dedication of Abbot Baldwin's crypt, led by Sir Richard Riche, the commissioners returned to the Abbey, which was in the middle of an outbreak of plague. That day the Abbot signed the deed of surrender, along with the prior, Thomas Dennis (alias Ringstead) and forty other monks. On the same day pensions were assigned to the remaining religious. The Abbot's was exceptionally large, at £333 6s 8d; the prior received only £30. Most of the other monks were awarded £6 13s 4d, but some of the older monks received slightly higher sums than their brethren, between £8 and £13.

On 7 November Sir Richard Riche and other commissioners who had received the

---

72 Pinner (2015), pp. 157–60.
73 See Young (2014), pp. 22–32.
74 Ibid., pp. 42–5.

surrender wrote to Henry that the ex-Abbot was 'very conformable and is aged', suggesting that Reeve had no more strength left to put up any kind of resistance. The commissioners recommended that Reeve should have 500 marks a year and a house. They reported that yearly revenues from the Abbey's lands and possessions would yield 4,000 marks for the crown, and informed the king that they had taken into custody the Abbey's plate and the best ornaments. The rest had already been sold. They estimated the value of the bells and the lead from the roof at 4,500 marks. The commissioners asked for instructions on whether they should deface the church and the rest of the monastery.[75]

The answer was evidently yes. A short while later the Abbey buildings were sold by the crown by letters patent for £412 19s 4d.[76] This was the buildings' value as a source of materials, and took into account the inconvenience and expense of demolishing England's greatest Romanesque church. The popular view held in Bury that the populace descended on the Abbey and robbed the stone is not accurate. In the first place, the entire site belonged to the Crown, so taking stone without authorisation would have been theft from the king; and second, the business of pulling down a monumental Romanesque church required specialist equipment. Richard Gilyard-Beer described the archaeological evidence for the destruction uncovered by investigations in the 1960s:

> The destructive activity immediately following the dissolution was illustrated by the nature of the great masses of masonry that had fallen from the higher parts of the church. Practically all these had been systematically stripped of their dressed stonework, even from the under surfaces, and as the very great weight of some of the masses makes it highly unlikely that they have ever been moved it may be inferred that much of the ashlar was robbed from scaffolding before the high walls of the church collapsed or were felled ... The only other indication of dissolution activity was the survival of thin patches of yellow sand here and there just above the medieval floor levels, containing a few minute fragments of window glass and traces of burned daub, and probably representing a layer of breakers' debris from the ransacking of the church.[77]

We ought to imagine an organised, official demolition operation involving scaffolding rather than robbing of the ruins over a longer period. Indeed, the oldest engravings of the Abbey ruins support this. They do not show significantly more ruins of the church standing then than are visible today, suggesting that the destruction was both sudden and soon after the dissolution. However, the commissioners must have arranged the removal of the altar-tomb of Mary Rose Tudor before the Abbey Church was completely destroyed. It was moved to the north-east corner of the chancel of St Mary's Church.[78]

On the Feast of the Translation of St Edmund to the rotunda, 31 March 1540, John

---

75 Page (1907), p. 67.
76 Whittingham (1952), p. 168.
77 Gilyard-Beer (1969), p. 257.
78 'Quarterly meetings', *Proceedings of the Bury and West Suffolk Archaeological Institute* 1 (1853), pp. 53–6, at p. 56. According to this description the coffin bore the date 1553, but since this date is given elsewhere in the article as the year of Mary's funeral it is likely to be an error of transcription rather than an indication that Mary was reinterred in St Mary's during the reign of Mary I. The original altar-tomb was replaced by a plain slab in 1784.

Reeve breathed his last in a house at the top of Crown Street, close to the present Dog and Partridge public house. Reeve was probably at least in his early sixties, since it is likely that he was over the age of 30 when he was elected Abbot in 1514. His epitaph implies that he died of grief, or at least that he never recovered from the shock of witnessing the destruction of everything to which he had devoted his life. The last guardian of the body of St Edmund was buried, as the saint had been in the reign of King Æthelstan, in front of the high altar of St Mary's Church. Reeve's grey marble ledger stone bore a brass depicting the Abbot in full pontificals with his mitre and crozier, with four coats of arms at each corner. Yates thought that the Abbot had it made some years before his death, although he would not of course have been able to prepare the epitaph:[79]

> Here lie buried the bones of that man whom Bury once knew as her Lord and Abbot, born at Melford in Suffolk, named John; his family and father Reeves. He was magnanimous, prudent, learned and kind, of integrity, and loving his vow of religion – who, when he had seen the thirty-first year of the reign of Henry VIII, and on the thirty-first day of March, by the blow was felled to the earth. O kind God spare his soul! – 1540.[80]

---

79 Yates (1843), pp. 222–3.
80 Ibid., p. 222: *Buria quem dominum ac Abbatem noverit olim, / Illius hic recubant osso sepulta viro, / Suffolce Melforda nomen nato Johannem / Dixerunt Kemis* (sic. for *Revis?*) *progenie, atque pater; / Magnanimus, prudens, doctus fuit atque benignus, / Integer, et voti religionis amans – / Regni cum Henrici octavi viderat annum / Ter decimum ac primum, Martius atque dies / Unum terque decem … flamine terras / Occidit. O animae parce benigne Deus! – 1540.*

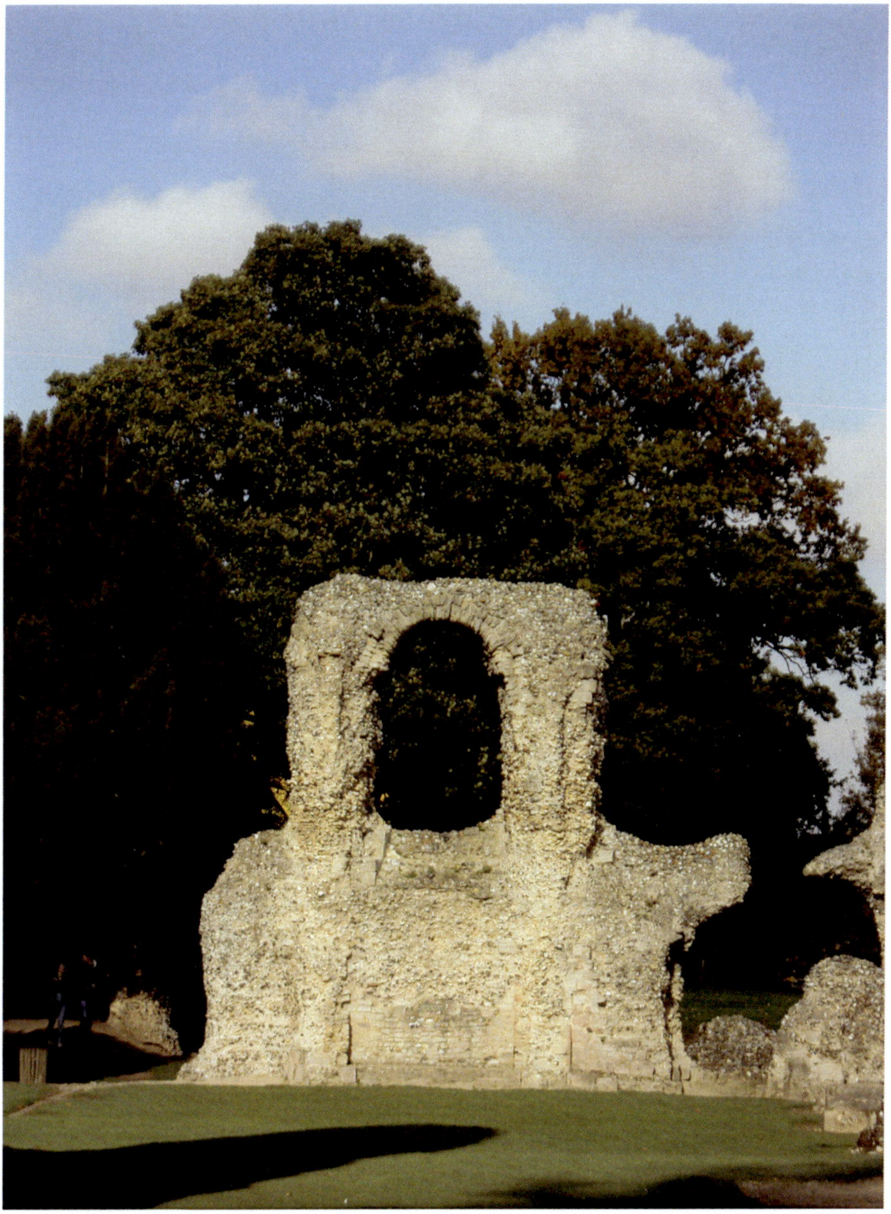

Figure 32 The ruins of the north transept of the Abbey Church. Photo by the author.

Chapter 7
Legacy

The dissolution removed the monks from the Abbey, destroyed the Abbey buildings and ended the line of Abbots, but in several ways the Abbey continued to exist. The Abbot's authority reverted to the king, while the privileges and exemptions of the *banleuca* of Bury St Edmunds and the Liberty of St Edmund, both in temporal and ecclesiastical affairs, remained. The townsfolk found themselves no better off than they had been under the Abbots, as crown officials replaced Abbey officials, and the townsfolk did not succeed in their struggle to have the town recognised as a borough until 1606, sixty-seven years after the dissolution. Meanwhile, the papacy did not recognise the dissolution of the Abbey, and in 1615 English Benedictine monks in exile in France picked up the threads of the Abbey's monastic inheritance. A new St Edmund's, claiming the lands and privileges of the old Abbey, was established in Paris in 1621. The result was that the idea of the Abbey, and the idea of the Abbey's special privileges, proved a great deal more difficult to kill than Thomas Cromwell had ever imagined.

The aftermath of dissolution

There is no reason to suppose that the town of Bury St Edmunds benefited in any way from the dissolution. Indeed, it is likely that the disappearance of the Abbey was the single most disastrous event, socially, economically and culturally, in the history of west Suffolk. The site of the Abbey, the materials of the Abbey buildings and all of the Abbey's possessions passed immediately into the ownership of the crown. Whereas hitherto the townsfolk had been forced to negotiate with an Abbot resident in Bury, they were now compelled to negotiate with a government bureaucracy in faraway London, claiming the same rights over them as Abbot Reeve. The town of Bury instantly lost its representation in parliament in the form of the Abbot as a spiritual peer, and the county of Suffolk lost its senior magnate. From being the site of a royal abbey of national significance, the site of parliaments and the resort of kings, Bury St Edmunds was reduced to a provincial backwater. As MacCulloch argued:

> With his seat in the House of Lords and his wide estates outside the Liberty, the late medieval Abbot of Bury was a person of great consequence; his disappearance left Bury suddenly 'provincial', the abbey ruins dominating the town as negatively as the Abbots had once done with positive authority. Administratively, the Liberty and Crown lessees who replaced the Abbot as Steward were shadows of the old regime.[1]

---

1   MacCulloch (1986), p. 22.

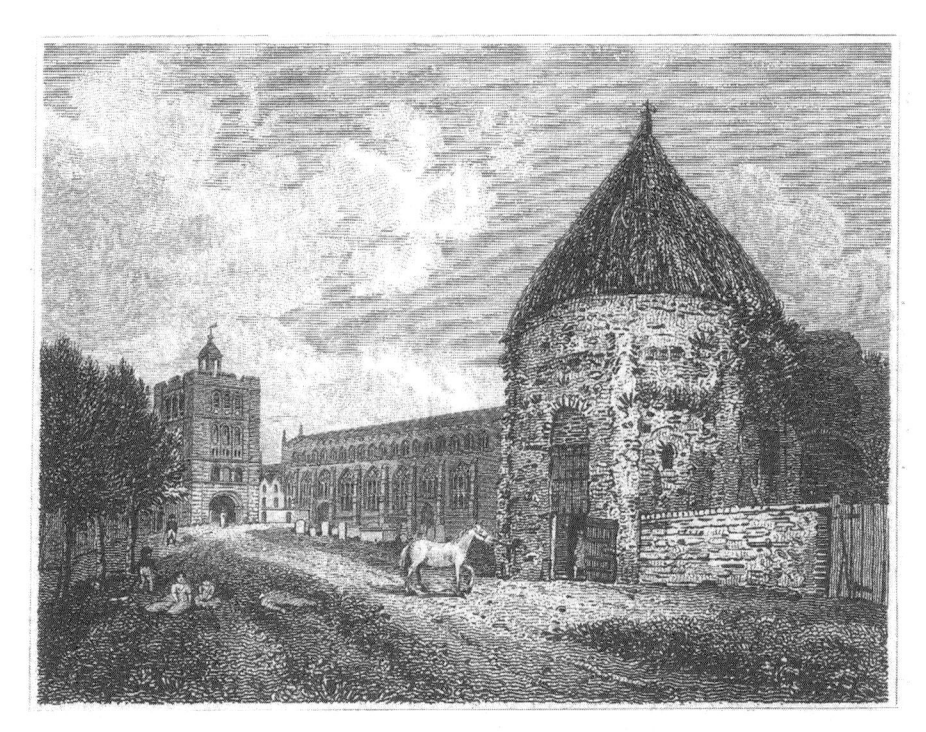

Figure 33 Samson's Tower in use as a stable (1818). Engraving from Thomas Higham, *Excursions in the County of Suffolk* (1818–19), plate facing p. 15.

Lobel likewise argued that the town's economy must have suffered significantly from the dissolution.[2] The townsfolk were freed from some of their traditional payments to the Abbey – notably the 'cope' paid on the election of a new Abbot – but this can hardly have made up for the disappearance of the pilgrims whose disposable income had made Bury a significant market town in the first place. Although the Abbots and sacrists had claimed to own the town, they had also paid for improvements and necessary works on the town's gates, streets and walls.

The end of the Abbey also meant an end to the alms routinely distributed by the monks to the poor and destitute, as occurred at the funeral of Mary Tudor in 1533, and an end to the free education established by Abbot Samson in the twelfth century (at least until Edward VI's re-foundation of the Grammar School in 1550). The Abbey had also been a great patron of various crafts that flourished in Bury, such as manuscript production and embroidery of ecclesiastical vestments, not to mention the stonemasonry of John Wastell and his apprentices. All these vanished overnight. It was not only the town that was affected: manors such as Elmswell were transformed from seasonal palaces for a great magnate to homes for insignificant provincial squires, or worse, the possessions of heedless absentee landlords.

The monks themselves seem to have adapted fairly successfully to the new conditions.

---

2   Lobel (1935), p. 168.

Eight of them retired on their pensions, while a large proportion of the remainder, twenty former monks, secured ecclesiastical benefices in Suffolk, Norfolk or Cambridgeshire. Four became chantry priests, two became schoolmasters, one worked as a notary in Bury and one was a weaver in 1555. The fate of eight monks is unknown. Of those monks who secured benefices, eight were appointed to them during the Marian restoration of Catholicism in 1553–58: Robert Hessett to Tostock in 1556; Humphrey Attleborough to Brinton in 1557; Thomas Diss to Thornham Parva in 1554, then Burgate in 1558; John Bradfield to Little Whelnetham in 1556; Aylott Hawstead to Norton in 1556; John Barton to Rushbrooke in 1555, then Horringer in 1558; Peter Dunwich to Thwaite in 1555; Ralph Warkton to Woodditton in 1554. A further eight, appointed before 1553, served into and through Mary's reign.[3]

This pattern is suggestive of religious conservatism amongst the former monks, although the fact that John Hadley alias King was appointed high master of the newly founded Bury Grammar School between 1550 and 1552 (during the reign of Edward VI) might suggest that he was content with the new religious teachings.[4] The Grammar School was a re-foundation, but several institutions continued to exist from the old regime without a break. In 1539 the two parish churches of St Mary and St James remained, along with the College of Jesus, the Candlemas Guild, the Guilds of St Botolph and St Nicholas, the hospitals of St Peter, St Nicholas and St Petronilla, and even the chantry attached to the Chapel of the Charnel in the Great Churchyard. In the period 1539–48, therefore, the town continued to enjoy a rich religious life in spite of the loss of the Abbey.

The Candlemas Guild, which before the dissolution had informally taken over most of the functions of the old Guild Merchant dissolved after the rebellion of 1327, proved especially important in the post-dissolution period. The Guild ended up arranging for watchmen at the town gates and for essential repair works. However, in 1548 an Act of Parliament of Edward VI finally outlawed chantries, dissolving the remaining colleges and hospitals of the town as well as outlawing religious guilds. Under this Act, on 12 November 1548, commissioners listed the property belonging to the newly dissolved chantries.[5] The Guildhall Feoffees eventually came into being in 1555 as a successor to the Candlemas Guild, managing the lands and income of the former chantries for the benefit of the parishes of St Mary and St James, based at the Guildhall in Guildhall Street, which effectively became Bury's town hall.[6] The dissolution of the Guilds of the Assumption and St Peter allowed a former guildhall in Eastgate Street to be taken over by the newly re-founded Grammar School in 1550.[7]

The Liberty of St Edmund and the Liberty of Bury St Edmunds

From a jurisdictional point of view, the *banleuca* of Bury St Edmunds was a grey area. Authority over the town's markets was claimed by the steward of the Liberty of St Edmund

---

3   Blackwood (2001), pp. 310–11.
4   On King see Elliott (1963), pp. 35–6.
5   Margaret Statham, (ed.), *Accounts of the Feoffees of the Town Lands of Bury St Edmunds, 1569–1622*, SRS 46 (Woodbridge: Suffolk Records Society, 2003), p. xxvi.
6   Ibid., p. xxvii.
7   Ibid., p. xxviii.

(sometimes known at this period as the 'Franchise of Bury'), but it had always been legally questionable whether the *banleuca* itself formed part of the Liberty. However, the local gentry '[took] up the threads of the Abbot's old authority' in the locality,[8] and both MacCulloch and John Craig have argued for a more or less seamless transition from the authority of the Abbot to the authority of local lessees, with no real transformation of the underlying structures of power.[9] The Liberty was administered, in effect, as a separate county. Bury hosted its own quarter sessions and summoned its own grand juries; not only that, but justices of the peace in west Suffolk attended only the quarter sessions at Bury.[10] In Elizabeth's reign, the under-steward of the Liberty claimed the right to serve writs in the name of the steward, who had inherited this right from the Abbot as sheriff of the Liberty – albeit this independence did not go uncontested by the sheriff of Norfolk and Suffolk.[11]

The secular post-dissolution administration of the Liberty of St Edmund was by officers who had already existed before 1539, and no new offices were invented. In 1535 the duke of Suffolk had been hereditary chief steward of the Liberty of St Edmund, and Sir John Cornwallis was steward of the cellarer's manors; both continued in office.[12] The privileges and responsibilities of the steward of the Liberty remained legally unchanged after the dissolution; the only difference was that he now acted on behalf of the king rather than the Abbot. On Henry VIII's death in 1547 the lord chamberlain, Thomas, Lord Darcy was appointed steward of the Liberty of St Edmund by Lord Protector Somerset in succession to the Howard dukes of Suffolk.[13]

Darcy was succeeded in 1555 by Sir Nicholas Bacon of Redgrave, who would go on to be Queen Elizabeth's first lord keeper of the great seal. The Bacons had served the Abbey before the Dissolution; Sir Nicholas's father, Robert Bacon, was sheepreeve and hundred bailiff of St Edmunds.[14] Bacon acquired the stewardship of seven-and-a-half of the Liberty's eight-and-a-half hundreds between 1555 and 1562, as well as monopolising most of the stewardships of the duchy of Lancaster within Suffolk. He was also appointed steward of the Honour of Eye, and on the death of Sir Clement Heigham in 1571 (the Abbot's old appointee), Sir Nicholas's eldest son was appointed chief bailiff of the Liberty of Bury St Edmunds (the *banleuca*).[15] Although the duke of Norfolk continued to claim the hereditary stewardship of the Liberty of St Edmund, Bacon and the duke agreed that the Liberty should be administered in the duke's name by servants of Bacon.[16]

Local government in the *banleuca* itself was divided between the governors of the new Grammar School, founded by Edward VI in 1550, the Guildhall feoffees who administered the old guild lands, and the justices of the peace for the Liberty of St Edmund. These bodies competed with the steward of the Liberty for control of the town, re-enacting on

---

8   MacCulloch (1986), p. 22.
9   See John Craig, *Reformation, Politics, and Polemics: The Growth of Protestantism in East Anglian Market Towns, 1500–1610* (Farnham: Ashgate, 2001), pp. 71–4.
10 MacCulloch (1986), pp. 35–7.
11 Ibid., p. 121.
12 Ibid., pp. 65–6.
13 Ibid., p. 78.
14 Ibid., pp. 137–8.
15 Ibid., p. 87–8.
16 Ibid., p. 92.

a smaller scale the contests between the townsfolk and the Abbot of the previous two centuries. Proposals for the establishment of a corporation for the town in 1562 were rebuffed by the steward, Sir Nicholas Bacon, who argued that there was no need for any more corporations. In 1601 the townsfolk made another attempt, and this time it was the county gentry, apparently orchestrated by Bacon's servant Roger Barber, who resisted reform. Sir Robert Jermyn and Sir John Higham wrote to Sir Robert Cecil explaining that the townsfolk were 'mechanical[s] and tradesmen' and claimed they were trying to avoid 'the common charges of the country', as well as intending to impose high tariffs on stallholders in the market that would impoverish the surrounding countryside. Most damningly of all, the gentry questioned the capacity of a future corporation to protect and maintain the Protestant faith in the town. Thus a 'tight ... oligarchy' of county gentry maintained as complete a control of the town as the Abbots ever had.[17]

By the end of Elizabeth's reign the 'Liberty of St Edmund' does not seem to have existed in strict legal terms. A royal grant of the stewardship of the Liberty to Thomas Howard, baron de Walden of 27 June 1602 contained no explicit mention of the stewardship. Instead, the individual rights of the steward were enumerated in relation to specific manors, and the Liberty itself referred to only obliquely, as the totality of the rights previously held by the duke of Norfolk:[18]

> And by these presents we give and concede to the aforesaid Lord Howard and Henry Howard, to their heirs and assigns, that the same aforesaid Thomas Lord Howard and Henry Howard, their heirs and assigns, should have, hold and enjoy in perpetuity of the rest, under the permissions conceded beforehand by these presents ... the court leets, frankpledges, law days, assizes and assays of bread, wine and beer ... and all other rights, jurisdictions, franchises, liberties, customs, privileges, profits, comforts, advantages, emoluments and hereditaments whatsoever, as much and as many and of whatever kind, and as fully, freely and entirely, and in as complete a manner and form as were had, held or enjoyed by the aforesaid Thomas recently Duke of Norfolk.

The situation was a complex one, in which Bacon was the lessee of most of the Abbot's former rights but the duke remained the hereditary steward, as his ancestors had been since before the dissolution.[19]

King James I finally granted Bury a royal charter on 3 April 1606,[20] erecting a corporation which was granted the right to display the arms of the Abbey. Nevertheless, even

---

17 Ibid., pp. 329–30.
18 'Appendix' in Yates (1843), pp. 11–12: *'ac per presentes damus et concedimus, prefat[o] D[omi]no Howard et Henr[ico] Howard, hered[ibus] et assign[atis] suis, quod ip[s]i prefat[o] Thomas D[omi]nus Howard et Henr[icus] Howard, heredibus et assignatis suis, de cetero imperpetuam habeant, teneant, et gaudeant, ac habere, tenere, et gaudere valeant et possint, infra permissionibus per presentes preconcessis ... curtis lettum, franc plegum, lawdayes, assisam et assaiam panis, vini, et cervisae ... ac omnia alia jura, jurisdictiones, franchesas libertates, consuetudines, privilegia, proficia, commoditates, advantagia, emolumenta, et hereditamenta quecunque, quot, quanta, qualis, ac adeo plene, libere, et integre, ac in tam amplis modo et forma, prout predictus Thomas nuper Dux Norfolciensis ... habuit, tenuit, vel gavisus fuit.'*
19 MacCulloch (1986), p. 92.
20 For the charter see 'Appendix' in Yates (1843), pp. 13–37.

as late as 1623 Bacon deliberately attempted to revive a dispute over stall-rents on Bury market 'in an attempt to maintain his old criminal jurisdiction as lessee of the Liberty of St Edmund against the new powers of the corporation'.[21] In 1627 the Liberty became enmeshed in a complex legal dispute arising from the fact that the right to collect arrears in taxation was granted to the Liberty rather than the farmers of post-fines who claimed the same right.[22] Long after the establishment of the Bury Corporation, the Liberty of St Edmund 'retained something of its old mystique', and it retained a separate grand jury at the assizes into the nineteenth century.[23]

Indeed, in many ways it was the Liberty's judicial independence that proved one of the Abbey's most enduring legacies. Before the dissolution, the Abbot had appointed justices for the Liberty and even, on occasion, served as a justice himself. After the dissolution justices of the Liberty of St Edmund were appointed by the crown. As a result of the dissolution the assizes for the Liberty were able to move into the town rather than being compelled, as they had been since 1469, to meet outside the *banleuca* at Great Barton or at a burial mound called Henhow on Shirehouse Heath.[24] The anomalous status of Bury's independent courts came to the fore in 1778 when a writ was issued by the great court of the Liberty to someone residing in the borough of Bury St Edmunds. This led to a legal dispute about whether Bury was in the Liberty or not – an old issue that had arisen in the Middle Ages. Sir Charles Davers, the chief steward of the Liberty of Bury St Edmunds, thought the town was in the hundred of Thingoe and therefore in the Liberty of St Edmund. The town's incorporation in 1606, however, suggested that it was free from the Liberty of St Edmund's jurisdiction. However the case was decided, the town of Bury St Edmunds retained its own courts (distinct from those of the Liberty of St Edmund) as late as 1835.[25]

The Archdeaconry of Bury St Edmunds

Bury St Edmunds and the Liberty of St Edmund retained their distinctiveness as secular jurisdictions, but the Abbot's old ecclesiastical privileges were also preserved. The bishop of Norwich was frustrated in his attempts to gain control of Bury after the Reformation, much as he had been in preceding centuries. The sacrist's old court of ecclesiastical causes, the Portmanmoot, continued to exist into the reign of Elizabeth and was only extinguished by the charter of 1606.[26] The town of Bury St Edmunds became a peculiar under the jurisdiction of the archbishop of Canterbury, outside the bishop of Norwich's jurisdiction, and in 1548 the reforming Archbishop Thomas Cranmer took advantage of his special authority in the town to appoint Rowland Taylor as archdeacon of Bury St Edmunds by letters patent.[27]

The archdeacon essentially assumed the old role of the sacrist (although without the

---

21 MacCulloch (1986), pp. 329–30.
22 Diarmaid MacCulloch (ed.), *Letters from Redgrave Hall: The Bacon Family, 1340–1744*, SRS 50 (Woodbridge: Suffolk Records Society, 2008), pp. 115–19.
23 MacCulloch (1986), p. 35
24 Ibid., pp. 23–4.
25 Lobel (1935), pp. 116–17
26 Ibid., p. 168
27 MacCulloch (1986), p. 168.

sacrist's secular authority over the government of the town), although the role was usually held in tandem with the position of archdeacon of Sudbury, whose jurisdiction covered the rest of the Liberty of St Edmund (apart from peculiars such as Hadleigh). The difference between the two posts was that the archdeacon of Sudbury was under the authority of the bishop of Norwich whereas the archdeacon of Bury St Edmunds answered only to the archbishop of Canterbury. MacCulloch noted that the archdeacon of Bury St Edmunds enjoyed 'an unusual degree of autonomy within his jurisdiction … issuing schoolmasters' licences in a quasi-episcopal manner, and his court was much more of a competitor with the diocesan court than was its fellow in the Archdeaconry of Suffolk'.[28] Rowland Taylor was also rector of Hadleigh, giving him enormous influence and power in west Suffolk to spread the evangelical message.

However, in July 1553 the religious balance shifted back in favour of Catholicism when Henry VIII's eldest daughter Mary, supported by the gentry of Suffolk and Norfolk, launched a successful bid for the throne from Framlingham Castle and unseated the Protestant pretender, Mary Rose Tudor's granddaughter Lady Jane Grey. Taylor was deprived of his offices and burned to death for heresy at Hadleigh on 9 February 1555. MacCulloch had argued that the decision of local gentry such as the Druries and Heighams to lend their support to Mary and her restoration of Catholicism may have been partly due to their fond memories of Abbot Reeve and the generous legacies he bequeathed to them.[29] However, it is possible that the loyalty of the gentry in the vicinity of Bury had nothing to do with the Abbey and more to do with the lingering influence of the Gardiner family. Stephen Gardiner, who was born in Bury and whose grandfather Robert was the alderman who drew up a protest against the Abbot in 1471, was bishop of Winchester and Mary's lord chancellor in 1553.[30] As such, he was one of the queen's most powerful counsellors as well as England's most powerful churchman until the appointment of Cardinal Reginald Pole as archbishop of Canterbury.

Gardiner owed his early political success at the court of Henry VIII to the clerk of the King's Council, Richard Eden, who was likewise a member of a prominent Bury family. In recognition of Richard Eden's patronage, Gardiner appointed his son George Eden as his secretary, and both George and Thomas Eden served as Suffolk magistrates during the period of Gardiner's chancellorship. Gardiner even secured the election of Thomas Eden as MP for Taunton (a seat controlled by the see of Winchester) in November 1554. Gardiner also continued to help out the Suffolk gentry, assisting Clement Heigham in obtaining the manor of Nedging.[31] Mary's restoration of Catholicism was not universally welcomed, but Peter Wickins has suggested that 'the comparative absence of dissent' in the Liberty of St Edmund during Mary's reign may have been connected to the duke of Norfolk's position as hereditary steward.[32] Mary consolidated the crown's control in Suffolk by annexing some of the former lands of the Abbey to the duchy of Lancaster, including the manor of Mildenhall, of which Mary's supporter Sir Clement Heigham had been steward since the

---

28 Ibid., p. 27.
29 Ibid., p. 210.
30 See C. D. C. Armstrong, 'Gardiner, Stephen (*c.*1495x8–1555)' in *ODNB*, vol. 21, pp. 433–45.
31 MacCulloch (1986), pp. 234–5.
32 Peter Wickins, *Victorian Protestantism and Bloody Mary: The Legacy of Religious Persecution in Tudor England* (Bury St Edmunds: Arena Books, 2012), pp. 281–2.

1520s.³³ Heigham acted continuously as chief bailiff of the Liberty of Bury St Edmunds from 1528 until his death.³⁴

The clearest sign of the restoration of the old Catholic order in Bury itself was the appointment of Dr Edmund (or Edward) Rougham as the second archdeacon of Bury St Edmunds, in succession to Rowland Taylor, in 1555. Rougham had been a friend of the Lutheran Robert Barnes in the 1520s, but by 1529 he was sacrist, an office he held until the dissolution.³⁵ During the latter part of Henry VIII's reign Rougham sided with the religious conservatives. In June 1546 he was sent by the Privy Council to report on a sermon preached at Bury by Rowland Taylor, which led to Taylor's arrest, and in November of that year he preached at the burning of another heretic, John Kirby of Mendlesham.³⁶ Rougham's appointment as archdeacon effectively restored to him many of his former powers, with complete authority over the inhabitants of the town in ecclesiastical matters.

Rougham's tenure was short-lived. He died in 1556 and was buried at Rougham, and thereafter the office of archdeacon of Bury St Edmunds was always held in tandem with that of archdeacon of Sudbury.³⁷ Mary's restoration of the sacrist to power in 1555–6 was the closest the queen came to restoring the Abbey. In the end, Mary's regime confined itself to the restoration of Westminster Abbey, uniquely among the Benedictine houses. The fact that St Edmunds had been systematically and comprehensively demolished in 1540 meant that it was never a likely candidate for restoration, and in any case the crown was still benefiting from the dissolution. However, Rougham's legacy was the sacrist's continued shadowy existence: the Court of the Commissary of the Sacrist of St Edmunds continued to have jurisdiction over probate of wills for all persons dying within the *banleuca* until its amalgamation with the archdeacon of Sudbury's Court in 1844.³⁸

In Elizabeth's reign, the town of Bury's status as an ecclesiastical peculiar allowed radical Puritans more freedom than they would otherwise have enjoyed. During the 'Bury Stirs' of the 1580s attempts were made by both Puritan and conservative factions to gain control of Bury's two parish churches. Anti-Puritan conformists allied with Catholic recusants to try to bring Bury under the bishop of Norwich's jurisdiction.³⁹ The town's ecclesiastical independence, which endured until the nineteenth century, may have been one factor behind the choice of one of the two ancient parish churches of Bury St Edmunds to serve as a cathedral for the new Anglican diocese of St Edmundsbury and Ipswich in 1914. By that date it was considered desirable for a diocese to cover the same territory as a county; West Suffolk and East Suffolk had formally been established as a separate counties in 1874, so the new diocese would cover two counties. This, rather than Bury's past history, was the

---

33 MacCulloch (1986), p. 237.
34 Wickins (2012), p. 274.
35 Thomson (1982), p. 95. Rougham was not, as MacCulloch and Wickins erroneously claimed, the Abbey's former sexton (MacCulloch (1986), p. 168; Wickins (2012), p. 231).
36 Wickins (2012), p. 231.
37 MacCulloch (1986), p. 168.
38 Peter Northeast (ed.), *Wills of the Archdeaconry of Sudbury 1459–1474*, SRS 44 (Woodbridge: Suffolk Records Society, 2001), pp. xxxix–xl.
39 MacCulloch (1986), p. 210. On the Bury Stirs see pp. 200–11 and John S. Craig, 'The Bury Stirs revisited: An analysis of the townsmen', *PSIAH* 37 (1991), pp. 208–24.

immediate reason why the bishop of the diocese was to live in Ipswich and the cathedral was to be St James' Church in Bury.

St Edmund's restored, 1615

By the beginning of 1540 there were officially no more Benedictine monks left in England – although the dissolution was not, of course, recognised by the papacy, which regarded Henry VIII's acts as illegal. However, when Mary I became queen in 1553, after a successful bid for the throne launched from East Anglia, the restoration of the monasteries did not follow automatically. Mary depended on the support of a gentry and aristocracy who had been immeasurably enriched by the dissolution, such as the Kytsons of Hengrave Hall, with whom she stayed on her way to Framlingham Castle in 1553. Mary was caught between political reality and her loyalty to the papacy, which regarded the patrimony of the monasteries as inalienable church lands. At Mary's request, on 20 June 1555 Pope Pius IV issued the bull *Praeclara*, dissolving the old monasteries and confirming the rights of owners of former monastic lands.[40] However, Mary restored Westminster Abbey as a token Benedictine house; whether other monasteries, including Bury, would have followed had she ruled for longer must remain pure speculation.

On St Edmund's day, 20 November 1556, a group of monks composed of former members of dissolved English monasteries and Italian Cassinese Benedictines took possession of Westminster Abbey. Their abbot was John Feckenham, a former monk of Evesham. J. C. H. Aveling suggested that the Bury monk Roger or Reginald Maldon, recorded as the vicar of Moulton in 1547, was one of the first to enter the restored Westminster.[41] According to some accounts, the life of the restored Abbey was more like that of a college of priests than a monastery.[42] The brief restoration came to an end on 12 July 1559, and Maldon apparently returned to his benefice at Moulton, where he was buried in 1564.[43] Monastic life in England was extinguished for a second time, and Englishmen seeking to enter the religious life were forced to go abroad. The first to do so was Robert Sayer (1560–1602) of Redgrave, where the Bacon stewards of the Liberty of St Edmund had moved into the Abbot's old lodge.[44] Sayer was professed at Monte Cassino in 1589.[45]

By the early years of the seventeenth century, the large number of Englishmen entering

---

40 David M. Lunn, *The English Benedictines 1540–1688* (London: Burns and Oates, 1980), p. 3.
41 'Appendix A' in J. McCann and C. Cary Elwes (eds), *Ampleforth and its Origins: Essays on a Living Tradition* (London: Burns, Oates and Washbourne, 1952), p. 278.
42 Lunn (1980), pp. 3–4.
43 C. S. Knighton, 'Westminster Abbey restored', in Eamon Duffy and David Loades (eds), *The Church of Mary Tudor* (Farnham: Ashgate, 2006), pp. 77–123, at p. 118 rejects the identification of Reginald Maldon, monk of Westminster with Roger Maldon, monk of Bury on the grounds that Archbishop Matthew Parker would not have given the living of Moulton to a man with his religious background. Moulton was a peculiar under the jurisdiction of the Archbishop of Canterbury (Joanna Martin, 'Ecclesiastical Jurisdictions' in David Dymond and Edward Martin (eds), *An Historical Atlas of Suffolk* (Ipswich: Suffolk County Council Planning Department, 1988), pp. 16–17).
44 MacCulloch (1986), p. 26.
45 Thompson Cooper (rev. D. D. Rees), 'Sayer, Robert [*name in religion* Gregory] (1560–1602)' in *ODNB*, vol. 49, p. 161.

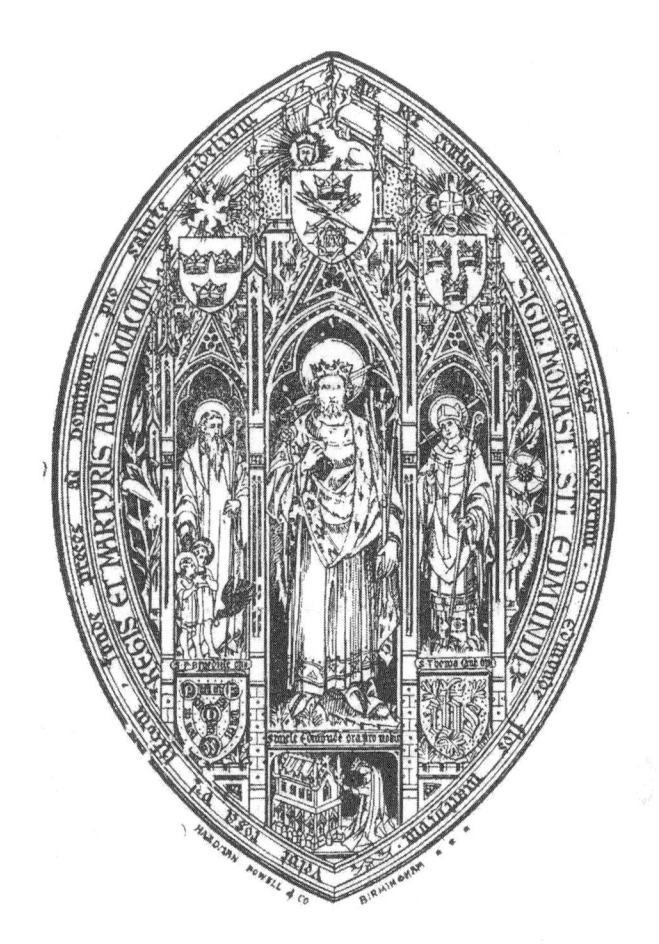

Figure 34 Seal of St Edmund's Abbey, Douai (now Woolhampton). From J. B. Mackinlay, *Saint Edmund King and Martyr* (1893), p. 411.

Spanish and Italian monasteries had created a demand for a distinct English Benedictine congregation that would be able to found English monasteries on the Continent. Many of those who entered Spanish and Italian monasteries did so after training at English seminaries, where they took a binding oath to return to England on mission which could not be set aside once they became monks. A new organisation of missionary Benedictines was needed for England, and on 21 November 1607, in the Gatehouse Prison in Westminster, a surviving monk of the re-founded Westminster Abbey, Sigebert Buckley, clothed two young Englishmen in the habit of St Benedict, thereby guaranteeing the continued existence of Westminster Abbey. However, English Benedictines argued that Westminster Abbey, as the last surviving Benedictine abbey, was the inheritor of *all* the rights and privileges of the medieval English Benedictine congregation. The restored English Benedictines regarded themselves as heirs of St Augustine of Canterbury as much as John Feckenham.

The English Benedictine priory at Douai, St Gregory's, became the first house of the new congregation. Within the year, St Gregory's boasted its first martyr: George Gervase, who had grown up in Bury St Edmunds, was executed at Tyburn on 11 August 1608. On the same day a devastating fire destroyed much of Bury, and according to the Benedictine historian Bede Camm, 'many noticed with awe' that the fire started on the same day and at the same hour that Gervase was executed.[46] St Gregory's was followed by the foundation of St Laurence's priory at Dieulouard in Lorraine in 1608.

In 1615 Marie of Lorraine, abbess of Chelles, sent six monks from Dieulouard to establish an English Benedictine house of studies in Paris. Accordingly, Clement Reyner, Nicholas Curre, George Gaire, Alban Roe, Placid Gascoigne and Dunstan Pettinger arrived in the French capital, where their superior, Augustine Bradshaw (d. 1618), was installed on 25 June 1615. The monks were a distinguished group. Bradshaw had already founded both St Gregory's, Douai in 1606 and St Laurence's, Dieulouard in 1608; Clement Reyner would go on to become the foremost historian of the English Benedictines, and both he and Placid Gascoigne would later serve as abbots of Lambspring, a monastery near Hildersheim in Germany which was assigned to the English Benedictines. Alban Roe achieved the greatest distinction of all, suffering martyrdom for the Catholic faith in 1642.

The original intention was that the community would be a house of studies of the University of Paris, allowing English monks to attend lectures in the university,[47] much as Gloucester Hall had served as a house of studies for English Benedictines in Oxford before the Reformation. In 1617 the English Benedictine congregation was formally established, allowing the house in Paris to become a priory, under its first prior William Gifford (1554–1629), known as Gabriel de Sancta Maria. In 1618 Gifford was consecrated coadjutor bishop to the archbishop of Rheims, and in 1622 he succeeded as archbishop-duke and premier peer of France – an impressive achievement for the son of an obscure Hampshire gentleman.[48]

In 1621 the second General Chapter of the restored English Benedictine congregation declared that 'for the preservation of the rights of the congregation to the monasteries of England, each of the communities should in future be appropriated to one of the English monasteries'. The Paris priory was accordingly assigned the 'right and title' of the Abbey of Bury St Edmunds.[49] The Chapter did this on the grounds that it claimed, through succession from Sigebert Buckley, the privileges of all pre-Reformation English monasteries, including Bury. In theory, the 'right and title' of the new St Edmund's meant that, in the event of the restoration of Catholicism as England's national religion, St Edmund's would repossess the site of the Abbey and all of its former lands.

This possibility did not seem as remote in the early seventeenth century as it does in hindsight. In 1623, there was widespread speculation that the prince of Wales (the future Charles I) would convert to Catholicism in order to marry the Spanish Infanta, and in the 1630s many Catholics believed that Charles inclined towards Catholicism. The Curia in

---

46   Bede Camm, *Nine Martyr Monks: The Lives of the English Benedictine Martyrs beatified in 1929* (London: Burns, Oates and Washbourne, 1931), p. 48.
47   Paul Arblaster, 'Paris 1615–1676' in Geoffrey Scott (ed.), *Douai 1903 Woolhampton 2003: A Centenary History* (Worcester: Stanbrook Abbey Press, 2003), pp. 1–36, at pp. 4–5.
48   Ibid., p. 14.
49   S. Marron, 'The early years at St Edmund's, Paris', *Douai Magazine* 3:4 (1925), pp. 258–65, at p. 258; Arblaster (2003), p. 18.

Rome even started drawing up lists of nominees to fill English sees when the time came.[50] As late as 1661, the Catholic owner of St Saviour's Hospital in Bury, Sir Edward Gage of Hengrave, was concerned that he would have to give up his property if the monks were restored, and reached an agreement with the English Benedictine congregation that his family would continue to hold St Saviour's for forty years after such a restoration.[51] Another reason for assigning titles to the monasteries was to allow Catholic owners of former monastic lands to give alms to the monastery whose lands they had appropriated,[52] and in doing so feel that they were salving their consciences. Alms offered to the Congregation as a whole could, in theory, be designated as alms offered to St Edmunds Abbey, if a landowner happened to be a beneficiary of that Abbey's dissolution.

A link existed between the Paris priory and old St Edmunds through one of its founders, Alban Roe, who was born Bartholomew Roe in the town in 1583 and was known in religion as *Albanus a Sancto Edmundo*, 'Alban of St Edmund'. Alban Roe imitated both of his saintly patrons in his martyrdom at Tyburn on 31 January 1642, and was canonised by Pope Paul VI in 1970.[53] However, the idea of restoration was a mere fantasy for St Edmund's in the first phase of its existence. The monks were briefly made homeless in 1619 when Marie of Lorraine withdrew her support, and were forced to rely on the charity of their former prior, the archbishop-duke of Rheims. It was not until 1642 that they were able to purchase any property, and they did not obtain letters of establishment from the king of France until 1650. Recognition as a monastery followed in 1656, but it was not until 1674 that the monks could afford to start building a priory church.[54]

The monks of St Edmund's were also riven with conflict over the interpretation of its own history. In 1619 John Barnes, an English monk who was a member of the Spanish Congregation, argued that the only true legally erected Benedictine congregation in England before the Reformation was that of Cluny, and therefore all of the rights of the English Benedictines reverted to the Cluniacs after the second dissolution of Westminster Abbey.[55] Barnes was supported by Francis Walgrave, a former monk of St Edmund's who was now a Cluniac.[56] In response to Barnes and Walgrave's allegations, the monks of the English Benedictine Congregation turned their attention to their own history, and Augustine Baker, the celebrated mystical writer, was despatched to Oxford to consult the annals of medieval England. His collections at Jesus College were a valuable resource for Benedictine historians for centuries thereafter. One document he preserved by transcribing it was the account of the fire of 1465 first published by James in 1895 (see Chapter 5).

In 1626 the St Edmund's monk Clement Reyner (1588–1651) published the fruits of Baker's research, the meticulous and compendious *Apostolatus Benedictinorum in Anglia* ('The apostolate of the Benedictines in England'), intended as a riposte to Barnes as well

---

50 Arblaster (2003), p. 20.
51 Young (2015a), pp. 38–9.
52 Lunn (1980), p. 110.
53 On Alban Roe see Geoffrey Scott, 'Three seventeenth-century Benedictine martyrs', in David H. Farmer (ed.), *Benedict's Disciples*, 2nd edn (Leominster: Gracewing, 1995), pp. 266–81, at pp. 275–8.
54 Arblaster (2003), pp. 1–2.
55 Lunn (1980), p. 109.
56 Arblaster (2003), pp. 18–24.

as an antidote to the anti-monasticism of Protestant antiquaries. *Apostolatus* argued that the black monks of the monastic cathedral churches of medieval England represented the authentic English church, since the monks were introduced by St Augustine of Canterbury himself, the apostle of the English.[57] Bury St Edmunds played an important role in Reyner's argument. He pointed out that when Cnut introduced monks to Beodricsworth in the eleventh century, the king chose English black monks, not the recently reformed Cluniacs, in order to placate the English who had been so useful to him in a war against Norway:

> Canute a Danish man, forasmuch as he was of the same kindred as the Anglo-Saxons, now very much desired to embrace and seek out the love of the English who had been most faithful and most courageous soldiers against the Norwegian rebels, and with whom he greatly desired to purge himself of the crime of St Edmund's murder, did not advocate Cluniacs, strange and foreign-born men for the monastery of St Edmund, once founded by Alfwin Bishop of the East Saxons and recently adorned by him with monks around the year of grace 1020, but without doubt he established English monks, fellow-citizens of their king, and most attached to the glory of the same martyr, so that the English might be more grateful through such a benefit accrued through the monks.[58]

According to Reyner, Cnut's choice of English monks to serve the cult of St Edmund was a recognition of the patriotic significance of the cult for the English. St Edmund was simultaneously a patriotic icon, a role he was to carry on fulfilling, but also a distinctly Benedictine preoccupation: the English monks were, naturally, 'most attached to the glory of the ... martyr' (*martyris gloriae addictissimos*) whose fellow-citizens (*concivis*) they were. St Edmund had become part of the modern English Benedictines' patriotic foundation myth.

Reyner went on to cite Abbot Samson's treatment of the Cluniacs as evidence for the superior claims of the English monks,[59] and noted that St Edmunds, amongst other abbeys, was always exempt from episcopal jurisdiction.[60] Reyner cited a speech by Cardinal Allen, the founder of the English Colleges at Douai and Rheims and a key figure of the English Counter-Reformation, in praise of the Benedictines. In an aside, Allen mentioned 'those noble monasteries of Westminster, St Albans, St Edmunds and Glastonbury, whose

---

57 Clement Reyner, *Apostolatus Benedictinorum in Anglia* (Douai, 1626), pp. 1–9. On Reyner see D. D. Rees, 'Reyner, Wilfrid' in *ODNB*, vol. 46, pp. 525–6.

58 Reyner (1626), p. 142: *Canutum hominem Danum, ac proinde eiusdem cum Anglo Saxonibus idiomatis, qui tunc cupidissime ambiebat et venabatur Angloru[m] amore[m] quos fidelissimos, fortissimosq[ue] milites co[n]tra rebelles Noruegos expertus fuisset, & apud quos maxime cupiebat se a caedis S. Edmundi crimine purgare, no[n] Cluniacenses homines externos & alienigenas ad coenobium S. Edmundi olim ab Alfwino Orientaliu[m] Saxonu[m] Episcopo fundatu[m], & recenter a se monachis ornatu[m] circa annum gratiae 1020. aduocasse, sed Anglicos sine dubio monachos, conciuis sui regis, & martyris gloriae addictissimos ibidem posuisse, vt et gratior esset Anglis per monachos tali beneficio cumulatos; & magis placeret martyri in caelis regnanti, qui sine dubio vt verus Christi cultor, maxime curaret domesticos suae fidei.*

59 Ibid., pp. 162–3.

60 Ibid., pp. 91–2.

Abbot, just like many others clearly shown was martyred in the time of Henry VIII'.[61] By joining the lustre of the martyrdom of Richard Whyting, the last abbot of Glastonbury, with the other three greatest abbeys of pre-Reformation England, Allen glossed over the crucial difference between Glastonbury and the other great abbeys (its resistance to the royal supremacy), and helped create the myth of a 'monastic golden age'.

However, Reyner made no explicit claims for the exemplary piety of the monks of Bury, and offered instead another explanation for their renown: 'The monks of St Edmundsbury were great in the estimation of England on account of the sacred body of Edmund, king and martyr, to which our kings often came on pilgrimage by reason of religion.'[62] Almost ninety years after its presumed destruction or reburial, the body of St Edmund still mattered to the English Benedictines, not so much as an object of devotion but as a link between the Benedictines and English royalty. It was this link that guaranteed the Abbey's exemptions from episcopal authority, which still mattered to Benedictines in the seventeenth century. Reyner's enthusiasm was not equalled by his antiquarianism – he erroneously claimed that St Edmund's reign began in 870[63] – but Reyner's work established the basic rationale for considering St Edmund a Benedictine saint. Thus the choice of St Edmund as patron of the Paris foundation was natural enough, and sent a message about the Congregation's patriotism and canonical legitimacy.

According to canon law, an abandoned monastery became dissolved by default a hundred years after the last monk left it.[64] The Abbey of Bury St Edmunds would therefore have ceased to exist canonically in 1639, but two factors complicated the Abbey's canonical status. One was Pope Pius IV's dissolution of *all* the monasteries in 1555, and the other was Pope Urban VIII's Bull *Plantata*, issued on 12 July 1633, which confirmed the English Benedictines as inheritors of the rights of all pre-Reformation Benedictine foundations. *Plantata* permitted the congregation to appoint 'cathedral priors' for the ancient Benedictine sees of England, who in theory could exercise ordinary jurisdiction in the absence of bishops. The Benedictines interpreted *Plantata* as confirming their assignment of the 'right and title' of ancient monasteries to new religious houses in 1621, so that although the Abbey of Bury St Edmunds was not mentioned by name in the bull, it was implicitly re-founded through the renewal of English Benedictine privileges. Because *Plantata* appeared before 1639 it saved the theoretical Abbey from theoretical dissolution, and the Abbey continued to exist as a canonical (if not a real) entity.

A long-standing association between St Edmund's and royalty began in 1661 when three Paris monks, Placid Adelham, Augustine Latham and Bennet Hankinson, were sent to Catherine of Braganza's Chapel Royal in Somerset House. Adelham remained there until he was expelled in 1675.[65] In 1677 the priory church next to the Val-de-Grâce

---

61 Ibid., p. 243: *Vt nihil dicamus de nobilissimis monasterijs, West-Monasteriensi, S. Albani, S. Edmundi, Glastenburiensi, cuius Abbas, sicut & plurimi alij claro perfuncti sunt martyrio tempore Henrici octaui.*
62 Ibid., p. 163: *Coenobium Edmundi burgense magnae erat in Angliae existimationis propter Sacrum corpus Edmundi Regis ac Martyris, ad quod saepe Reges nostri peregrinationis religiosae causa veniebant.*
63 Ibid., p. 58.
64 Ibid., p. 115.
65 Arblaster (2003), pp. 33–4.

on the Faubourg St Jacques was finally completed and dedicated to St Edmund.[66] The monastery is now numbers 268 and 269 Rue St Jacques and houses a music school, the *Schola Cantorum*.[67] The possibility of the monks' return to Bury became very real in 1685, when the Catholic James II succeeded to the throne. Many believed that the restoration of the monasteries was imminent, including John Halls, owner of the old Abbot's Palace in Bury. Perhaps hoping to pre-empt confiscation by the crown, he offered to sell the site to the monks of St Edmund's, as the community's chronicler recorded:

> When the king (James II.) was on the crown, as our house here in Paris bare the name of the Holy Martyr, St. Edmund, king of the East Angles; those who had the land of our old great abbey of St. Edmund's in England, frivolously and vainly apprehensive th[a]t we should again re-enter into all, they proposed to our the sale of 'em.

However, James II himself advised the monks against the purchase, 'th[a]t they might not give occasion to publick clamours and noises th[a]t would be seditiously made under pretext th[a]t the monks were a going to be put into possession of all again'.[68] In the event, the Jesuits stole the march on the Benedictines and bought the property instead.

On 13 December 1686, in an effort to reassure Protestant landowners, the Benedictine monk Phillip Michael Ellis formally renounced all of the rights of the old Benedictine congregation to the pre-Reformation monasteries in a sermon preached before James in the Catholic Chapel of the Palace of Whitehall. In David Lunn's view, 'This formal act, which had every appearance of being perfectly valid, provides an exact date beyond which all the old monastic houses of England were well and truly extinct.'[69] As a consequence of Ellis's renunciation, St Edmund's in Paris ceased formally to claim the right to be the inheritor of the pre-Reformation property and privileges of the Abbey of Bury St Edmunds, but it was still the symbolic successor of the medieval St Edmunds.

In 1701 King James II died in exile at St Germain-en-Laye and his funeral took place in St Edmund's Priory Church. Because it was expected that the Stuarts would one day be restored to the English throne, the king's body was not buried but remained in a catafalque in the Lady Chapel and became a place of pilgrimage for Jacobites.[70] In the eighteenth century St Edmund's became renowned as a centre of scholarship and Enlightenment scientific endeavour. The Society of St Edmund became a focus for scientific demonstrations and papers delivered by English emigrés resident in Paris, and its members corresponded with the Royal Society.[71] However, the French Revolution resulted in the confiscation of the monks' property. The *sans culottes* opened the catafalque of James II and discovered that the body of the king, regarded as saintly by Jacobites, was incorrupt. In events that strangely mirrored Abbot Samson's behaviour in 1098, the imprisoned prior of St Edmund's, William Parker, touched the king's hand and found it

---

66 Scott (2003), p. 37.
67 Ibid., p. 39.
68 Benet Weldon, quoted in Joseph Boniface Mackinlay, *Saint Edmund King and Martyr* (London: Art and Book Company, 1893), pp. 405–6. See also Young (2006), p. 213.
69 Lunn (1980), p. 139.
70 Ibid., p. 37.
71 Ibid., pp. 46–9.

to be as supple as the hand of a sleeping man. The *sans culottes* charged people a fee to view the body.⁷²

In the summer of 1794 the monks were allowed to return to the Paris monastery, but in 1818 the community made the decision to move to Douai in northern France.⁷³ By this time the monks of St Edmund's were one of the few English communities to remain on the Continent. Most had returned to England, now ironically a place of safety for Catholics from the anti-Catholic violence of the French revolutionaries. There was a certain appropriateness to the monks settling at Douai, which was a city with strong medieval associations with Bury St Edmunds. In the Middle Ages there was a street in Bury called *Frenkysmanestrete* ('Frenchman Street'), now the eastern end of Abbeygate Street, where traders from Douai settled in order to sell their wares at Bury Fair in November and December every year.⁷⁴ At Douai the monks became more aware of their monastic lineage, and one of them, Joseph Mackinlay (in religion Boniface), carried out extensive research on St Edmund and Bury.⁷⁵ Unfortunately, Mackinlay sometimes wrote with more enthusiasm than concern for historical accuracy. His book *Saint Edmund King and Martyr* appeared in 1893.

During the course of the nineteenth century the English Benedictine houses, which had always (with the exception of Lambspring in Hanover) been priories, acquired the status of abbeys. By this time the titular cathedral priories created by Urban VIII in *Plantata* had become honorific titles bestowed on senior or retired priors. The creation of abbeys meant that titles were also required for retired abbots, and so the Holy See approved the creation of titular abbacies named after the great Benedictine abbeys of medieval England. One of these was Bury St Edmunds, and the first titular Abbot of St Edmundsbury was Thomas Paulinus Heptonstall (1798–1869), a monk of St Gregory's, Downside, who was given this honour in 1862.⁷⁶ Heptonstall acted for many years as agent in England of the Australian bishops, and was buried at Little Malvern. The present titular Abbot is Dom Stephen Ortiger, who retired as abbot of Worth, Sussex in 2002.

In 1900 St Edmund's, Douai became an abbey, and on 4 November 1900 Dom Laurence Larkin was blessed as Douai's first abbot by Archbishop William Scarisbrick, a monk of Douai and a former bishop of Mauritius.⁷⁷ The enthronement of Abbot Larkin took place 361 years to the day after the surrender of the Abbey of Bury St Edmunds by Abbot Reeve, and 4 November was surely chosen to emphasise the status of St Edmund's, Douai as Bury's symbolic successor. However, in 1903 anti-Catholic laws made it impossible for the community to remain in France, and the monks returned at long last to England where they made their home at Woolhampton, near Reading. In the 1930s one of the monks, Aloysius Bloor, did all he could to revive the medieval offices for the Feast of St Edmund.⁷⁸

---

72   Ibid., p. 59.
73   See Alban Hood, 'Douai 1818–1903' in Geoffrey Scott (ed.), *Douai 1903 Woolhampton 2003: A Centenary History* (Worcester: Stanbrook Abbey Press, 2003), pp. 61–97.
74   Statham (1998), p. 101.
75   Hood (2003), pp. 86–7.
76   Henry Norbert Birt, *Obit Book of the English Benedictines, 1600–1912* (Edinburgh: Mercat Press, 1913), p. 160.
77   Hood (2003), p. 93.
78   Geoffrey Scott, 'Woolhampton 1903–2003' in Geoffrey Scott (ed.), *Douai 1903*

The monks of St Edmund's seventeenth-century ambition to return to Bury St Edmunds was never fulfilled. Between 1731 and 1755 there was a Catholic mission in the town led by Benedictine monks, but they were drawn from St Gregory's, Douai, St Laurence's, Dieulouard, and Lambspring Abbey.[79] Nevertheless, the abbey of St Edmund at Woolhampton maintains its historic connection with Bury St Edmunds, and on 20 November 2015, at celebrations of the community's 400th anniversary, the Anglican bishop of St Edmundsbury and Ipswich was invited to preach at Vespers. In 2020 both the monks of St Edmund's and the town of Bury St Edmunds will celebrate the millennium of the foundation of the Abbey by King Cnut, and it is to be hoped that such an important anniversary will be suitably marked.

Woolhampton 2003: A Centenary History (Worcester: Stanbrook Abbey Press, 2003), pp. 98–173, at p. 126.
79   See Young (2015a), pp. 109–23.

Chapter 8
Discovery

In the centuries since the dissolution, the ruins of the Abbey of Bury St Edmunds excited ridicule and admiration in equal measure, as Protestant England struggled to come to terms with its Catholic past. On the one hand, the Abbey Church was a splendid achievement containing the tombs of famous past worthies, but on the other hand it was a monument to what later generations regarded as a superstitious belief in the miraculous efficacy of St Edmund's body. Over time, however, as the controversies of the Reformation receded into memory, the study of medieval monastic history became more acceptable, although historians were slow to turn their attention to Bury, and the first book on the Abbey was not published until 1745. John Battely's posthumous and incomplete work stands at the head of a long line of scholarly studies of the Abbey's surviving manuscripts, which were complemented in the nineteenth century by the beginnings of modern archaeological investigations of the ruins. It was only by a long and slow process, and by the hard work of investigators who did not have the advantage of the sources readily available today, that we were able to achieve our current level of knowledge of the history of East Anglia's greatest Abbey.

John Leland and the early antiquaries

Antiquarian interest in the historical value of the Abbey of Bury St Edmunds began even before its dissolution, as the visits paid to the Abbey by John Leland demonstrate. A surviving letter from one of Leland's agents at Barnwell in Cambridgeshire to the commissioners in Bury may have been written on 9 November 1539, just five days after Abbot Reeve's surrender to the crown. Leland, who operated without an overt religious agenda, belonged to a Humanist tradition of historiography that emphasized the importance of consulting original sources. At the same time, however, the Reformation generated a demand for antiquarian studies proving the independence of the ancient British church from Rome.[1] Leland's primary interest was in the Abbey's library, and his agent wrote ahead of his arrival:

> And whereas Master Leland at this present time cometh to Bury to see what books be left in the library there, or translated thence into any other corner of the said monastery, I shall desire you upon just consideration right readily to further his cause, and to permit him to have the use of such as may further him in setting forth such matters as

---

1   Graham Parry, *The Trophies of Time: English Antiquarians of the Seventeenth Century* (Oxford: Oxford University Press, 1995), p. 2.

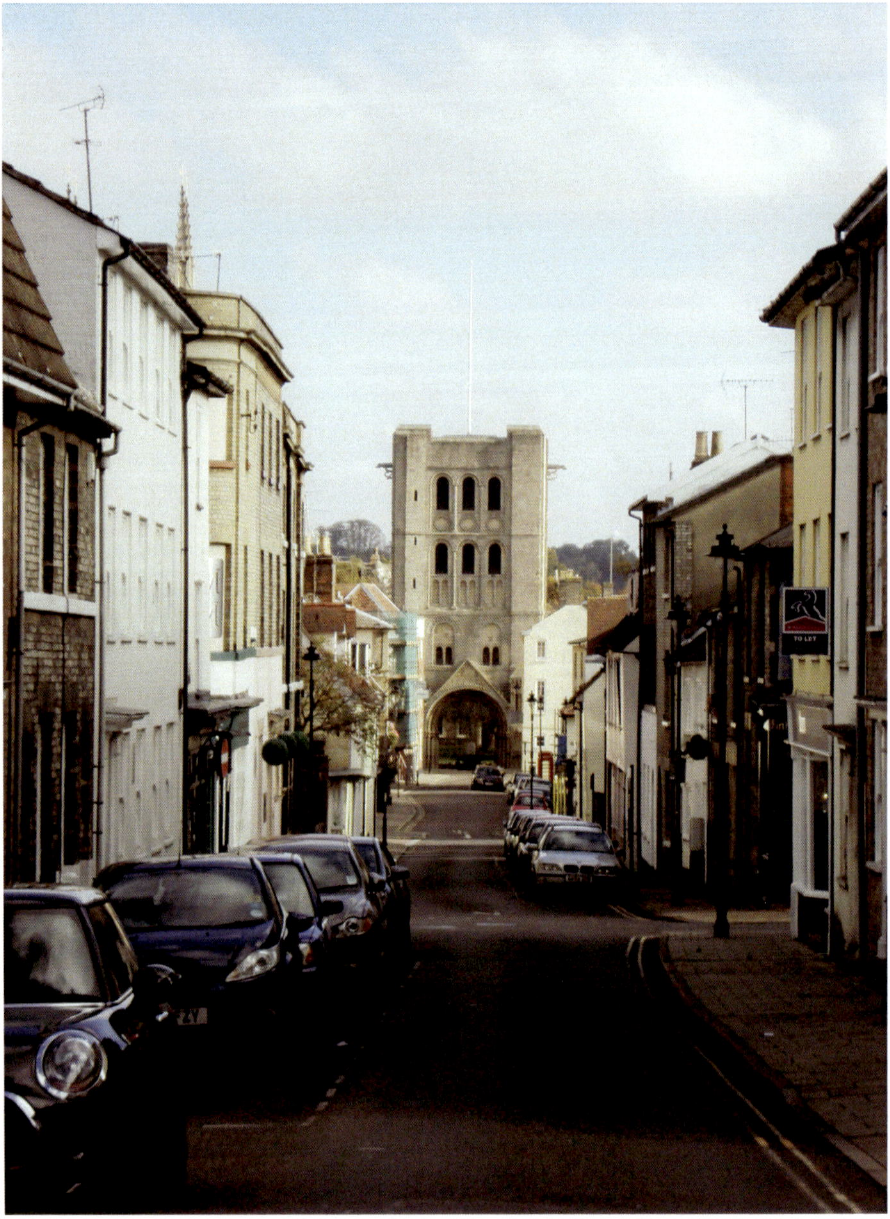

Figure 35 The 'great axis' today: the Norman Tower from the west end of Churchgate Street. Photo by the author.

he writeth for the King's Majesty. In so doing ye shall bind me to show unto you at all times like gratitude: for if I were present at this time with you I would gladly myself fulfil this honest request.[2]

As noted in Chapter 6, in 1535 the Abbey had begun disposing of its books, both to ensure their survival and to raise income. Leland, as royal librarian, was claiming the remainder as the King's property, although it is unclear how many he found on arrival. Most of the surviving books from Bury were probably disposed of in 1535, and only a fraction of Bury's charters and registers survive: 176 extant Bury charters compared with Lincoln Cathedral's 4200.[3] However, in comparison with other dissolved monasteries that were not erected into cathedral churches by Henry VIII, Bury's archives fared remarkably well. One reason for this was the continued existence of the Liberty of St Edmund as an administrative unit of local government; cartularies and manorial rolls, in particular, remained significant documents for those who had acquired monastic lands after the Dissolution.[4] Unfortunately, the significance of these documents also led to their being damaged; the Curteys Register, for instance, listed the cellarer's manors in alphabetical order, and the post-dissolution owners of these manors tore out the quires referring to their lands.[5] However, Sir Nicholas Bacon's status as steward of the Liberty meant that more of the Abbey's financial documents were concentrated in the hands of the Bacon family than anyone else's.[6]

The extent of John Leland's contribution to the survival of documents from St Edmunds is difficult to assess. Leland's manuscript collections, which were organised by Thomas Hearne in the eighteenth century, suggest that he merely made notes on matters that interested him. These were the lands and property donated to the monastery over the course of the centuries, preserved in various registers, and those gifts and donations recorded 'Out of the little book of the funerals of noble men and Abbots buried in the Monastery of St Edmund' (*Ex libello de Exequiis nobilium virorum et Abbatum sepultorum in monasterio S. Edmundi*).[7] Leland also produced an account of the story of St Edmund which remained unpublished in his lifetime, but which was accompanied by a detailed account of benefactions to the Abbey.[8] It is possible that the Elizabethan archbishop of Canterbury, Matthew Parker, who obtained the twelfth-century illuminated Bury Bible for Corpus Christi College, Cambridge, was able to do this as a result of the documents preserved by Leland.

In addition to those families who desired to retain documents from the Abbey as evidence

---

2   John Leland, (ed. Lucy Toulmin Smith), *The Itinerary of John Leland in or about the Years 1535–1543* (London: G. Bell, 1907), vol. 2, p. 148.
3   Thomson (1980), p. 3.
4   Ibid., p. 2.
5   Ibid., p. 35.
6   These included the *Registrum Rubrum, Registrum Sacristae, Registrum Pynchbeck, Registrum Alphabeticum* and *Registrum Nigrum*, all now in Cambridge University Library (James (1895), p. 97).
7   Leland (1907), vol. 2, pp. 148–50.
8   John Leland (ed. Thomas Hearne), *Joannis Lelandi antiquarii de rebus Britannicis collectanea* (London, 1770), vol. 1, pp. 220–26. See also vol. 6, pp. 138–45.

of their land rights, local antiquaries also contributed to the survival of documents, most notably Sir Simonds D'Ewes of Stowlangtoft and Thomas Eden. D'Ewes, descended from a family of Flemish printers, was an antiquary and moderate Parliamentarian during the Civil War.[9] The Eden family were major landowners in the Sudbury area and acquired the Dominican priory in the town at the dissolution. Their connections with Bishop Stephen Gardiner have already been mentioned.[10] D'Ewes was in possession of a 'little register of the monastery of Bury' (*registrum parvum monasterii de Bury*), while Eden owned the *registrum Swaffham* of the fifteenth-century sacrist John Swaffham.[11]

The only book from the Abbey that was preserved in the town itself was the so-called 'psalter of St Edmund', a relic originally kept close to (or inside) the shrine, which was supposed to be the book from which St Edmund learned the psalms during a sojourn at Attleborough shortly after his coronation. This manuscript was part of the parish library of St James' Church, and the survival of this 'relic' was somewhat ironic given the library's reputation as an impressive collection of Protestant theological works. However, even the most enthusiastic of Protestant antiquaries, such as the former Carmelite friar John Bale and William Lambarde, the chorographer of Kent, voiced mixed feelings over the destruction of monastic libraries that accompanied the extirpation of superstition.[12]

In 1586 William Camden published his *Britannia*, the first attempt at a complete description of the antiquities of England, adopting a chorographical (county by county) approach. Camden mentioned the removal of the body of St Edmund to Bury St Edmunds,[13] although his account of the saint's martyrdom came under his treatment of the village of Hoxne.[14] Camden openly lamented the destruction of the Abbey, condemning those who 'under a goodly pretense of reforming religion preferred their private respects and their owne enriching before the honour of Prince and Country, yea and before the Glory of God himselfe'. However, he seemed as much captivated by the Abbey's great wealth and the famous tombs that were lost as he was horrified by the sacrilege of the dissolution:

> If you demand how great the wealth of this Abbey was, a man could hardly tell, and namely how many gifts and oblations were hung upon the tomb alone of St Edmund: and besides, there came in, out of lands and revenues, a thousand five hundred and three score pounds of old rent by the year .... But as great a piece of work as this was, so long in building and still increasing, and as much riches as they gathered together for so many years with St Edmund's shrine, and the monuments of Alan Rufus Earl of Brittany and Richmond, Sir Thomas of Brotherton son to King Edward the First, Earl of Norfolk, and Marshal of England, Thomas of Beaufort, Duke of Exeter, W[illiam] Earl of Stafford, Mary Queen Dowager of France, daughter to King Henry the Seventh, and many other worthy personages there entombed; were by King Henry

---

9   John M. Blatchly, 'D'Ewes, Sir Simonds' in *ODNB*, vol. 16, pp. 1–4.
10 MacCulloch (1986), p. 325.
11 Thomson (1980), p. 5.
12 Duffy (2012), p. 235.
13 William Camden, *Britannia siue Florentissimorum regnorum, Angliae, Scotiae, Hiberniae, et insularum adiacentium ex intima antiquitate chorographica descriptio* (London, 1590), p. 359.
14 Ibid., p. 366.

the Eighth utterly overthrown. What time as at one clap he suppressed all monasteries … And yet there remaineth still lying along the carcass, as one would say, of that ancient monument, altogether deformed, but (for ruins I assure you) they make a fair and goodly show, which whosoever beholdeth, he may both wonder thereat, and withal take pity thereof.[15]

Camden also acknowledged that the legacy of the Abbey lingered in the jurisdictional peculiarity of the town of Bury's status as a peculiar of the archbishop of Canterbury: 'The Bishop of Rome … granted, That the said place should bee subject to no Bishop in any matter, and in matters lawfull depend upon the pleasure and direction of the Archbishop. Which is yet observed at this day.'[16]

Camden was the earliest author to describe the ruins of the Abbey, and it is likely that a great deal more was standing in the 1580s than is visible today. A royal grant of the site of the Abbey to John Eyre of 14 February 1560 mentioned a 'mansion-house', which was probably the old Abbot's Palace, along with 'the Dorter Court', 'the Garners', the Abbot's Stables, the 'Hay-house', the Gate House and Great Court, and the 'Pallaies Garden'. The grant also mentioned the King's Hall, the Chamberlain's office and Bradfield Hall as if they were still standing edifices.[17] Eyre did not remain long in possession, and on 1 March 1560 the site passed to Thomas Badby, who hosted Queen Elizabeth in the old Abbot's Palace in 1578 and supported the Puritan faction in town politics.

In 1580 Thomas Andrews, a leading governor of the Bury Grammar School, brought a Bill of Complaint against Badby in the Court of Chancery. Andrews complained that Badby had misused the churchyard and outbuildings of St James' and St Mary's 'in front of the ruined west front of the abbey church'. Badby was eventually dismissed as a justice of the peace from the county bench in 1582, which was a major setback for the Puritan faction.[18] In November 1581 Badby conveyed the Abbey site to Henry Blagge, Henry Grys and Richard Hunt, who in turn passed the property to Sir Robert Jermyn of Rushbrooke, a powerful member of the county gentry, in January 1592. In 1594 the Jermyns sold the property to the Cope family, who held it until 1623.[19]

The seventeenth-century antiquaries: Henry Spelman, John Weever and William Dugdale

In an age when the very memory of the past was charged with religious significance, it was almost inevitable that antiquaries contributed to the preservation of a reverence for the material remains of pre-Reformation religion. Antiquarianism was an activity that united as well as divided Catholics and Protestants. Duffy has drawn attention to the conformist authorship of several works that defended the monks and condemned the Reformation,[20] and during the Civil War and Interregnum (1642–60) Royalists rallied

---

15 Camden (1637), pp. 460–1.
16 Ibid., p. 60.
17 Yates (1843), pp. 245–6.
18 MacCulloch (1986), pp. 201–2.
19 Yates (1843), pp. 247–8.
20 Duffy (2012), pp. 247–50.

around antiquarian projects such as William Dugdale's *Monasticon*, since 'antiquaries did not believe that tradition was a deadening force in religion'.[21]

In the first half of the seventeenth century the Laudian party within the Church of England was increasingly embracing the medieval past in order to extend the church's authority over land and property. The most notable example of this development was the work of the antiquary Henry Spelman (c.1562–1641), whose *History and Fate of Sacrilege* condemned the owners of former monastic property and described their grisly fates. In addition to including ancient examples such as the death of the thegn Leofstan, punished for displaying the body of St Edmund,[22] Spelman described how a man he met while travelling in Suffolk recounted the violent deaths without issue of owners of monastic property.[23] These may well have included the owners of the Abbey precincts in Bury; between 1560 and 1720 only two owners managed to pass the property on to a son.[24] So controversial was Spelman's *History* that it did not appear in print until 1698.[25]

Spelman's principal contribution to the discovery of the Abbey's history, however, was his detailed description in verse of a painted copy of a stained glass window from the cellarer's lodgings. Spelman's Latin poem, entitled *Iconotypicon Buriense* ('the copy of the Bury picture'), was written in 1621 at the behest of the archbishop of Armagh, James Ussher, who was interested in the Antichrist. The window depicted the pope, whom seventeenth-century English Protestants identified as the Antichrist. According to Spelman, he saw the painted copy of the stained glass window at the shop of a London 'cutter' (engraver). 'A right honest old gentleman' told Spelman that he had seen the stained glass window in the Abbey itself, 'and the painter that took it out, did often tell me about forty years since'.[26] This would mean that the original window was still *in situ* in the early 1580s, suggesting that the cellarer's offices were still standing at that date.

Richard Yates paraphrased Spelman's poem:

> On this window was painted in a prophetic representation the true and false church, each distinguished by appropriate marks. On the upper part of the left compartment the Pope is seated on a splendid throne, robed in gold and purple, crowned with his triple diadem, the token of his threefold kingdom, Heaven, Earth, and Hell; and, lest he should appear a mortal, rays, the indication of Divinity, surround his temples. With his right hand he grasps the subjected world with its conquered kings, and with his left eagerly receives gifts. He is surrounded by the Church; Monks, Friars, Abbots, Priests, Anchorets, and those who admire the Roman trifles, bearing globes and crosses: the Cardinal alone is absent, because this order was then unknown. Kings and Peers kneel before his footstool; one presents a splendid gift, another money, and a third driven from his government resigns his crown. On another part they are paying gold, that their ancestors, redeemed from the dead, may enter Heaven, who therefore are seen

---

21 Parry (1995), p. 18.
22 Henry Spelman, *The History and Fate of Sacrilege* (London, 1698), p. 107.
23 Parry (1995), p. 282. On Spelman's *History* see Graham Parry, *The Arts of the Anglican Counter-Reformation* (Woodbridge: Boydell, 2006), pp. 171–6.
24 See Yates (1843), pp. 245–9.
25 On Spelman's attitudes to church property see Parry (1995), pp. 159–68.
26 Yates (1843), p. 182.

rising from the sepulchres. At his feet stands an executioner crowned with garlands and exulting in slaughter: near him a stupid friar preaching his impious dogmas; those around him, astonished, admire his inspiration with uplifted hands and eyes; an active demon flutters around his head, and applauds the lying prophet. Lower down, on the other side, is seen the aged Elias, in the open fields, on foot, uncovered, without pomp, without attendants, without flattery; he gives to the people the pure word received from Heaven, and brings back the erring flock to the fold of his Lord; he points out the causes of error, and declares the Scriptures to be the only way to salvation. The Romanists, lower down, oppose; one beats the ground with his feet, and, with his nose turned up, pretends that a stench proceeds from the holy lips; another stops his ears; and a third disregards the words of the Prophet. On the right stands the Apostle Paul, and below him Malachi, each with a label, and the passage from the Epistle to the Thessalonians, foretelling the falling away of True Religion and the appearing of the Man of Sin.[27] At the top, over the triple head of Antichrist, ascribed to the Pope, that a deceiving Church should make the world drunk with lascivious cups. Below, the hoary Malachi the ambassador of divine love foretells that the great day shall come, when the Almighty shall overwhelm the world with flames;[28] but first that a little flock shall be saved, and points to Elias, and under that form, a church separated from the Roman and giving the people the doctrines of a Reformed word.[29]

Spelman regarded the copy of the medieval stained glass window as 'prophetic' (*praescia*) because he chose to apply a seventeenth-century Protestant interpretation to scenes that cannot possibly have been intended to represent what Spelman saw. There is no reason to suppose, from what Spelman describes, that the maker of the window intended to represent the pope negatively, even if the preaching friar is inspired by a demon (and this would hardly be surprising given the Abbey's antipathy to the friars). Nor did Spelman have any good reason to believe that the figure of Elijah was intended as a contrast to the pope, nor that the people objecting to Elijah are 'Romanists'. It is more probable that they were supposed to be Jews failing to heed the words of their own prophet. However, in spite of his bizarre interpretation of the window as a confirmation of Protestant doctrine, Spelman preserved some idea of what it was like.

Another example of Latin literature inspired by the remains of the Abbey was a poem written some time before 1634 by William Hawkins, master of Hadleigh Grammar School, describing his experience as a juror at the Bury St Edmunds quarter sessions (then held in the old St Margaret's Church at the southeast corner of the churchyard). During a lull in the proceedings, Hawkins took a stroll in the ruins of the Abbey:[30]

---

27 II Thessalonians 2:3: 'Let no man deceive you by any means: for that day shall not come, except there come a falling away first, and that man of sin be revealed, the son of perdition'.
28 Perhaps Malachi 3:2: 'But who may abide the day of his coming? and who shall stand when he appeareth? for he is like a refiner's fire, and like fullers' soap'.
29 Yates (1843), p. 181.
30 William Hawkins, 'Musae Juridicae' in *Corolla Varia* (Cambridge, 1634), pp. 47–50: *Interea ... / A turbis quoties horamque animumq[ue] vacantem / Sevocat, in clausi spatiatur proxima campi. / Heu campos ubi Troja fuit! Ferit undiq[ue] squalor / Saxorum miserorum, & lamentabile funus. / Nec satis est lustrasse semel : meditatus easdem / Itque reditque vias. Oculo miserante ruinas*

> Meanwhile ... as often as he calls away an unoccupied hour and mind from the crowd, he strolls into the nearby area of the enclosed open space .... The squalor of wretched stones and lamentable destruction strike the eye .... 'This once flourished, he said, as the most revered among the honoured seats of the monks'. Behold, what remnants of a seat so conspicuous, so powerful with land and wealth ... fragments that would not give admission to the stone-breaking pickaxe. So great a task was it to demolish the close-knit mass. Along with the entrances but little else remains, but it does survive so that the spectator may estimate the limbs of Hercules from his foot ... instead of columns constructed with such Daedalean art, instead of so many tombs of noblemen and abbots [lit. wearers of the mitre], he finds nothing but nettles. Above all, he seeks what is the place of the bones of King Edmund. The bones, visited by so many prayers of their worshippers and enriched by so many gifts are nowhere .... Flame has devoured them: the winds that sweep all things away have blown them away. Blind superstition has thus been duly buried. But why should horrid devastation, an impious avenger, have ruined temples well-adapted for sacred rites, which pious minds and generous hands constructed in great numbers throughout the whole kingdom?[31]

Hawkins's moralistic tone was typical of post-Reformation commentators on monastic ruins, and his poem should be seen in a tradition of stylised neo-Latin poetry inspired by melancholy remains of antiquity. As such, its usefulness for shedding any light on the state of the ruins at the time is limited.

Another likely antiquarian visitor to the Abbey ruins in the 1620s was John Weever, whose *Ancient Funerall Monuments* was published in 1631. As the title of Weever's book suggests, his primary interest was in the great men and women buried in the Abbey Church, whose destruction he deplored on account of the fact that it included the destruction of their resting places.[32] Weever was a native of Lancashire who toured the dioceses of Canterbury, Rochester, London and Norwich in search of monumental inscriptions to illuminate English history. Duffy has noted that while Weever was well disposed towards the monks in general, he regarded their later history as one of decline and therefore had little interest in the last phase of monasticism, but rather what the monks preserved of an earlier, purer age.[33]

Weever's concern about the desecration of tombs is poignant, given that the outbreak

---

/ *Antiquati operis, Monachoru[m] haec floruit, inquit,* / *Inter honoratas olim Augustissima Sedes.* / *De tam conspicua, fundisque opibusque potenti,* / *En quas relliquias! Quam pauca cadaveris ossa* / *Fragmina murorum, scopulis aequanda marinis,* / *Fragmina saxifragum non admissura ligonem!* / *Tantae molis erat compactam excindere molem.* / *Cum prothyris pauxilla manent. Sed & illa supersunt,* / *Ex pede ut Herculeos spectator judicet artus.* / ... / *Pergit & indagans magnivestigia Templi,* / *Pro tam Daedaleâ fabricatis arte columnis,* / *Pro tot Nobilium Mitratorumque sepulchris,* / *Urticas reperit. Quaerit super omnia, Regis* / *Ossibus Edmundi quisnam locus. Ossa colentum* / *Tot votis ambita diu, tot ditia donis* / *(Ipsum Ubi vix restat) nusquam sunt. Flamma momordit:* / *Diffla[ver]unt cinerem, qui verrunt omnia, venti.* / *Caeca superstitio sic rite sepulta. Quid autem* / *Commoda Templa sacris, toto plurima regno* / *Mens pia, larga manus construxerat, improba vindex* / *Vastities uno pessundaret horrida flatu?*

31 I am indebted to John Trappes-Lomax for his advice on this translation.
32 John Weever, *Ancient Funerall Monuments* (London, 1631), pp. 721–5.
33 Duffy (2012), pp. 251–3. On Weever see Parry (1995), pp. 190–216.

of Civil War and the enforcement of Puritan worship in East Anglia led to renewed attacks on supposedly 'superstitious' monuments. Pre-Reformation brasses in Suffolk churches were a particular target of iconoclasts if they featured inscriptions asking for prayers for a person's soul or figures in Catholic vestments. In 1643 the brass of Abbot Reeve in his pontifical vestments, along with his epitaph, was removed for these reasons, and a further indignity was perpetrated against the Abbot in around 1745 when a ship's purser, 'one Sutton', was buried in his place in front of the high altar of St Mary's. The antiquary William Cole, walking in the churchyard with James Burrough in 1746, was horrified to discover the Abbot's new tomb 'laid by the entrance into the South porch'.[34] The Victorians put a new ledger stone commemorating the Abbot before the high altar, and presumably restored his remains to their original position as well.

If Spelman and Weever had shown some sympathy for the medieval past, William Dugdale was the first antiquary to take 'an unprejudiced view of the Middle Ages', approaching medieval sources largely on their own terms.[35] He served as a herald in the College of Arms, devoting his time to antiquarian research, and his crowning achievement was an immense three-volume survey of all the monastic houses of England, the Latin *Monasticon Anglicanum* (1655–73). Begun before the restoration of the monarchy in 1660, Dugdale's work was at least partly an antiquarian protest against the Reformation and the further destruction of England's churches wrought by the Puritans.

Dugdale relied heavily on the manuscript collections of a fellow high churchman, Roger Dodsworth, as the basis for the *Monasticon*, which did not follow any particular geographical order but proceeded by religious order, starting with the Benedictines. The key materials reproduced and cited in the *Monasticon* were monastic charters, although other documents also featured including accounts of the lives of the English saints to whom the monasteries were dedicated. The *Monasticon*'s unprejudiced presentation of the evidence caused considerable controversy, leading to accusations that it was intended to make Catholicism palatable.[36] St Edmunds featured in the second volume.

In contrast to other Protestant antiquaries, who tended to view the arrival of the monks as a sign of decline, Dugdale's assessment of the secular clerks who originally ran the shrine of St Edmund was a negative one. He made no mention of the fact that in 1010, they were sufficiently concerned for the safety of the saint's body that they moved it to London. Dugdale was the first historian to quote the supposed charter of King Edmund granting the *banleuca* to the Abbey in 945, even correctly transcribing the Old English sections from the manuscript in the Bodleian Library. Further charters followed, along with the *Testes corporis S. Edmundi incorrupti* ('Witnesses of the incorrupt body of St Edmund') copied from Leland's collections.[37] The lists of donations to the monastery and Abbots came from the same source,[38] and Dugdale's collection concluded with a lengthy charter of Edward III concerning the rights of the Abbot and convent, a list of sacrists and a document on the rights of the cellarer.[39]

---

34 Yates (1843), p. 223.
35 Parry (1995), p. 217.
36 On Dugdale's *Monasticon* see Parry (1995), pp. 227–36.
37 William Dugdale, *Monasticon Anglicanum* (London, 1655–73), vol. 2, pp. 293–4.
38 Ibid., pp. 294–6.
39 Ibid., pp. 297–302.

Antiquitates S. Edmundi Burgi.

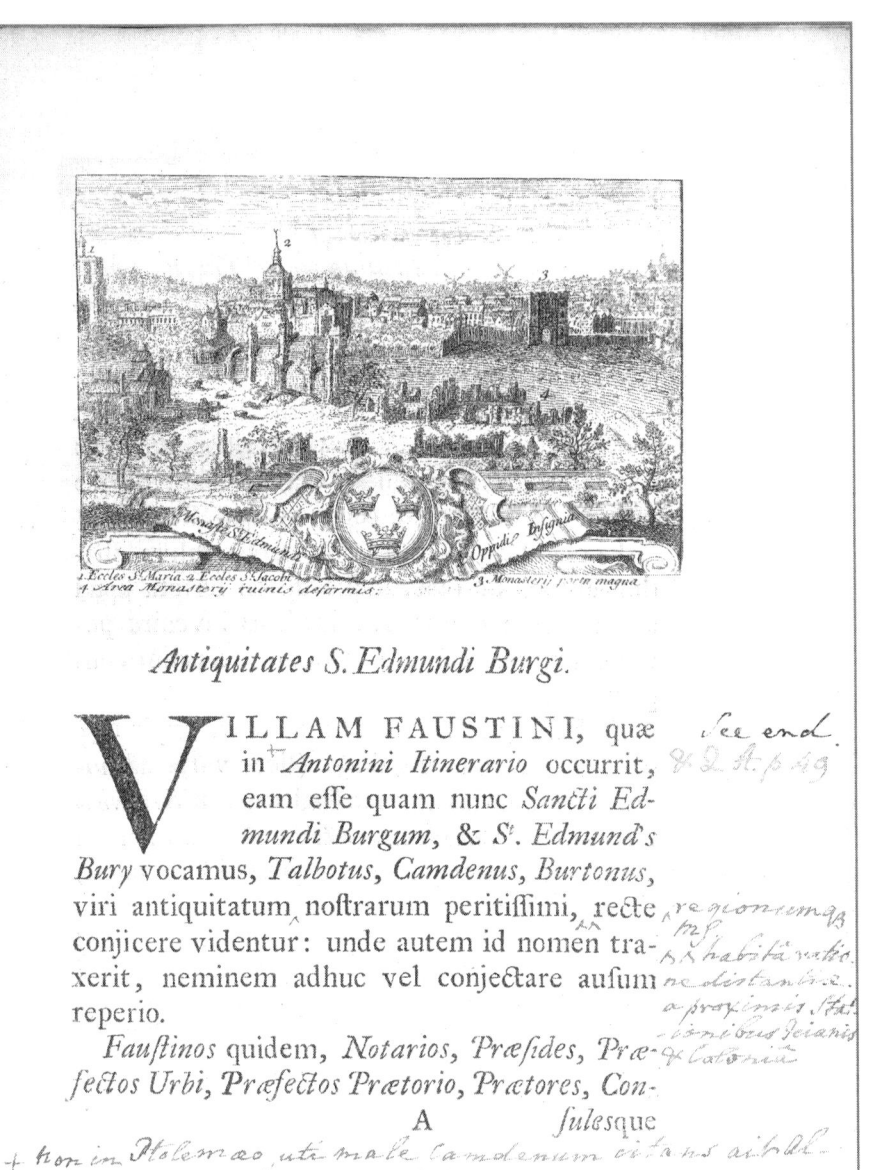

VILLAM FAUSTINI, quæ in †*Antonini Itinerario* occurrit, eam esse quam nunc *Sancti Edmundi Burgum*, & *S*ᵗ. *Edmund's Bury* vocamus, *Talbotus, Camdenus, Burtonus*, viri antiquitatum nostrarum peritissimi, recte conjicere videntur: unde autem id nomen traxerit, neminem adhuc vel conjectare ausum reperio.

Faustinos quidem, *Notarios*, *Præsides*, *Præfectos Urbi*, *Præfectos Prætorio*, *Prætores*, *Consulesque*

Figure 36 Opening page of John Battely's *Antiquitates S. Edmundi Burgi* (1745) with annotations in the hand of George Ashby

John Battely

John Battely (1646–1708) can be considered the father of the historical study of the Abbey of Bury St Edmunds, although his important contribution was not published until long after his death. Battely was born in Bury and his family was native to Suffolk. He enjoyed the patronage of William Sancroft, who was archbishop of Canterbury between 1677 and 1691 and who also came from an old Suffolk family related to the Battelys. Both men attended the Bury Grammar School. In 1688 Battely was appointed archdeacon of Canterbury. His Suffolk connections and association with Archbishop Sancroft and his successor, Archbishop Thomas Tenison, gave him access to archival material in a number of different locations in the late 1680s and early 1690s when he is likely to have conducted most of his research on the Abbey. Battely was a founding member of the Society of Antiquaries of London, and his work on the Roman forts of Kent, *Antiquitates Rutupinae*, was well received when it appeared in 1711.

Battely died before he had a chance to complete his Latin work on Bury, entitled *Antiquitates S. Edmundi Burgi ad Annum MCCLXXII perductae*. The unfinished work eventually appeared in print in 1745 under the joint editorship of Battely's nephew Oliver Battely and the master of Gonville and Caius College, Cambridge, James Burrough (1691–1764). Burrough, who was also a native of Bury and is best known for his design of the Senate House in Cambridge, provided the illustrations for *Antiquitates* and commissioned George Vertue (1686–1756) to engrave them.[40] I have argued elsewhere that Battely stopped work on his *Antiquitates* in 1691–92.[41] He was writing, therefore, at a time of crisis for the Church of England, when the clergy were being forced to choose between swearing a new oath of allegiance to William and Mary (who were crowned king and queen in 1689) and maintaining the sanctity of an oath they had already taken to a still-living monarch, James II.

Archbishop Sancroft, Battely's patron, chose to give up everything to maintain the sacredness of his oath, and ended his life stripped of his honours, living in retirement in rural Suffolk. Battely himself proved more flexible; to support his antiquarian interests he needed a guaranteed income from the benefices and offices he held in plurality. Battely's St Edmund, like William and Mary, is an elected monarch,[42] and in another echo of the age, Battely portrayed the introduction of Benedictine monks to the management of St Edmund's shrine as its downfall, although he praised the secular clergy for their care of the saint's body.[43]

After an extensive introductory chapter examining the earliest origins of Bury St Edmunds and the veracity of the story of St Edmund's martyrdom (Battely was an early sceptic), Battely then gave brief accounts of the first fifteen Abbots from Ufi to Simon of Luton, although it was the appendices Battely's editors provided that were most valuable to subsequent authors.[44] The editors even provided a list of the remaining Abbots and an account of the manuscripts used and their current owners.[45] Vertue provided the first

---

40 Young (2008), pp. 472–3.
41 Ibid., p. 468.
42 Battely (1745), pp. 21–2.
43 Ibid., pp. 36–8.
44 Ibid., pp. 115–60.
45 Ibid., pp. 161–3.

published ground plan of the Abbey Church, which was based on a fifteenth-century description by William Worcestre,[46] as well as a large engraving of the old Abbot's Palace. However, the utility of Battely's contribution to local history was limited because he wrote in Latin for a learned academic audience.

The old Abbot's Palace was one of the last surviving buildings of the monastic complex, since it was turned into a private house after the Reformation. In 1685 the Palace passed into the possession of the Jesuits after the monks of St Edmund's, Paris turned down the chance to buy it. The Jesuits established a school, which existed until late November 1688 when a mob attacked 'the Mass house in the Abby Yard' and pulled it down following news of the Prince of Orange's landing in England.[47] However, although the Palace was damaged on this occasion it was not completely destroyed. James Burrough made a drawing of it in 1720 which was later reproduced as an engraving in Battely's *Antiquitates*, and as late as 1728 the Jesuits returned to Bury in search of books left behind in the Palace. However, it likely that the Palace had been pulled down by this time.[48]

Popular antiquarianism

The eighteenth century was the golden age of English antiquarianism, and although a taste for Classical antiquities predominated, there was also a great deal of interest in England's medieval past. By the second half of the century, an increasingly educated middle class with the freedom and means to travel was creating a considerable demand for affordable vernacular guidebooks. The man who responded to this demand in Bury was George Ashby (1724–1808), the rector of Barrow. The first edition of his *Description of the Ancient and Present State of the Town and Abbey of Bury St. Edmund's, in the County of Suffolk* appeared in 1769, and since it ran to only 82 pages it was easily portable. Ashby took Battely's *Antiquitates* as his starting point,[49] but continued a narrative of the history of town and Abbey down to the plague of 1636. The second half of the book featured an account of benefactions to the Abbey,[50] a list of famous persons buried there,[51] and a list of the Abbots.[52] Finally, the book featured descriptions of the two parish churches and other buildings,[53] and an account of modern benefactors to the town.[54]

In spite of antiquarian interest in the ruins, their deliberate destruction continued into the eighteenth century. On 20 February 1772 workmen demolishing part of the church accidentally discovered the body of Thomas Beaufort, the third son of John of Gaunt

---

46   For this description see William Worcestre (ed. John H. Harvey), *Itineraries of William Worcestre* (Oxford: Clarendon Press, 1969), pp. 161–3.
47   Young (2015a), p. 66.
48   Young (2006), p. 217.
49   Ashby's heavily annotated copy of Battely's *Antiquitates* is in the present author's possession; Ashby disagreed primarily with Battely's interpretation of the evidence for a Roman settlement at or near Bury.
50   George Ashby, *A Description of the Ancient and Present State of the Town and Abbey of Bury St. Edmund's, in the County of Suffolk*, 2nd edn (Bury St Edmunds, 1771), pp. 24–35.
51   Ibid., pp. 35–6.
52   Ibid., pp. 37–40.
53   Ibid., pp. 43–58.
54   Ibid., pp. 58–78.

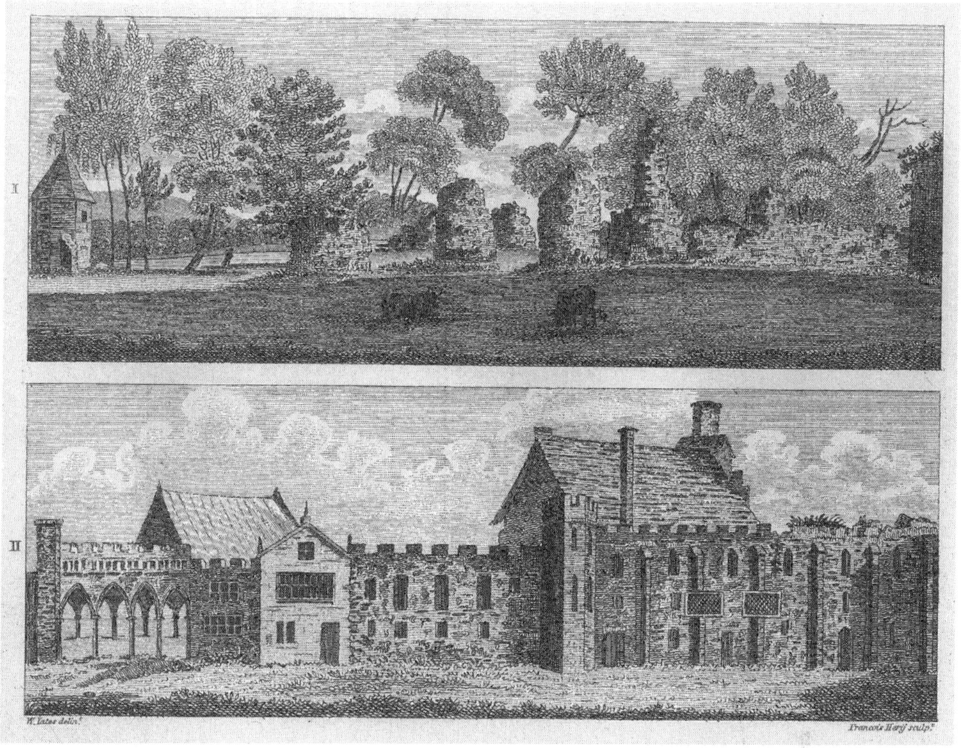

Figure 37 The hand of time: the Abbot's Palace in 1804 (top) and 1720 (bottom). Engraving from Richard Yates, *An Illustration of the Monastic Antiquities of the Town and Abbey of St Edmund's Bury* (1843), plate facing p. 44.

(d. 1427), 'near the wall on the left-hand side of the Choir of the Chapel of the Blessed Virgin, not enclosed in a vault, but covered over with common earth'. Thomas Beaufort, as Exeter, is a key character in Shakespeare's plays *Henry V* and *Henry VI Part 1*. It seems likely that he was buried at Bury because he was an honorary member of the confraternity. The workmen realised they could sell the lead coffin, and removed the body and 'threw it promiscuously amongst the rubbish'. However, the body was unusually well preserved, and a local surgeon and antiquary, Thomas Gery Cullum, took an interest and sawed up the skull and cut the arms off below the elbows. The remains were eventually reburied among the ruins, but Beaufort's hands, preserved by Cullum in alcohol, are still in the collection of the Royal College of Surgeons.[55] The discovery even attracted the attention of the Royal Society.[56]

The discovery of Beaufort's body was fortuitous, as it seems to have stimulated the

---

55 C. J. S. Thompson, 'The hands of Thomas Beaufort, third son of John of Gaunt', *British Medical Journal* 1:3562 (13 April 1929), pp. 701–2.

56 Charles Collignon, 'Some account of a body lately found in uncommon preservation, under the ruins of the Abbey, at St. Edmund's-Bury, Suffolk; with some reflections upon the subject', *Transactions of the Royal Society* 62 (1772), pp. 465–8.

antiquary Edward King into making a thorough examination of the ruins in order to correct errors in the plan drawn up by Sir James Burrough included in the 1745 edition of Battely's *Antiquitates*. King read his paper to the Society of Antiquaries on 3 February 1774. He indicated that some sort of surface excavations, at the very least, took place in the summer of 1772, since he remarked that the ruins 'were laid quite open to the view the summer before last'. Simon of Luton's Lady Chapel was discovered: 'a large chapel on the north side of the choir', where Beaufort was found buried.[57] On 26 January 1775 King read a second paper to the Society of Antiquaries, reporting on a lead seal discovered in the ruins and a fragment of an inscription, apparently from the tomb of John Lydgate, discovered in the area of the crypt.[58]

In 1804 a stationer and bookseller from Harleston, Edmund Gillingwater (1736–1804), published *An Historical and Descriptive Study of St. Edmund's Bury, in the County of Suffolk*, which was considerably longer than Ashby's brief guide (at 311 pages). However, as John Blatchly observed, the book 'breaks little new ground',[59] although it featured such fashionable additions as a list of plants found in the vicinity of the town.[60] Both Ashby and Gillingwater relied almost exclusively on Battely and other historical sources for their account of the Abbey and made little or no effort to consider its physical remains, a task that was left to Richard Yates (1769–1834).

Yates was born in one of the seventeenth-century houses built into the Abbey's west front. His father Richard Yates the elder (1741–1803) was an employee of the Marquess of Bristol, the owner of the ruins, and showed visitors around for a small fee. However, Richard the elder was also an amateur historian and, on his death in 1803, his son (by now a clergyman of the Church of England) 'undertook to enlarge, edit, and publish his father's extensive drawings and notes on the history of the abbey'. Richard was assisted by his younger brother William (1774–1830), who was also a clergyman and a schoolmaster at Shacklewell. It was William who measured out the ruins of the Abbey Church and created the first ground plan of the building based on observation.[61] Richard Yates's *Illustration of the Monastic History and Antiquities of the Town and Abbey of St. Edmund's Bury* appeared in 1805, but was incomplete, and when Richard died in 1834 the rest of his work was still unpublished.

Yates's *History and Antiquities of the Abbey of St. Edmund's Bury* finally appeared in 1843, with the earlier work published as an addendum. It was the first attempt at a truly comprehensive history of the Abbey, although at the time of its publication Yates's historical scholarship had already been superseded in some respects by that of another Suffolk antiquary, John Gage-Rokewode (1786–1842). Gage-Rokewode was the fourth son of Sir Thomas Rookwood Gage, sixth baronet of Hengrave, the leading Catholic gentleman of Suffolk. He trained as a barrister but never practised, and in 1829 he became drector of the

---

57 Edward King, 'Remarks on the Abbey Church of Bury St. Edmund's in Suffolk', *Archaeologia* 3 (1775), pp. 311–15, at p. 312.
58 Edward King, 'An account of the Great Seal of Ranulph Earl of Chester; and of two ancient inscriptions found in the ruins of St. Edmund Bury Abbey', *Archaeologia* 4 (1786), pp. 119–31.
59 John M. Blatchly, 'Gillingwater, Edmund (*bap.* 1736, *d.* 1813)' in *ODNB*, vol. 22, pp. 287–8.
60 Edmund Gillingwater, *An Historical and Descriptive Study of St. Edmund's Bury, in the County of Suffolk* (Bury St Edmunds: J. Rackham, 1804), pp. 283–97.
61 Yates (1843), facing p. 34.

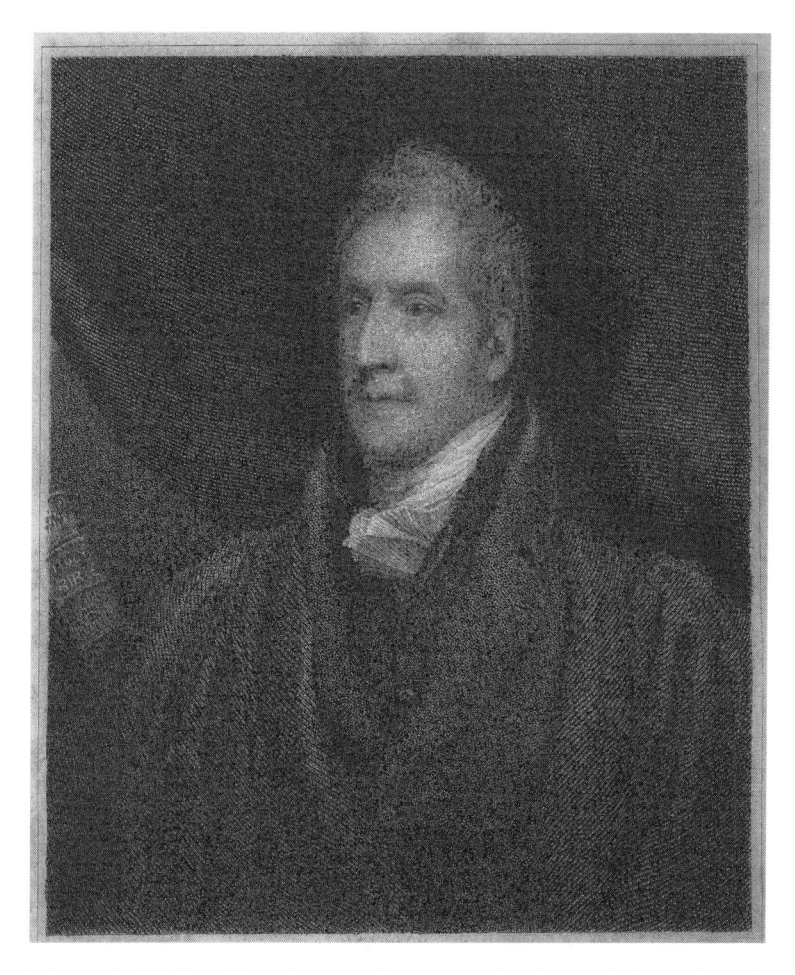

Figure 38 Portrait of Richard Yates, from *An Illustration of the Monastic Antiquities of the Town and Abbey of St Edmund's Bury* (1843), facing frontispiece

Society of Antiquaries of London. On the death of his elder brother Thomas Gage, seventh baronet, John inherited his extensive papers on the history of Suffolk and Hengrave Hall in particular, and eventually created a book from them, *The History and Antiquities of Hengrave*, in 1822. However, Gage-Rokewode's abiding ambition was to produce a multi-volume history of Suffolk by hundreds – although he only completed the first volume, on Thingoe Hundred, which was published in 1838. In the same year Gage-Rokewode inherited Hengrave Hall from his brother Robert.[62]

Although Gage-Rokewode's *Thingoe Hundred* was an important contribution to the Abbey's history, including as it did a comprehensive account of the Abbey's landholdings in the area, his edition of Jocelin de Brakelond's *Chronicle* (1840) for the Camden Society

---

62 Thompson Cooper (rev. John M. Blatchly), 'Rokewode, John Gage' in *ODNB*, vol. 47, pp. 605–6.

attracted more attention. As Yates's cursory treatment of Abbot Samson shows, Bury's most famous Abbot was little known before Gage-Rokewode's publication, which enthralled the essayist Thomas Carlyle with its lifelike and characterful portrayal of Tottington's greatest son. Carlyle accordingly visited Bury, where he was greatly impressed by the ruins, and his volume *Past and Present* (1843) included an extended historico-political meditation on Jocelin.[63] Carlyle was uncomplimentary of Gage-Rokewode's 'dryasdust' antiquarianism, and seemed surprised that he himself had enjoyed reading Jocelin's *Chronicle* so much. More than anything else, however, Carlyle was determined to emphasise that the modern town of Bury St Edmunds was a mere remnant in comparison with the Abbey's former glory:

> All this that now thou seest, and namest Bury Town, is properly the Funeral Monument of Saint or Landlord Edmund. The present respectable Mayor of Bury may be said, like a Fakeer (little as he thinks of it), to have his dwelling in the extensive, many-coloured Tombstone of St. Edmund; in one of the brick niches thereof dwells the present respectable Mayor of Bury.[64]

Carlyle felt the immense weight of history as he looked upon the Abbey ruins: 'Alas, how like an old osseous fragment, a broken blackened shin-bone of the old dead Ages, this black ruin looks out, not yet covered by the soil; still indicating what a once gigantic Life lies buried there!'[65] Carlyle gave his account a political edge, portraying St Edmund as a ruler determined to uphold tradition and order against 'certain Heathen Physical-Force Ultra-Chartists',[66] thereby comparing the Danes to political radicals of the early nineteenth century. In Alice Chandler's view, Carlyle admired Abbot Samson's capacity for hero-worship of Edmund even if he could not share Samson's faith.[67] *Past and Present*, reprinted numerous times, was far more widely read than the work of antiquaries like Yates and Gage-Rokewode would ever be, and it made Samson famous. It seems likely that it was Carlyle's effusive prose rather than the painstaking work of the Yates family that set the stage for the expansion of historical interest in the Abbey in the second half of the nineteenth century.

Archaeology and imagination

In 1849 John Darkin, clerk of works to the restoration of St James' Church, carried out excavations of the east end of the Abbey and monastic buildings near the river,[68] creating a plan which was supplemented in 1865 when Graham Hills made and published new measurements of the ruins,[69] which were the private property of the marquess of Bristol. However, Hills undertook no excavations. Meanwhile, the history of the Abbey became the inspiration for more fanciful speculations by Margaretta Katherine Greene, who lived

---

63   Carlyle (1843), pp. 34–116.
64   Ibid., p. 49.
65   Ibid., p. 42.
66   Ibid., pp. 46–7.
67   Alice Chandler, *A Dream of Order: The Medieval Ideal in Nineteenth Century English Literature* (London: Routledge & Kegan Paul, 1971), pp. 141–4.
68   Whittingham (1952), p. 169.
69   Hills (1865), pp. 32–46, 104–40.

in one of the houses built into the Abbey's west front. Greene was born in the west front on 29 May 1837, the daughter of John Greene (d. 1867). After her father's death she carried on living in the Abbey ruins until 1883, when her failing health obliged her to move to Clifton. She died at Bulmer on 13 February 1889 and her body was brought back to Bury for a funeral at St James's Church. Her obituary noted that 'many of our readers will remember the clever story called *The Secret Disclosed*, which, though only privately printed, was largely circulated, and invested the ancient Abbey Ruins with a romance, which has never since left them.'[70]

The Secret Disclosed: A legend of St Edmund's Abbey, by 'an Inmate', was privately (and anonymously) printed for Greene by the Bury printer Samuel Gross in 1861. Following the romantic narrative fashion of the time, Greene presented her work of fiction as a genuine historical narrative, and it was quickly accepted into local folklore. Greene began with an account of her family's ghostly experiences in the west front:

> The nave of the once splendid church of St. Edmund is now a garden, in which the old remains form a most interesting feature. The ancient refectory in which so many historical scenes have been presented, contains at the present time chiefly gooseberry bushes and vegetables. Within the remains of the West front of the church, stands the old rambling house, which is called 'The Abbey Ruins.' From its situation it might reasonably be supposed to be haunted, and I can assert as facts several strange phenomena connected with it. Every night, at eleven o'clock, a deep, dull sound is heard repeated several times, like a foot heavily stamping on the ground. No cause which might account for it has ever been discovered. But it is a still more remarkable fact that, at times the numerous family, who occupy the house have, when assembled, been startled by the sound of a footstep flitting across the room, and become conscious that something was passing, although nothing whatever could be seen.[71]

Greene's story then turned into fiction, as she recounted her imaginary discovery of a manuscript in a hidden recess:

> In the house is a secret chamber, the existence of which has long been known to the inhabitants of the dwelling. We all remember a vague sense of mystery connected with it in our childhood. A few weeks ago, in the course of some necessary repairs this secret room was opened, and we all explored it. One visit I paid to it alone. The carpenter had gone to his dinner, but had left his tools. I felt an irresistible impulse to examine carefully every part of the ruinous walls and dark recesses. My eye was caught by a cavity in the wall, which had been disclosed by the workmen having knocked off a projecting stone. I peeped in, and thinking I saw something which was neither stone nor mortar, I took up the hammer and with some difficulty enlarged the hole and extracted from it

---

70 A copy of Greene's obituary from an unidentified newspaper is pasted into the flyleaf of the copy of *The Secret Disclosed* in the Rare Books Room of Cambridge University Library, classmark 1861.8.108.

71 [Margaretta K. Greene], *The Secret Disclosed: a legend of St Edmund's Abbey* (Bury St Edmunds: Samuel Gross, 1861), pp. 4–5.

a small metal box. My delight and curiosity may be imagined; I hurried away with my treasure to my own room. I feared I might not be able to open it, but it yielded at once to a slight pressure, and contained – not money or jewels as I had hoped – but an old manuscript clearly written and beautifully illuminated. It was in antiquated English, but by slow degrees I read and understood it all.[72]

The story, set in 1447, features a nun called Maud Carewe who is duped by Cardinal Beaufort into killing Duke Humphrey and then herself. The Abbey ruins finally had their own ghost: 'There is but one day and one hour in the year when [Maud's] form will sometimes be perceived. It is on the 24th of February, *one hour before midnight*. She will be seen wandering restlessly through the ruins of the old church where she was buried.'[73]

Modern investigations

In 1886 a rather more factual account of the Abbey Church than Greene's was published by Edward M. Dewing, *Saint Edmund's Bury: The Abbey Church and Monastery*, although at 44 pages it was little more than a short guide.[74] A crucial contribution to the history of the Abbey came in 1890 when the first two volumes of Thomas Arnold's *Memorials of St Edmund's Abbey* appeared as part of *Rerum Britannicarum Medii Aevi Scriptores*, known as the 'Rolls Series'. The aim was to provide authoritative editions of medieval texts, most of them in Latin. Arnold (1823–1900), who was the third son of the celebrated headmaster of Rugby School whose name he shared, converted to Catholicism in 1856, and by 1890 was living in Dublin as a retired professor of University College.[75] Arnold drew attention to the shortcomings of Carlyle's exclusive focus on Jocelin's *Chronicle*, and explained the rationale for his own project:

> I propose to use the more varied materials here offered to the reader in the same general spirit, and while describing – or rather allowing them to speak for themselves, – the founders and continuators, the ruling ideas and cardinal institutions of St. Edmund's Abbey, to trace the deeply interesting historic sequence connecting by an unbroken chain the age of our great Alfred with the times of Luther and Sir Thomas More.[76]

The final volume of Arnold's *Memorials* appeared in 1896. Meanwhile, the Cambridge antiquary Montague Rhodes James was engaged in ground-breaking work on the Abbey in the public library of Douai, in northern France. In addition to being the home of the refounded monastery of St Edmund's, the town of Douai had been the home of the English College since the 1560s, an institution founded by Cardinal William Allen for the education of English Catholic priests. It was also the home of another English Benedictine monastery, St Gregory's, from 1606, together with a number of other English Catholic

---

72 Ibid., p. 5.
73 Ibid.
74 Edward M. Dewing, *Saint Edmund's Bury: The Abbey Church and Monastery* (Bury St Edmunds: F. T. Groom, 1886).
75 Bernard Bergonzi, 'Arnold, Thomas (1823–1900)' in *ODNB*, vol. 2, pp. 505–7.
76 Arnold (1890–96), vol. 1, p. iv.

institutions. As a consequence of its status as a centre for English Catholic exiles, many medieval English manuscripts found their way to Douai, and on the suppression of the colleges and religious houses in 1793, these manuscripts ended up in the public library.

James was apparently the first English antiquary who thought of looking for previously undiscovered material on the Abbey in France. He had a longstanding interest in Bury, having spent his early years at the rectory in Great Livermere. James was elected a fellow of King's College, Cambridge in 1886; in the same year he became deputy director of the Fitzwilliam Museum, and director in 1889. In 1892 he published the first attempt to elucidate the mutilated sculpture cycle in the Lady Chapel of Ely Cathedral. James's first Bury-related breakthrough came when he discovered, in the College of Arms in London, 'a miscellaneous collection of material from the tenth to the fourteenth centuries made by the Bury monk, John of Everisdun' (College of Arms, Arundel MS xxx). James noticed that in the early fourteenth century someone had copied down inscriptions from wall-paintings, altar pieces, stained glass windows and tapestries in English churches. Most were from the Abbey of St Edmund, and therefore this document gave a very good indication of the layout of the Abbey as well as the treasures it contained.[77]

Then, in Douai's municipal archives, James discovered the *Liber coenobii S. Edmundi* ('Book of the Monks of St Edmunds'), dating from around 1424, which contained the *Registrum Coquinarie* (Douai, Bibliotheque Publique 553), a register compiled by the obedientary in charge of the Abbey's kitchens (the kitchener), Andrew Astone.[78] Using this document, James was able to reconstruct an imaginary tour of the Abbey as well as pinpointing the burial places of eighteen Abbots. In 1895 the Cambridge Antiquarian Society published a two-volume monograph by James, *On the Abbey of S. Edmund at Bury*, which featured a preliminary catalogue of surviving books from the monastic library in the first volume, and James's 'tour', based on the *Registrum Coquinarie* and other sources, in the second.

James's work immediately attracted the attention of a local historian, Sir Ernest Clarke (1856–1923), who had been appointed the University of Cambridge's first lecturer in agricultural history in 1896.[79] Clarke was especially intrigued by James's identification of the tombs of Abbots in the Chapter House, concluding that if the site of the Chapter House could be successfully identified, the bodies of the Abbots (including the famous Samson) could be found. Accordingly, in 1902 Clarke negotiated with the owner of the site, the marquess of Bristol, for permission to excavate with the help of the Suffolk Institute of Archaeology (although the latter body 'was rather inclined to drag its feet').[80] As director of the Fitzwilliam Museum James was formally in charge of the excavations, but he did not see them until Christmas 1902.

Then, early in 1903, the excavators discovered the tombs of six Abbots arranged perpendicularly along the middle of the Chapter House floor. The discovery was announced in *The Times* on 3 January 1903, and it excited so much interest that the marquess of Bristol's agent had the remains removed from the coffins in which they were found and placed in

---

77 Richard W. Pfaff, *Montague Rhodes James* (London: Scolar Press, 1980), p. 137.
78 James (1895), p. 95. The manuscript contained the names of two later owners, Robert Wode and John Smith of London.
79 'Obituary: Sir Ernest Clarke', *The Times* 43282 (6 March 1923), p. 16E.
80 Pfaff (1980), p. 139.

secure numbered boxes. The bones were reinterred on 27 January, at which point some of them were very nearly mixed up.[81] James identified the Abbots based on their position of burial, and ledger slabs inscribed with their names were eventually placed over the reinterred remains, which can still be seen by visitors to the Abbey ruins today. A mount of silver-gilt recovered from Abbot Samson's crozier can also be seen in the treasury of St Edmundsbury Cathedral.

Buoyed up by the success of the Chapter House excavation, the Abbey Excavating Committee pushed for a full investigation of the east end of the Abbey, but it seems likely that funds ran out. In March 1905 Clarke was still hoping that James might explore the crypt, but James's biographer Richard Pfaff concluded that the two men fell out. James found Clarke 'increasingly tiresome', and he was annoyed that Clarke's new translation of Jocelin's *Chronicle* (1903), which James himself had suggested, contained so many errors.[82] In 1912 St Edmundsbury Borough Council leased the Abbey ruins from the marquess of Bristol, but no further excavations took place for decades, even though James observed in 1936, the year of his death, that 'no monastic site in England needs investigation more or, probably, would repay it better'.[83]

In the absence of archaeology, one local amateur fell back on less conventional methods. During the 1930s the rector of Risby, Archibald Webling, employed a psychic medium in order to communicate with the souls of dead monks, and thought he had discovered the final resting place of St Edmund as well as much new 'information' about the layout of the Abbey. Based on the 'communications' he received, Webling wrote an historical novel based on the life of Abbot Reeve, *The Last Abbot* (1944).[84] The Council commissioned excavations of the Prior's House and part of the Infirmary in 1933–34,[85] but the Second World War then intervened, and it was not until December 1948 that the curator of Moyse's Hall Museum, H. J. M. Maltby, investigated the west end of the crypt.[86] In April 1951 the archaeologist Arthur Whittingham, for whom the site had long been 'too unintelligible', began working on a new plan of the Abbey buildings by examining the Chapter House, the only building whose location was then known with certainty.[87] Slowly but surely, Whittingham pieced together what is still the definitive plan of the entire Abbey.[88]

In 1953 St Edmundsbury Borough Council finally acquired the freehold of the Abbey Gardens. At long last, the townsfolk were in possession of the Abbey, although the houses built into the west front are still private dwellings. The contemporary visitor to the Abbey ruins may not find them especially impressive, but he or she is nevertheless the beneficiary of centuries of discovery and investigation that began with the tentative explorations of Edward King in the eighteenth century and culminated in Whittingham's plan. At the

---

81 Ibid., p. 140.
82 Ibid.
83 James (1930), p. 36.
84 See Young (2014), pp. 61–5.
85 Whittingham (1952), p. 169.
86 H. J. M. Maltby, 'Excavations of the Abbey ruins, Bury St Edmunds', *PSIAH* 24 (1948), pp. 256–7.
87 Whittingham (1952), p. 169.
88 Ibid., foldout plan facing p. 172.

time of writing, plans are under way to open the newly built tower of St Edmundsbury Cathedral to the public, which should make it possible for more people to appreciate the extent and grandeur of the ruins by viewing them from above. Perhaps the approaching millennium of the Abbey's foundation in 2020 will also stimulate local archaeologists to attempt a geophysical survey of the site, which surely has many secrets still to yield.

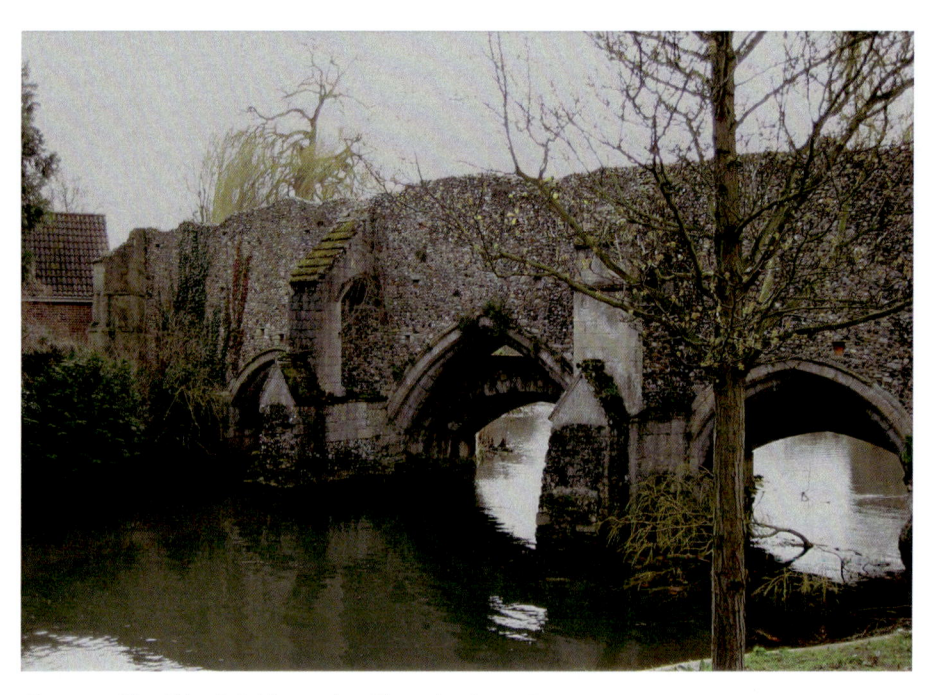

Figure 39 The Abbot's Bridge today. Photo by Susan Curran.

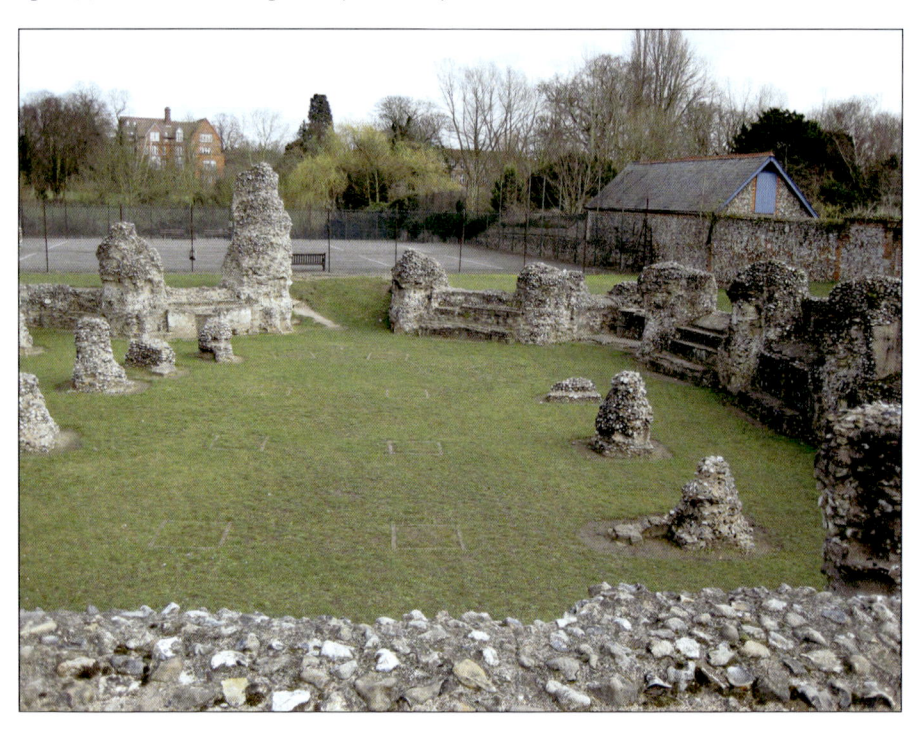

Figure 40 The ruins of Abbot Baldwin's crypt today. Photo by Susan Curran.

Appendix I
Abbots, priors and sacrists of the Abbey of Bury St Edmunds[1]

Abbot	Years	Prior	Years	Sacrist	Years
Ufi[1]	*1020–44?*				
LEOFSTAN	1044–65	Brihtric	1044–65		
BALDWIN	1065–97	Eadric	1065–87	Thurstan	1065–95
		Benedict Saxo	1087–94	Toli	1095–96
		William	1095–96		
ROBERT I	1100–02				
ROBERT II	1102–07	Ælfer	1102–07, 1108–?	Geoffrey	1102–07
		Baldwin[2]	1107–08		
ALEBOLD	1114–19				
ANSELM	1121–48	Talbot	1125–36	Hervey	1121–36
		Ording of Stow	1136–38	Ralph	1136–48
Ording of Stow[3]	*1138*	William	1138		
ORDING of Stow	1148–56	Sihtric	1148–53	Elias	1148–53
HUGH I	1157–80			Frodo	1156–60
		Theobald	1160–?	William Schuch	1160–80
		Hugh	?–1173	William Wiardel	1173–82
		Robert	1173–1200		
SAMSON of Tottington	1182–1211	Herbert	1200–10	Samson	1182–86
				Hugh	1186–88
				Walter of Banham	1206–11
				William of Diss	Dates unknown
HUGH II of Northwold	1214–29	Richard of the Isle	1220–22	Robert of Graveley	1211–17

1   The Abbot, prior and sacrist were the three most important officials of the Abbey. The list of priors and sacrists is based on the research of Thomson (1982). Some dates are approximations. Reigns of Abbots are dated from election in Chapter rather than papal or royal confirmations.

Abbot	Years	Prior	Years	Sacrist	Years
		Henry of Rushbrook	1222–33	Richard of the Isle	1217–20
				Richard of Newport	1220–34
RICHARD I of the Isle	1229–34			Gregory of St Albans	1234
HENRY I of Rushbrook	1235–48	Gregory of St Albans	1234–42		
		Daniel	1242–44	Nicholas of Warwick	1242–44
		Richard du Bois	1244–54		
EDMUND of Walpole	1248–56			Simon of Luton	1251
		Simon of Luton	1252–57	Richard of Horringer	1251–59
SIMON of Luton	1257–79	Robert Russel	1258–80	Richard of Colchester	1259
JOHN I of Northwold	1279–1301	Stephen Ixworth	1280–87	Simon Kingston	1259–80
				William of Hoo	1280–94
				John Snailwell	1294–96
				Richard de Brunne	1296–98
THOMAS I of Tottington	1302–12	William Rockland	1287–1312	Reginald of Denham	1298–1312
RICHARD II of Draughton	1312–35	Richard Denham	*fl.* 1318	William of Stow	*fl.* 1318
		Peter of Clopton	1325–27	Ralph Castone	*fl.* 1327
		Geoffrey Hemlington	1328–33	Hugh of Saxham	*fl.* 1334
WILLIAM I Bernham	1335–61	William of Stow	1333–41	Nicholas Wortham	1354–57
		Edmund Brundish	1341–61	Simon Langham	1358–61
HENRY II of Hunstanton	1361	Henry Kirkstead	1362–63		
JOHN II of Brinkley	1361–78	John of Cambridge	1374–81	John Lavenham	1361–83
Edmund Bromefield[4]	*1379*				

Abbot	Years	Prior	Years	Sacrist	Years
JOHN III Timworth	1379–1389	John Gosford	1382–1405	Thomas Rudham	1383–90
WILLIAM II Cratfield	1390–1415	Robert Icklingham	1405–26		
WILLIAM III Exeter	1415–29	William Curteys	1426–29	William Barrow	1407–26
WILLIAM IV Curteys	1429–46	John Bohun	*fl.* 1437	John Cranewys	1426–41
WILLIAM V Babington	1446–53			Thomas Derham	1441–67
JOHN IV Bohun	1453–69	Richard Ringstead	1461–64	John Woolpit	1467–69
		Robert Ixworth	1468–69	Robert Ixworth	1469
ROBERT III Coote (alias Ixworth)	1469–74	Richard Ingham	1474–75	Thomas Rattlesden	1469–70
				John Kirtling	1470–72
RICHARD III Ingham	1475–79			John Swaffham	1472–89
THOMAS II Rattlesden	1479–97	Thomas	*fl.* 1492	John Hawstead	1491–97
WILLIAM VI Bunting (alias Coddenham)	1497–1513	Robert Mildenhall	1497–1517	Christopher Ockham	1497–1503
				William Dersham	1503–04
				Richard Fouldon	1505–10
JOHN V Reeve (alias Melford)	1513–39	Thomas Dennis (alias Ringstead)	1517–35	John Eye	1510–20
				Thomas Knettishall	1520–28
				Edmund Maltward (alias Rougham)	1529–39

Notes

1. The supposed first Abbot is historically doubtful (see Chapter 1).
2. Consecrated bishop of Rochester in 1108, after which his predecessor Ælfer resumed the office.
3. Ording was first elected Abbot in 1138 when Anselm was nominated bishop of London, but Anselm was not confirmed by the king so came back to Bury as Abbot.
4. An anti-Abbot, never elected by Chapter.

Appendix II
A guided tour of the Abbey Church in 1465

The idea of a descriptive tour of the building for an imaginary visitor originated with M. R. James, who adopted this technique as the best way to convey the medieval state of the building.[1] *This tour is largely based on James's, with the addition of later insights from Arthur Whittingham, John Crook and Rebecca Pinner, and it guides the visitor around the church and the buildings in its immediate vicinity as they would have appeared in 1465. On 20 January 1465 the Abbey Church was seriously damaged by a devastating fire, and it is unclear how much of the original furnishings survived this and were still in situ at the time of the dissolution in 1539 (see Chapter 5). Much of what follows is educated guesswork based on scholarly speculation rather than a factual description.*

St James's Gate

The visitor should approach the Abbey from Churchgate Street in order to appreciate the full magnificence of the building. The main entrance to the 'sacred' side of the Abbey precincts is St James's Gate, built in the reign of Abbot Anselm (1121–48); to either side, stretching as far as St Mary's Church in the south and as far as the new Abbey Gate in the north (broken for the front of St James's Church) is the tall and insurmountable precinct wall. The visitor will pass under a great round-headed arch, and beneath this is a carved stone tympanum featuring Christ in glory, surrounded by angels and the symbols of the four evangelists.[2]

The West Front and West Transept

The visitor now stands about a hundred yards away from the west front of the Abbey Church, which is visible for the first time. Three huge portals are flanked to north and south by large octagonal towers; these were built under Abbot Samson (1182–1211) and are unique in Christendom. The West Tower, as well as the flanking smaller and lower octagonal towers, are topped by leaded spires. The longest and highest west front of any church in Christendom (at 246 feet long) is most famous for the cast bronze doors in the central portal that the visitor is about to enter. These date from the reign of Anselm, when Ralph and Hervey were sacrists, and were the work of the celebrated Master Hugo. It is said of Hugo that 'as in his other works he surpassed everyone else, so in the making of these gates [he] did surpass himself'. The doors are gilded so that they shine brightly when struck by the evening sun.

Above the central doorway is a carved depiction of the Last Judgement (the Doom).[3] Inside the west front, the visitor is in the west transept, standing beneath the crossing of

---

1 James (1895), pp. 127–50.
2 St James' Gate still exists as the 'Norman Tower', but the tympanum was destroyed in 1788 to give 'a freer access for loads of hay and straw' (James (1895), p. 127).
3 A fragment of this Doom may still survive, a very worn carved angel on display at Moyse's Hall Museum (Whittingham (1952), p. 171).

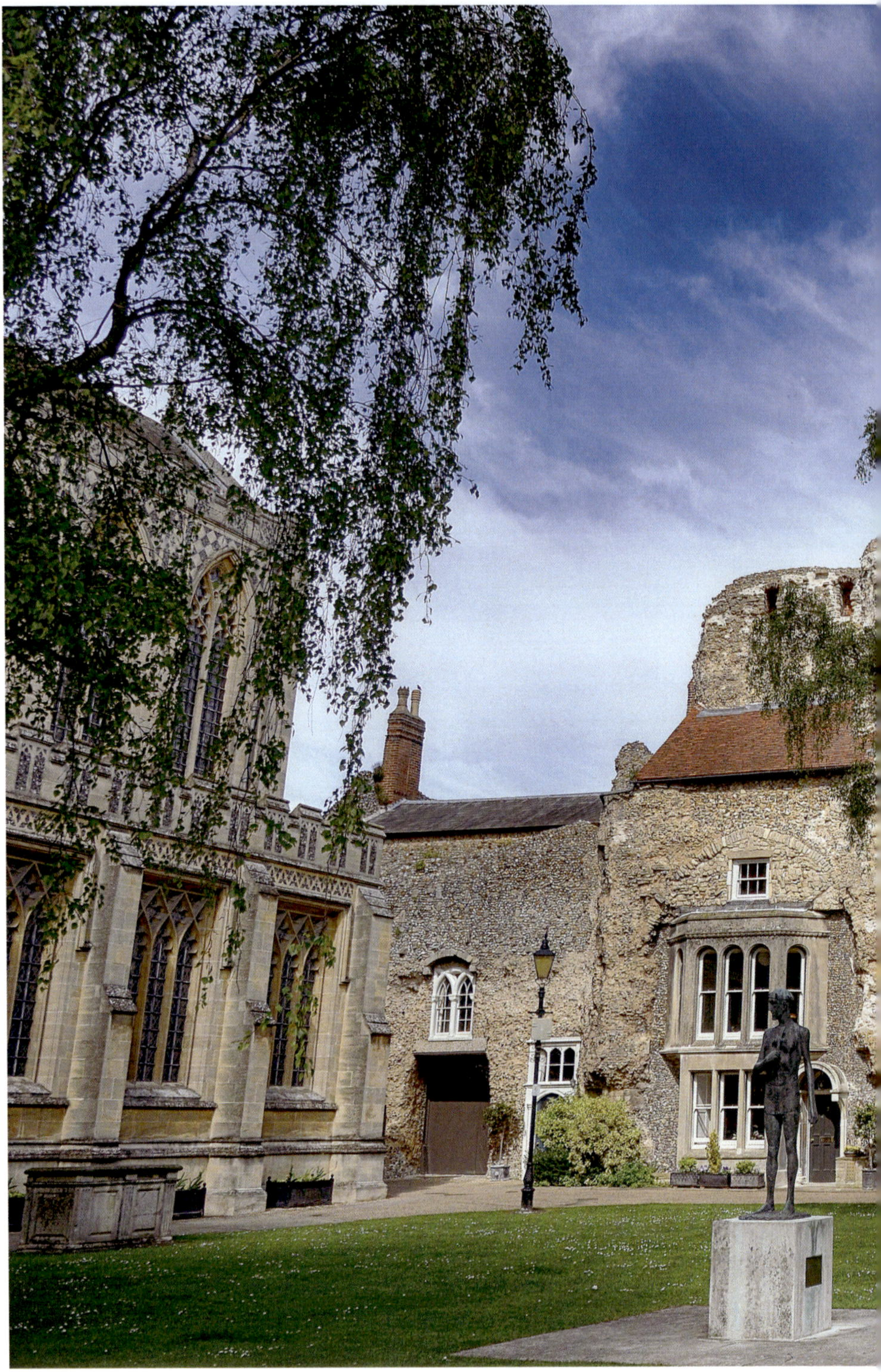

Figure 41 The ruins of Abbot Samson's west front of the Abbey Church today. Photo by Clive Dunn.

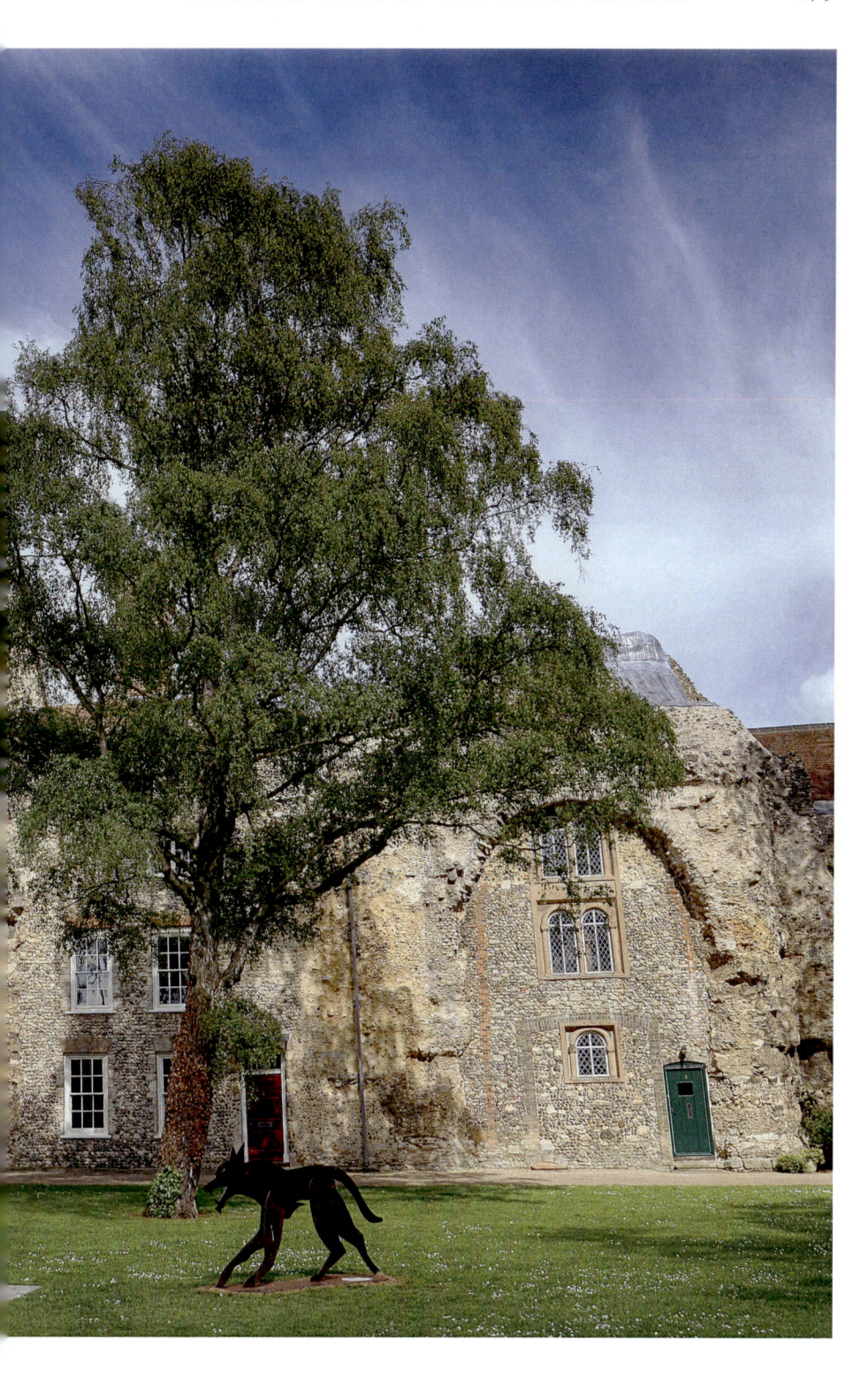

the west tower, where two massive piers mark the start of the nave. To south and north are the entrances to two sets of double-storied chapels: on the left hand side is the chapel of St Denis, with the chapel of St Faith above it accessed by a spiral stairway. This is a reminder that the north end of the west front was built over the old church of St Denis, built by Abbot Baldwin. To the south is the chapel of St John the Baptist, containing the baptistery, with the chapel of St Catherine above it.

The Nave

The visitor should now turn east and look down the nave, which is twelve bays long, each one formed by a rounded Norman arch and the stonework decorated in bands of bright colour. All of this was completed under Abbot Anselm. Above is a clerestory of plain glass windows and above that a wooden roof, magnificently painted in the fourteenth century under the sacrist John of Lavenham, at a cost of £100. The visitor should walk up the south aisle, which features twelfth-century stained glass in the twelve rounded Norman windows; the windows of the north aisle are plain, because the cloister lies on that side and the windows have to admit as much light as possible. The windows depict sixty-seven scenes from the life of Christ, including the Nativity, the Temptation in the Wilderness, the Marriage at Cana, Christ's encounter with the Woman of Samaria, and the Raising of Lazarus. The series ends at the south transept (by the altar of St Nicholas) with the Bearing of the Cross.

Crossing over the nave to the north aisle, the visitor will see a larger version of an image common on the north walls of parish churches: a painting of St Christopher. Further to the east, the visitor will see lights burning before an image of the Virgin Mary at the crossing with the north transept, and in front of this the tombs of two Abbots, Thomas of Tottington (d. 1312) and Richard of Draughton (d. 1335). Moving back to the centre of the nave and facing east, the visitor's view of the east end of the church will be blocked by an enormous stone choir screen or *pulpitum*, richly decorated with statues, which was made under Hugo the Sacrist in Abbot Samson's time, and restored under John of Northwold. On top of the screen are huge figures of the Virgin Mary and St John, flanking the enormous hanging rood (crucifix) that was likewise set up by Hugo the Sacrist.

The South Transept

The transepts of the church are unusually wide, and each one has an eastern aisle of three bays. The south transept features two apsidal chapels on the east side, beginning with the chapel of St John the Evangelist to the north, with the chapel of St Giles in the triforium above it. This chapel was dedicated by Geoffrey, bishop of St Asaph.

Next to this is the chapel of St Nicholas, and in front of this chapel is the tomb of Alan, count of Brittany, who was originally buried in the old rotunda of St Mary and St Edmund before the present church was built, but was later moved to this location.

The North Transept

The North Transept contains the monks' entrance to the church, connecting with their dormitory, as well as the entrance to the Lady Chapel. At the south-east corner is an entrance to the crypt, while at the north-east corner is the apsidal chapel of St Martin, which has a fine window depicting the life of the saint. To the south of this used to stand the old chapel of St Mary, before it was demolished in 1275. This in turn had replaced the rotunda of St Mary and St Edmund, consecrated in 1032.

The Choir Enclosure

The visitor should return to the centre of the church and walk through the narrow entrance beneath the choir screen and into the choir enclosure, an area formed by the arms of the screen extending eastwards towards the nave altar. On either side are eighty richly carved stalls occupied by the monks for the daily offices, with playfully decorated misericords under the seats. On the south side, and most elaborately carved of all, is the abbot's throne. Behind the stalls, both to north and south, hang giant painted cloths or *dorsaria*, which were the work of John Wodecroft, a royal painter of the thirteenth century. The *dorsaria*, already two centuries old and therefore grimy with smoke from candles, feature ninety painted scenes from the Book of Genesis, beginning with the creation of Adam and ending with Jacob blessing the sons of Joseph. On the south side another *dorsarium* depicts the Parable of Dives and Lazarus and the Miracle at Cana, and verses above the abbot's throne warn against the sin of pride.

Approaching closer to the abbot's throne, the visitor will be able to see some detailed carvings of miracles attributed to St Edmund. Turning to the east, the visitor will see the four monumental piers supporting the crossing beneath the central tower and, beyond them, the choir altar. This has a small retable behind it, allowing access around it on both sides.

The Presbytery and High Altar

Immediately behind the choir altar, in front of the high altar, is the alabaster tomb of the church's founder, Abbot Baldwin (d. 1097), with a great candelabrum on top of it. This tomb was made under the subsacrist Thomas Rudham in the fourteenth century. Also between the choir altar and the high altar is the tomb of Abbot John of Northwold (d. 1301).

The high altar is adorned with two painted pictures given by Edmund of Brundish in the fourteenth century, and behind it is a silver-gilt retable given by Abbot Richard I (1229–34). Hanging in front of the high altar is a pyx containing the Blessed Sacrament, and above it is an intricately carved and painted wooden beam, featuring thirteen scenes from the Passion, beginning with the entry into Jerusalem and ending with the incredulity of St Thomas. Hanging below the beam is another painted cloth, bearing an image of Christ in majesty with earth, sea and sky under his feet, surrounded by angels carrying the instruments of the Passion. On top of the carved beam rests the famous cross commissioned by Elias, sacrist under Abbot Ording (1148–56), flanked by figures of the Virgin Mary and St John and carved by the great Master Hugo. Also on top of the beam, beside the images, are chests containing relics. Immediately behind the beam is a solid wall of masonry, which the sacrist Walter of Banham built under Abbot Samson, after the fire of 17 October 1198 which damaged the shrine of St Edmund.

Next to the high altar stands the great seven-branched candlestick, which holds the Pasch or Easter Candle, lighted first on the vigil of Easter and relit for the major festivals of the year, along with six other candles of 4 lb each. The famous candlestick is decorated with scenes of the creation and fall of Adam, and was regilded by Walter of Banham. In front of the great candlestick is a large painted panel depicting the future punishment in hell of wicked monks, usurers and lawyers, as well as the Five Works of Mercy and the Last Judgement.

The Shrine of St Edmund

Behind the high altar, surrounded by a semi-circular ambulatory, is the presbytery, in the centre of which stands the shrine containing the incorrupt body of St Edmund himself. Above is the splendid stone vaulting of the apse, which was painted under Robert of Graveley, sacrist in Samson's reign. John of Lavenham was responsible for installing traceried windows in the decorated style around the apse, after the damage done to the church in the riots of 1327. There are thirteen windows in the clerestory of the presbytery, and four on each side in the ambulatory.

The base of the shrine was originally of simple construction, renewed in the time of Abbot Samson as a stone coffin raised on a decorated slab supported on three wide piers. In the fourteenth century the base was refaced with the present shrine base, which is of purple marble at the base and green above. On top of the shrine base, which has cavities to allow pilgrims to crawl in and out, is the feretory, a wooden casket covered in silver-gilt plating. Above the open shrine the *furnus*, a richly decorated wooden canopy, is suspended by ropes. The sacrist John of Lavenham paid £12 13s 4d for it to be painted. At the west end of the shrine, facing the high altar, is a relief of Christ in glory in beaten gold, known as the 'majesty'. The entire shrine is plated with panels of beaten gold, depicting the miracles of St Edmund. Around the top of the shrine is a cresting of gold, given by Abbot Samson. On top of the shrine stands the cross of gold given by Henry Lacy, earl of Lincoln; another jewelled golden cross, also given by Lacy, hangs on the right-hand side of the shrine, and a huge carbuncle can be seen beneath this cross.

Above the painted canopy, and almost touching it, is suspended another rood. This carries reliquaries containing the blood-stained *camisia* (shirt), spear, sword and nail-clippings of St Edmund. The *camisia* is the main relic of the saint displayed to the faithful on great festivals. Close by is the banner of St Edmund, depicting Adam and Eve eating from the tree of knowledge, which was borne by St Edmund into battle against the Danes and has many times ensured victory when carried by the Knights of St Edmund. The other banner in the shrine area is the standard of Isaac Comnenus, ruler of Cyprus, given to St Edmund by King Richard I.

The shrine is surrounded by a metal railing, and four candles of 3 lb each are burning perpetually at the four corners. On great feasts these are joined by twenty-four candles of 1 lb each. At the east end of the shrine, between the tops of two columns, are three reliquary chests containing the bones of Abbot Leofstan (d. 1065), the holy woman Oswin, who clipped the martyr's nails and hair when he was first laid to rest at Beodricsworth, and Æthelwine the sacrist, who took the body of the saint to London for safekeeping in 1010. The stained glass windows around the presbytery depict the story of King Sweyn's punishment by St Edmund, and rich fabric hangings adorn the area, one of which features nine scenes from the life of St Edmund, concluding with the death of Sweyn. The altars of St Thomas, St Botolph and St Jurmin attend the shrine of St Edmund; the altars of St Thomas and St Jurmin were plated with silver in Abbot Baldwin's time.

The Ambulatory Chapels

At the easternmost extremity of the church, off the ambulatory, are three apsidal chapels. The chapel of St Saba on the north side is where novices are instructed, and was dedicated by Abbot Anselm, who had been abbot of the monastery of St Saba in Rome. The wall paintings in the chapel date from Anselm's time. In the centre is the Chapel of the Martyrs or of St Nicasius, which was formerly the chapel of the Virgin Mary until Abbot Simon of Luton built a new Lady Chapel on the north side of the choir. Next to this, on the south side, is the chapel of the Cross, formerly St Peter's Chapel. The chapel was rededicated by Alberic, bishop of Ostia and papal legate during Anselm's reign, at which time the replica of the 'Holy Face of Lucca' commissioned by Abbot Leofstan (or more probably Abbot Baldwin) was placed there. However, there is also another cross in the chapel called the great cross, which was commissioned by Godfrey the sacrist during the reign of Robert II (1102–7) from a painter called Wohancus. Relics are incorporated into the back of this cross, which was dedicated by St Anselm, archbishop of Canterbury.

In the south side of the ambulatory (or choir aisle) is the entrance to the chapel of St Botolph, built by Abbot John of Northwold as an addition to the church. This houses the relic of the arm of St Botolph which is regularly carried in procession on festival days.

The Crypt

There are two entrances to the crypt, at the north end of the south transept's eastern aisle and the south end of the north transept's eastern aisle. The crypt is the oldest part of the church built by Abbot Baldwin, and is vaulted in stone, with twenty-four columns. The whole area is 100 by 80 feet in size. The dedication of the crypt is celebrated on 5 November every year; it was consecrated by Ralph, bishop of Rochester and afterwards archbishop of Canterbury. A natural spring at the east end of the crypt provides holy water for pilgrims, while seats line the walls. The crypt is only partially underground, and is lit by windows set high up in the walls. Three chapels at the east end are dedicated to St Anne, St Mary and St Robert (there is also an altar of St Edward the Confessor in St Robert's Chapel).

The Lady Chapel

The Lady Chapel was built under Abbot Simon of Luton (1257–79) and measures 80 by 42 ft. The chapel is richly decorated. An ornate wooden screen, for which the Sacrist John of Lavenham paid £22, divides the Lady Altar from the body of the chapel. The richly embroidered altar frontal depicts Christ in majesty surrounded by the four evangelists. On the retable behind the Lady Altar the following eight scenes are depicted in eight medallions:

> The unveiling of the synagogue
> Aaron's rod, the vines of Jericho and the Annunciation
> Allegory of the meeting of Righteousness and Peace and the Visitation
> The Coronation of the Virgin
> The Nativity
> The Burning Bush

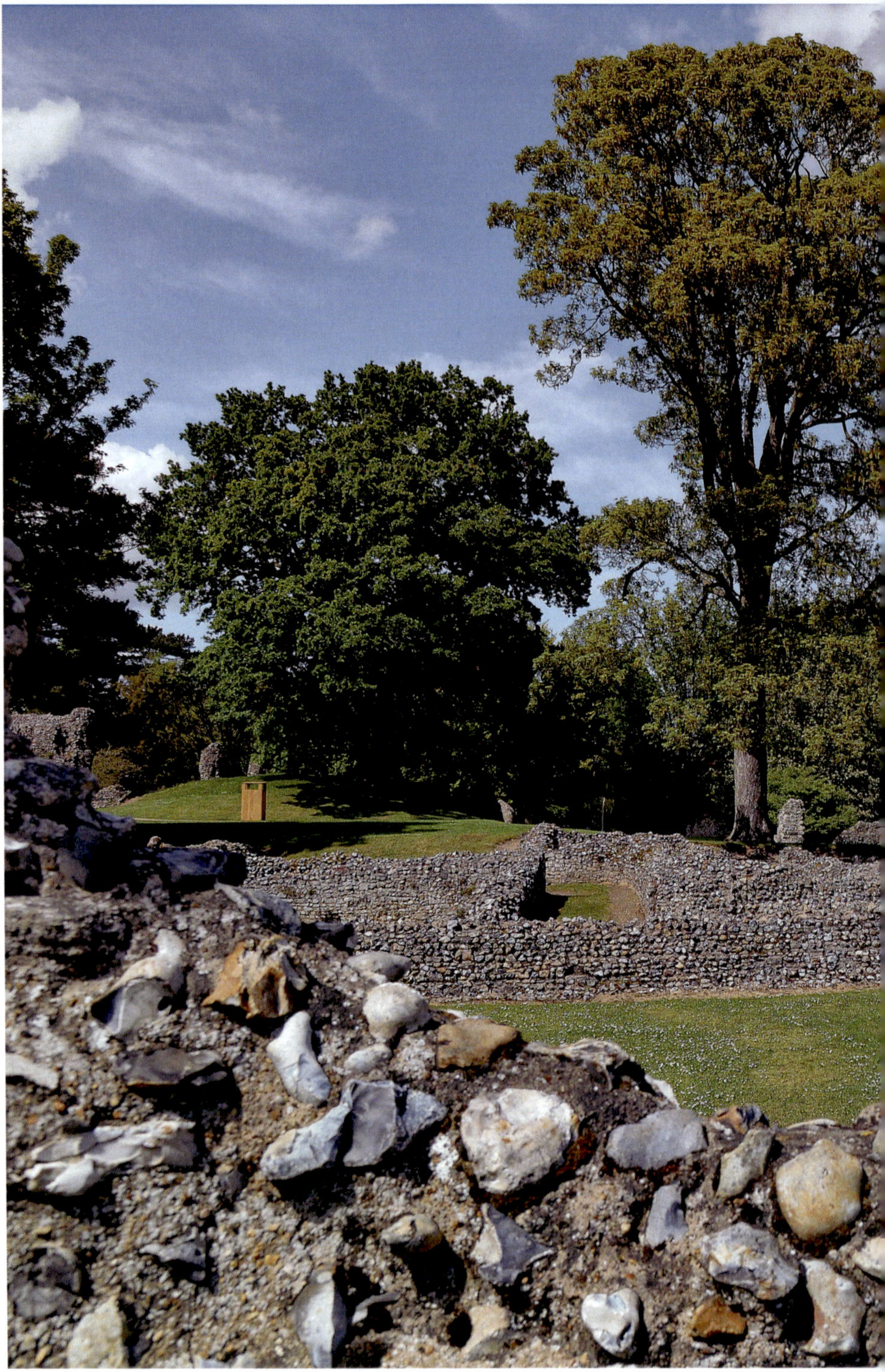

Figure 42 The ruins of Abbot Simon's Lady Chapel, looking north towards the site of the Abbot's Palace. Photo by Clive Dunn.

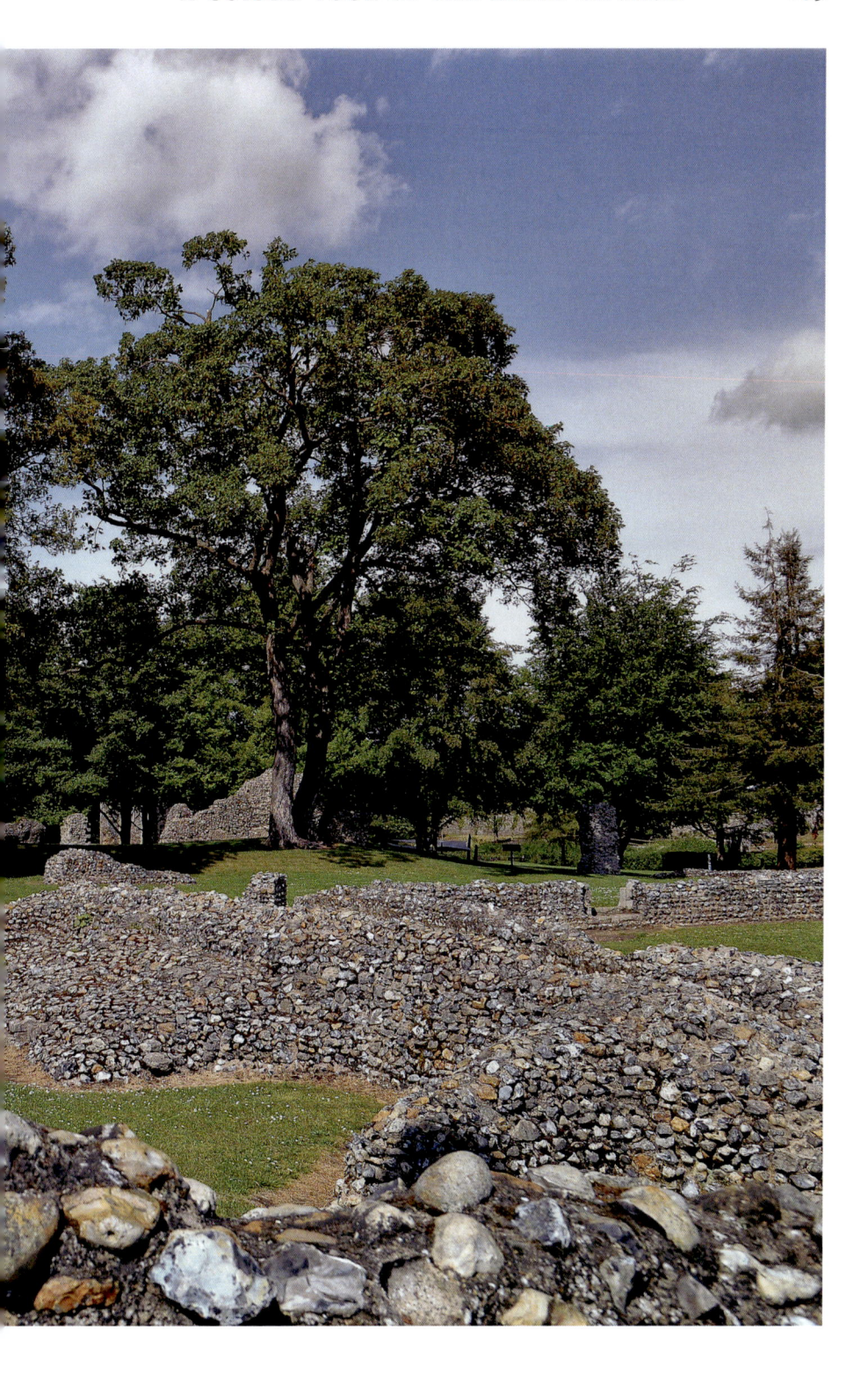

The sign given to Ahaz
Gideon's fleece

Above the retable is a depiction of Christ in majesty calling the blessed to him, and a wall painting depicting two of the miracles of the Virgin: saving a monk from drowning and saving the son of a Jew from a burning oven.

Another retable in the Lady Chapel contains more medallions depicting:

Elijah and the widow of Zarephath
Christ's deposition from the cross
Jonah swallowed by the great fish
Jonah vomited up by the great fish
The lion raising its whelp to life
The Resurrection
The women at the tomb and the angel

The embroidered frontal of a side altar depicts the church and synagogue. The ceiling is painted with medallions depicting the story of St Peter's contest with Simon Magus and the martyrdoms of St Peter and St Paul.

One stained glass window in the Lady Chapel depicts the Passion, while others contain scenes associated with the miracles and life of the Virgin: the story of Theophilus, who sold his soul to the devil but managed to redeem his contract by prayer to the Virgin, the death of Herod, and the healing of a clerk.

A freestanding image of the Virgin is surrounded by *tabulae*, painted boards depicting the healing of a sick clerk, the Assumption, the Annunciation, the Visitation, the visit of the Magi, the massacre of the innocents, the presentation of Christ in the Temple, the death of Herod, the story of Theophilus, and the rescue of the Jew's son from an oven.

In front of the altar are the tombs of three Abbots: Simon of Luton (d. 1279), William of Bernham (d. 1361) and John of Brinkley (d. 1379). On the north side of the chapel can be seen the tomb of Prior John Gosford, while Thomas Beaufort is buried in the north-east corner.

The Great Tower

The central tower of the Abbey Church is topped with a spire, with a sort of lantern built into it. The tower is famed for its nine bells, including Godefridus, Newport, the Sacrist's bell, Luton, Clopton and Master Hugo's bell. Godefridus is reputedly the largest bell in England, and was cast by one Hailfieus under Godefridus, sacrist under Abbot Robert II, from whom it derives its name. The other bells are similarly named after their donors.

The Cloister

On the north side of the church, and accessed via the north aisle of the nave, is the monastic cloister, which is a total of 160 ft across. The cloister was heavily damaged during the riots of 1327, when the townsmen broke forty 'carrels' (wooden desks for the monks), broke open chests and presses, and carried off books of liturgy and canon law. Prior John Gosford rebuilt the cloister entirely at his own expense. In the cloister there is a statue of

Abbot Anselm, and the Refectory is located on the north side and the Chapter House on the east. Above the east walk of the cloister is the Dormitory. The Lavatory, where the monks wash their hands before eating, is located by the Refectory door, and a series of stained glass windows here represent the sun, moon and stars and the seasonal occupations of the months.

The Chapter House

Prior Richard of Newport entirely rebuilt the first Chapter House, which was the work of Godefridus, following the 1327 riots. There is a *pulpitum* at the east end, and in the centre a lectern, while stone seats for the monks run around the walls. The tombs of six Abbots can be seen running down the centre of the Chapter House. They are, from east to west: Ording (d. 1156), Samson (d. 1211), Richard I (d. 1234), Henry of Rushbrook (d. 1248), Edmund of Walpole (d. 1256) and Hugh I (d. 1180). Of these tombs Ording's and Samson's are the most impressive, being made of marble, and they were restored by Abbot William Exeter in 1424.

The Infirmary

The Infirmary, located to the north-east of the Abbey Church and south of the Prior's House, incorporates what remains of the oldest building in the monastic complex, the church of St Benedict, which was paid for by Ælfric in Abbot Leofstan's time (or perhaps even earlier). It consisted of a tower and portico, and was the burial place of several abbots. For this reason the Infirmary altar is dedicated to St Benedict. The first Infirmary was built by Elias, sacrist in Ording's time, but a new one was constructed by Hugo and William in Samson's reign.

The chapel of St Stephen

The chapel of St Stephen and St Edmund, dedicated in 1276, adjoins the Prior's House and is an important site of pilgrimage because it contains the bier of St Edmund, on which Æthelwine carried the body of the saint to London and back in the eleventh century. The bier was originally housed in the rotunda of St Mary and St Edmund, which was demolished by Abbot Simon of Luton in 1275 to make way for the Lady Chapel. The first chapel of St Stephen was built by Abbot Baldwin in the south part of the monks' cemetery to house bones disturbed during his construction of the Abbey Church, and a new one was built in stone nearby by Abbot Anselm. Pilgrims leave offerings in this chapel in a pyx.

Bibliography

Robert Andrews, *The Rough Guide to Britain* (London: Rough Guides, 2001).
Paul Arblaster, 'Paris 1615–1676', pp. 1–36 in Geoffrey Scott (ed.), *Douai 1903 Woolhampton 2003: A Centenary History* (Worcester: Stanbrook Abbey Press, 2003).
C. D. C. Armstrong, 'Gardiner, Stephen (*c.*1495x8–1555)', *ODNB*, vol. 21, pp. 433–45.
Thomas Arnold (ed.), *Memorials of St Edmund's Abbey*, 3 vols (London: HMSO, 1890–96).
George Ashby, *A Description of the Ancient and Present State of the Town and Abbey of Bury St. Edmund's, in the County of Suffolk*, 2nd edn (Bury St Edmunds, 1771).
Ian Atherton, 'Salisbury, John (1501/2–1573), bishop of Sodor and Man', *ODNB*, vol. 48, pp. 710–11.
Mark Bailey, *Medieval Suffolk: An Economic and Social History, 1200–1500* (Boydell: Woodbridge, 2007).
Anthony Bale, 'Introduction', pp. 1–25 in Anthony Bale (ed.), *St Edmund, King and Martyr: Changing Images of a Medieval Saint* (York: York Medieval Press, 2009).
Debby Banham, 'Medicine at Bury in the time of Abbot Baldwin', pp. 226–46 in Tom Licence (ed.), *Bury St Edmunds and the Norman Conquest* (Woodbridge: Boydell Press, 2014).
David Bates, 'The Abbey and the Norman Conquest: an unusual case?' pp. 5–21 in Tom Licence (ed.), *Bury St Edmunds and the Norman Conquest* (Woodbridge: Boydell Press, 2014).
John Battely, *Antiquitates S. Edmundi Burgi ad annum MCCLXXII perductae* (Oxford, 1745).
Gordon Beattie, *Gregory's Angels: A History of the Abbeys, Priories, Parishes and Schools following the Rule of Saint Benedict in Great Britain, Ireland and their Overseas Foundations* (Leominster: Gracewing, 1997).
Bernard Bergonzi, 'Arnold, Thomas (1823–1900)', *ODNB*, vol. 2, pp. 505–7.
Paul Binski and Stella Panayatova (eds), *The Cambridge Illuminations: Ten Centuries of Book Production in the Medieval West* (Turnhout, Netherlands: Brepols, 2005).
Henry Norbert Birt, *Obit Book of the English Benedictines, 1600–1912* (Edinburgh: Mercat Press, 1913).
Gordon Blackwood, *Tudor and Stuart Suffolk* (Carnegie: Lancaster, 2001).
John Blair, 'Spearhafoc (*fl.* 1047–1051), abbot of Abingdon', *ODNB*, vol. 51, pp. 761–2.
E. O. Blake (ed.), *Liber Eliensis*, Camden 3rd Series 92 (London: Camden Society, 1962).
John M. Blatchly, 'D'Ewes, Sir Simonds', *ODNB*, vol. 16, pp. 1–4.
— 'Gillingwater, Edmund (*bap.* 1736, *d.* 1813)', *ODNB*, vol. 22, pp. 287–8.
Pamela Z. Blum, 'The St Edmund Cycle in the Crypt at Saint-Denis', pp. 57–68 in Antonia Gransden (ed.), *Bury St Edmunds: Medieval Art, Architecture and Economy* (London: British Archaeological Association, 1998).
James Bond, *Monastic Landscapes* (Stroud: Tempus, 2003).
William Camden, *Britannia siue Florentissimorum regnorum, Angliae, Scotiae, Hiberniae, et insularum adiacentium ex intima antiquitate chorographica descriptio* (London, 1590).
— *Britain, or A chorographicall description of the most flourishing kingdomes, England, Scotland, and Ireland* (London, 1637).
Bede Camm, *Nine Martyr Monks: The Lives of the English Benedictine Martyrs beatified in 1929* (London: Burns, Oates and Washbourne, 1931), p. 48.
Thomas Carlyle, *Past and Present* (London: Chapman and Hall, 1843).
David Carpenter (ed.), *Magna Carta* (London: Penguin Classics, 2015).
Matthew Champion, *Medieval Graffiti: The Lost Voices of England's Churches* (London: Ebury Press, 2015).

Alice Chandler, *A Dream of Order: The Medieval Ideal in Nineteenth Century English Literature* (London: Routledge and Kegan Paul, 1971).
T. M. Charles-Edwards, *Wales and the Britons, 350–1064* (Oxford: Oxford University Press, 2013).
Ernest Clarke, 'Yates, Richard (1769–1834)', rev. J. M. Blatchly, *ODNB*, vol. 60, pp. 751–2.
Charles Collignon, 'Some account of a body lately found in uncommon preservation, under the ruins of the Abbey, at St. Edmund's-Bury, Suffolk; with some reflections upon the subject', *Transactions of the Royal Society* 62 (1772), pp. 465–8.
Thompson Cooper, 'Rokewode, John Gage', rev. John M. Blatchly, *ODNB*, vol. 47, pp. 605–6.
— 'Sayer, Robert [*name in religion* Gregory] (1560–1602)', rev. D. D. Rees, *ODNB*, vol. 49, p. 161.
H. Copinger Hill, 'S. Robert of Bury St. Edmunds', *PSIAH* 21 (1932), pp. 98–107.
John S. Craig, 'The Bury Stirs revisited: an analysis of the townsmen', *PSIAH* 37 (1991), pp. 208–24.
— *Reformation, Politics, and Polemics: The Growth of Protestantism in East Anglian Market Towns, 1500–1610* (Farnham: Ashgate, 2001).
John Crook, 'The architectural setting of the cult of St Edmund at Bury 1095–1539', pp. 34–44 in Antonia Gransden (ed.), *Bury St Edmunds: Medieval Art, Architecture and Economy* (London: British Archaeological Association, 1998).
R. H. C. Davis (ed.), *The Kalendar of Abbot Samson and related Documents* (London: Camden Society, 1954).
Edward M. Dewing, *Saint Edmund's Bury: The Abbey Church and Monastery* (Bury St Edmunds: F. T. Groom, 1886).
Charles R. Dodwell, *The Pictorial Arts of the West, 800–1200* (New Haven, Conn.: Yale University Press, 1993).
D. C. Douglas, 'Fragments of an Anglo-Saxon Survey from Bury St Edmunds', *English Historical Review* 43 (1928), pp. 376–83.
— (ed.), *Feudal Documents from the Abbey of Bury St. Edmunds* (Oxford: Oxford University Press, 1932).
P. L. Drewett and Ian W. Stuart, 'Excavations in the Norman Gate Tower, Bury St. Edmunds Abbey', *PSIAH* 33 (1975), pp. 241–50.
William Dugdale, *Monasticon Anglicanum*, 3 vols (London, 1655–73).
Eamon Duffy, *The Stripping of the Altars* (New Haven, Conn.: Yale University Press, 1992).
— *Saints, Sacrilege and Sedition: Religion and Conflict in the Tudor Reformations* (London: Bloomsbury, 2012).
— 'Devotion to the Mother of God in the Medieval English cathedral', lecture delivered at Ely Cathedral, 1 September 2014.
Dee Dyas and Rodney M. Thomson, *The Bury Bible* (Woodbridge: Boydell & Brewer, 2008).
Christopher Dyer, 'The rising of 1381 in Suffolk: its origins and participants', *PSIAH* 36 (1988), pp. 274–87.
Robin J. Eaglen, *The Abbey and Mint of Bury St Edmunds to 1279* (London: British Numismatic Society, 2006).
— *The Abbey and Mint of Bury St Edmunds from 1279* (London: British Numismatic Society, 2014).
R. W. Elliott, *The Story of King Edward VI School Bury St. Edmunds* (Bury St Edmunds: Foundation Governors of the School, 1963).
G. R. Evans, 'Anselm (*d.* 1148), Abbot of Bury St Edmunds and hagiographer', *ODNB*, vol. 2, p. 258.
Eric Fernie, 'Baldwin's church and the effects of the Conquest', pp. 74–93 in Tom Licence (ed.), *Bury St Edmunds and the Norman Conquest* (Woodbridge: Boydell Press, 2014).
A. Finlay, 'Chronology, genealogy and conversion: the afterlife of St Edmund in the north', pp. 45–62 in Anthony Bale (ed.), *St Edmund, King and Martyr: Changing Images of a Medieval Saint* (York: York Medieval Press, 2009).

Sarah Foot, *Monastic Life in Anglo-Saxon England, c. 600–900* (Cambridge: Cambridge University Press, 2006).
— 'The Abbey's Armoury of Charters', pp. 31–52 in Tom Licence (ed.), *Bury St Edmunds and the Norman Conquest* (Woodbridge: Boydell Press, 2014).
John Foxe, *The Acts and Monuments of John Foxe*, 8 vols (London: George Seeley, 1870).
John Freely and Ahmet S. Çakmak, *Byzantine Monuments of Istanbul* (Cambridge: Cambridge University Press, 2004).
John Gage, *The History and Antiquities of Suffolk: Thingoe Hundred* (London, 1838).
Richard Gem and Laurence Keen, 'Late Anglo-Saxon finds from the site of St Edmund's Abbey', *PSIAH* 35 (1981), pp. 1–30.
Edmund Gillingwater, *An Historical and Descriptive Study of St. Edmund's Bury, in the County of Suffolk* (Bury St Edmunds: J. Rackham, 1804).
R. Gilyard-Beer, 'The eastern arm of the Abbey Church at Bury St. Edmunds', *PSIAH* 31 (1969), pp. 256–62.
Albert Goodwin, *The Abbey of St. Edmundsbury* (Oxford: Blackwell, 1931).
Robert S. Gottfried, *Bury St Edmunds and the Urban Crisis: 1290–1539* (Princeton, N.J.: Princeton University Press, 1982).
— *The Black Death: Natural and Human Disaster in Medieval Europe* (New York: Free Press, 1983).
Timothy Graham, 'Bury St Edmunds, Hugo of (*fl. c.*1130–*c.*1150)', *ODNB*, vol. 9, pp. 71–2.
Antonia Gransden (ed.), *The Letter-Book of William of Hoo 1280–1294*, SRS 5 (Ipswich: Suffolk Records Society, 1963).
— (ed.), *The Chronicle of Bury St. Edmunds 1212–1301* (London: Nelson, 1964).
— (ed.), *The Customary of the Benedictine Abbey of Bury St Edmunds in Suffolk* (London: Henry Bradshaw Society, 1973).
— *Historical Writing in England c. 550 to c. 1307*, 2 vols (London: Routledge & Kegan Paul, 1974).
— 'A democratic movement in the Abbey of Bury St Edmunds in the late twelfth and early thirteenth centuries', *Journal of Ecclesiastical History* 26 (1975), pp. 25–39.
— 'Baldwin, Abbot of Bury St Edmunds, 1065–1097', *Proceedings of the Battle Conference on Anglo-Norman Studies* 4 (1981), pp. 65–76.
— 'The legends and traditions concerning the origins of the Abbey of St Edmund', *English Historical Review* 100 (1985), pp. 1–24.
— 'The alleged incorruption of the body of St Edmund, king and martyr', *Antiquaries Journal* 74 (1994), pp. 135–68.
—'Abbo of Fleury's *Passio sancti Eadmundi*', *Revue Bénédictine* 105 (1995), pp. 20–78.
— 'The composition and authorship of the *De miraculis Sancti Eadmundi* attributed to "Hermann the archdeacon"', *Journal of Medieval Latin* 5 (1995), pp. 33–9.
— 'Some manuscripts in Cambridge from Bury St Edmunds Abbey: Exhibition Catalogue', pp. 228–85 in Antonia Gransden (ed.), *Bury St Edmunds: Medieval Art, Architecture and Economy* (London: British Archaeological Association, 1998).
— 'The cult of St Mary at Beodericsworth and then in Bury St Edmunds Abbey to c. 1150', *Journal of Ecclesiastical History* 55 (2004), pp. 627–53.
— 'The separation of portions between Abbot and Convent at Bury St Edmunds: the decisive years, 1278–1281', *English Historical Review* 119 (2004), pp. 373–406.
— 'Babington [Babyngton], William (*d.* 1453), abbot of Bury St Edmunds', *ODNB*, vol. 3, pp. 88–9.
—'Cratfield, William (*d.* 1415), abbot of Bury St Edmunds', *ODNB*, vol. 14, p. 48.
— 'Curteys, William (*d.* 1446), abbot of Bury St Edmunds', *ODNB*, vol. 14, pp. 760–1.
— 'St Edmund', *ODNB*, vol. 17, pp. 754–5.

— 'Hermann (*fl.* 1070–1100), Benedictine monk and hagiographer', *ODNB*, vol. 26, pp. 787–8.
— 'Luton, Simon of (*d.* 1279), abbot of Bury St Edmunds', *ODNB*, vol. 34, pp. 804–5.
— 'Samson (1135–1211), abbot of Bury St Edmunds' , *ODNB*, vol. 48, pp. 809–11.
— *A History of the Abbey of Bury St Edmunds 1182–1256* (Woodbridge: Boydell, 2009).
— *A History of the Abbey of Bury St Edmunds 1257–1301* (Woodbridge: Boydell, 2015).
Douglas Gray, 'Lydgate, John (*c.*1370–1449/50?)', *ODNB*, vol. 34, pp. 843–8.
[Margaretta K. Greene], *The Secret Disclosed: A Legend of St Edmund's Abbey* (Bury St Edmunds: Samuel Gross, 1861).
Ralph A. Griffiths, *King and Country: England and Wales in the Fifteenth Century* (London: Hambledon, 1991).
Robert Halliday, 'Moyse's Hall, Bury St Edmunds', *Suffolk Review* 25 (1995), pp. 27–44.
Cyril Hart and Anthony Syme, 'The earliest Suffolk charter', *PSIAH* 36 (1987), pp. 165–81.
William Hawkins, *Corolla Varia* (Cambridge, 1634).
Martin Heale, 'Training in superstition? Monasteries and popular religion in late Medieval and Reformation England', *Journal of Ecclesiastical History* 58 (2007), pp. 417–39.
Francis Hervey (ed.), *Corolla Sancti Eadmundi: The Garland of Saint Edmund King and Martyr* (London: John Murray, 1907).
T. A. Heslop, 'The production and artistry of the Bury Bible', pp. 172–85 in Antonia Gransden (ed.), *Bury St Edmunds: Medieval Art, Architecture and Economy* (London: British Archaeological Association, 1998).
Stephen Heywood, 'Aspects of the Romanesque Church of Bury St Edmunds Abbey in their regional context', pp. 16–21 in Antonia Gransden (ed.), *Bury St Edmunds: Medieval Art, Architecture and Economy* (London: British Archaeological Association, 1998).
Graham M. Hills, 'The antiquities of Bury St Edmunds', *Journal of the British Archaeological Association* 21 (1865), pp. 32–46, 104–40.
Richard Hoggett, *The Archaeology of the East Anglian Conversion* (Woodbridge: Boydell, 2010).
J. C. Holt, *Magna Carta*, 3rd edn (Cambridge: Cambridge University Press, 2015).
Alban Hood, 'Douai 1818–1903', pp. 61–97 in Geoffrey Scott (ed.), *Douai 1903 Woolhampton 2003: A Centenary History* (Worcester: Stanbrook Abbey Press, 2003).
M. R. James, *On the Abbey of S. Edmund at Bury*, 2 vols (Cambridge: Cambridge Antiquarian Society, 1895).
— 'Bury St. Edmunds manuscripts', *English Historical Review* 41 (1926), pp. 251–60.
— *Suffolk and Norfolk: A Perambulation of the Two Counties with Notices of their History and Their Ancient Buildings* (London: Dent, 1930).
Jocelin de Brakelond, *Chronica Jocelini de Brakelond*, ed. J. Gage Rokewode (London: Camden Society, 1840).
— *The Chronicle of Jocelin of Brakelond*, ed. H. E. Butler (Oxford: Oxford University Press, 1949).
Julie Kerr, *Monastic Hospitality: the Benedictines in England, c. 1070–c. 1250* (Woodbridge: Boydell, 2007).
Edward King, 'Remarks on the Abbey Church of Bury St. Edmund's in Suffolk', *Archaeologia* 3 (1775), pp. 311–15.
— 'An account of the Great Seal of Ranulph Earl of Chester; and of two ancient inscriptions found in the ruins of St. Edmund Bury Abbey', *Archaeologia* 4 (1786), pp. 119–31.
Henry of Kirkstead, *Catalogus de libris autenticis et apocrifis*, ed. R. H. and M. A. Rouse (London: British Library and British Academy, 2004).
C. S. Knighton, 'Batteley, John (*bap.* 1646, *d.* 1708)', *ODNB*, vol. 4, pp. 371–2.
— 'Westminster Abbey restored', pp. 77–123 in Eamon Duffy and David Loades (eds), *The Church of Mary Tudor* (Farnham: Ashgate, 2006).

Lisa Lampert, 'The once and future Jew: The Croxton 'Play of the Sacrament', Little Robert of Bury and historical memory', *Jewish History* 15 (2001), pp. 235-55.

John Leland, *Joannis Lelandi antiquarii de rebus Britannicis collectanea,* ed. Thomas Hearne, 6 vols (London, 1770).

— *The Itinerary of John Leland in or about the Years 1535–1543*, ed. Lucy Toulmin Smith, 2 vols (London: G. Bell, 1907).

C. P. Lewis, 'Avranches, Hugh d', first earl of Chester (*d.* 1101)', *ODNB,* vol. 3, pp. 1–3.

Tom Licence, 'The cult of St Edmund', pp. 104–30 in Tom Licence (ed.), *Bury St Edmunds and the Norman Conquest* (Woodbridge: Boydell Press, 2014).

V. D. Lipman, *The Jews of Medieval Norwich* (London: Jewish Historical Society of England, 1967).

Mary D. Lobel, 'A detailed account of the 1327 rising at Bury St. Edmund's and the subsequent trial', *PSIA* 21 (1933), pp. 215–31.

— *The Borough of Bury St. Edmunds: A Study in the Government and Development of a Monastic Town* (Oxford: Clarendon Press, 1935).

David M. Lunn, *The English Benedictines 1540–1688* (London: Burns & Oates, 1980).

Korey D. Maas, *The Reformation and Robert Barnes: History, Theology and Polemic in Early Modern England* (Woodbridge: Boydell, 2010).

Joseph Boniface Mackinlay, *Saint Edmund King and Martyr* (London: Art and Book Company, 1893).

F. W. Maitland, *Domesday Book and Beyond: Three Essays in the Early History of England*, 2nd edn (Cambridge: Cambridge University Press, 1987).

H. J. M. Maltby, 'Excavations of the Abbey ruins, Bury St Edmunds', *PSIAH* 24 (1948), pp. 256–7.

S. Marron, 'The early years at St Edmund's, Paris', *Douai Magazine* 3:4 (1925), pp. 258–65.

Joanna Martin, 'Ecclesiastical jurisdictions', pp. 16–17 in David Dymond and Edward Martin (eds), *An Historical Atlas of Suffolk* (Ipswich: Suffolk County Council Planning Department, 1988).

George May, *A Descriptive History of the Town of Evesham* (Evesham: George May, 1845).

J. Philip McAleer, 'The west façade complex at the Abbey Church of Bury St Edmunds: a description of the evidence for its reconstruction', *PSIAH* 39 (1998), pp. 127–50.

Liz Herbert McAvoy, *Medieval Anchoritisms: Gender, Space and the Solitary Life* (Woodbridge: D. S. Brewer, 2011).

J. McCann and C. Cary Elwes (eds), *Ampleforth and its Origins: Essays on a Living Tradition* (London: Burns, Oates & Washbourne, 1952).

Diarmaid MacCulloch, *Suffolk and the Tudors: Politics and Religion in an English County 1500–1600* (Oxford: Clarendon Press, 1986).

— (ed.), *Letters from Redgrave Hall: The Bacon Family, 1340-1744*, SRS 50 (Woodbridge: Suffolk Records Society, 2008).

Elsie McCutcheon, *Bury St Edmunds: Historic Town* (Bury St Edmunds: Alastair Press, 1987).

Frank Meeres, *A History of Bury St Edmunds* (Stroud: History Press, 2010).

Irina Metzler, *Disability in Medieval Europe: Thinking about Physical Impairment During the High Middle Ages, c. 1100–1400* (Abingdon: Routledge, 2006).

J. Brian Milner, *Six Hospitals and a Chapel: The Story of the Medieval Hospitals of Bury St Edmunds, Suffolk* (Bury St Edmunds: St Nicholas Hospice/Suffolk Institute of Archaeology and History, 2013).

Alfred W. Morant, 'On the Abbey of Bury St. Edmund's', *PSIA* 4 (1872), pp. 376–404

William of Newburgh, 'The history of England', pp. 347–403 in David C. Douglas and George W. Greenaway (eds), *English Historical Documents, 1042–1189*, 2nd edn (London: Routledge, 1981).

William Noel, 'The lost Canterbury prototype of the 11th-Century Bury St Edmunds Psalter', pp.

161–71 in Antonia Gransden (ed.), *Bury St Edmunds: Medieval Art, Architecture and Economy* (London: British Archaeological Association, 1998).

Peter Northeast (ed.), *Wills of the Archdeaconry of Sudbury 1459–1474*, SRS 44 (Woodbridge: Suffolk Records Society, 2001).

'Obituary: Sir Ernest Clarke', *The Times* 43282 (6 March 1923), p. 16E.

William Page (ed.), *The Victoria History of the County of Suffolk*, 2 vols (London: Constable, 1907).

Clive Paine, 'The Chapel and Well of Our Lady of Woolpit', *PSIAH* 38 (1993), pp. 8–12.

Elizabeth C. Parker, 'Master Hugo as sculptor: a source for the style of the Bury Bible', *Gesta* 20 (1981), pp. 99–109.

Elizabeth C. Parker and Charles T. Little, *The Cloisters Cross: Its art and meaning* (New York: Metropolitan Museum of Art, 1994).

Graham Parry, *The Trophies of Time: English Antiquarians of the Seventeenth Century* (Oxford: Oxford University Press, 1995).

— *The Arts of the Anglican Counter-Reformation* (Woodbridge: Boydell, 2006).

Richard W. Pfaff, *Montague Rhodes James* (London: Scolar Press, 1980).

— *Liturgy in Medieval England* (Cambridge: Cambridge University Press, 2009

Carl Phelpstead, 'King, martyr and virgin: *Imitatio Christi* in Ælfric's *Life of St Edmund*', pp. 27–44 in Anthony Bale (ed.), *St Edmund, King and Martyr: Changing Images of a Medieval Saint* (York: York Medieval Press, 2009).

John D. Pickles, 'Ashby, George (1724–1808)', *ODNB*, vol. 2, pp. 620–1.

Rebecca Pinner, *The Cult of St Edmund in Medieval East Anglia* (Woodbridge: Boydell, 2015).

Steven Plunkett, *Suffolk in Anglo-Saxon Times* (Stroud: Tempus, 2005).

'Quarterly meetings', *Proceedings of the Bury and West Suffolk Archaeological Institute* 1 (1853), pp. 53–6.

D. D. Rees, 'Reyner, Wilfrid' in *ODNB*, vol. 46, pp. 525–6.

Richard Rex, 'Wentworth, Jane [Anne; *called* the Maid of Ipswich] (*c.*1503–1572?)', *ODNB*, vol. 58, pp. 127–8.

John Ridgard, 'From the rising of 1381 in Suffolk to the Lollards', pp. 9–28 in David Chadd (ed.), *Religious Dissent in East Anglia III* (Norwich: Centre of East Anglian Studies, 1996).

Susan J. Ridyard, *The Royal Saints of Anglo-Saxon England: A Study of West Saxon and East Anglian cults* (Cambridge: Cambridge University Press, 1988).

R. H. Rouse, 'Bostonus Buriensis and the authors of the *Catalogus Scriptorum Ecclesiae*', *Speculum* 41 (1966), pp. 471–99.

Rebecca Rushforth, 'The Bury Psalter and the descendants of Edward the Exile', *Anglo-Saxon England* 34 (2005), pp. 255–61.

Erin A. Sadlack (ed.), *The French Queen's Letters: Mary Tudor Brandon and the Politics of Marriage in Sixteenth-Century Europe* (New York: Palgrave Macmillan, 2011).

E. R. Samuel, 'Was Moyse's Hall, Bury St Edmunds, a Jew's house?', *Transactions of the Jewish Historical Society of England* 25 (1977), pp. 43–7.

Susanne Saygin, *Humphrey, Duke of Gloucester (1390–1447) and the Italian Humanists* (Leiden, Netherlands: Brill, 2002).

Norman Scarfe, 'The Bury St Edmunds Cross: the work of Master Hugo', *PSIAH* 33 (1973), pp. 75–85.

— *Suffolk in the Middle Ages* (Woodbridge: Boydell, 1986).

— 'Jocelin of Brakelond's identity: a review of the evidence', *PSIAH* 39 (1997), pp. 1–5.

Walter F. Schirmer, *John Lydgate: A Study in the Culture of the XVth Century* (Berkeley, Calif.: University of California Press, 1961).

Geoffrey Scott, 'Three seventeenth-century Benedictine martyrs', pp. 266–81 in David H. Farmer (ed.), *Benedict's Disciples*, 2nd edn (Leominster: Gracewing, 1995).

— 'Woolhampton 1903–2003', pp. 98–173 in Geoffrey Scott (ed.), *Douai 1903 Woolhampton 2003: A Centenary History* (Worcester: Stanbrook Abbey Press, 2003).

Richard Sharpe, 'Reconstructing the medieval library of Bury St Edmunds Abbey: the lost catalogue of Henry of Kirkstead', pp. 204–18 in Antonia Gransden (ed.), *Bury St Edmunds: Medieval Art, Architecture and Economy* (London: British Archaeological Association, 1998).

David Sherlock and William Zajac, 'A fourteenth-century monastic sign list from Bury St Edmunds Abbey', *PSIAH* 26 (1988), pp. 251–73.

Henry Spelman, *The History and Fate of Sacrilege* (London, 1698).

Kay Staniland, 'Bury St Edmunds, Mabel of (*fl.* 1239–1265)', *ODNB*, vol. 9, p. 72.

Margaret Statham, *Yesterday's Town: Bury St Edmunds* (Whittlebury: Baron Birch, 1992).

— *The Book of Bury St Edmunds*, 2nd edn (Whittlebury: Baron Birch, 1996).

— 'The Medieval Town of Bury St Edmunds', pp. 98–110 in Antonia Gransden (ed.), *Bury St Edmunds: Medieval Art, Architecture, Archaeology and Economy* (London: British Archaeological Association, 1998).

— (ed.), *Accounts of the Feoffees of the Town Lands of Bury St Edmunds, 1569–1622*, SRS 46 (Woodbridge: Suffolk Records Society, 2003).

C. J. S. Thompson, 'The hands of Thomas Beaufort, third son of John of Gaunt', *British Medical Journal* 1:3562 (13 April 1929), pp. 701–2.

J. R. Thompson, *Records of Saint Edmund of East Anglia King and Martyr* (Bury St Edmunds: F. T. Groom, 1890).

Rodney M. Thomson, 'The Library of Bury St Edmunds Abbey in the eleventh and twelfth centuries', *Speculum* 47 (1972), pp. 617–45.

— (ed.), *The Chronicle of the Election of Hugh, Abbot of Bury St Edmunds and Later Bishop of Ely* (Oxford: Oxford University Press, 1974).

— (ed.), *The Archives of the Abbey of Bury St Edmunds*, SRS 21 (Woodbridge: Suffolk Records Society, 1980),

— 'Obedientiaries of St Edmund's Abbey', *PSIAH* 35 (1982), pp. 91–103,

Véronique Thouroude, 'Medicine after Baldwin: the evidence of BL, Royal 12. c. xxiv', pp. 247–57 in Tom Licence (ed.), *Bury St Edmunds and the Norman Conquest* (Woodbridge: Boydell Press, 2014).

Norman M. Trenholme, *The English Monastic Boroughs: A Study in Medieval History* (Columbia, Mo.: University of Missouri Press, 1927).

Elisabeth van Houts, 'The women of Bury St Edmunds', pp. 53–73 in Tom Licence (ed.), *Bury St Edmunds and the Norman Conquest* (Woodbridge: Boydell Press, 2014).

Thomas of Walsingham, *The Chronica Maiora of Thomas of Walsingham, 1376–1422*, ed. David Preest and James G. Clark (Woodbridge: Boydell, 2005).

A. F. Wareham, 'Baldwin (*d.* 1097), abbot of Bury St Edmunds', *ODNB*, vol. 3, pp. 441–2.

David Watkin, 'Burrough, Sir James (1691–1764)', *ODNB*, vol. 8, pp. 1008–9.

Teresa Webber, 'The provision of books for Bury St Edmunds Abbey in the 11th and 12th centuries', pp. 186–93 in Antonia Gransden (ed.), *Bury St Edmunds: Medieval Art, Architecture and Economy* (London: British Archaeological Association, 1998).

John Weever, *Ancient Funerall Monuments* (London, 1631).

Bridget Wells-Furby (ed.), *The 'Bohun of Fressingfield' Cartulary* (Woodbridge: Suffolk Records Society, 2011).

Stanley West, 'A new site for the martyrdom of St Edmund', *PSIAH* 35 (1983), pp. 223–5.

Dorothy Whitelock, 'Fact and fiction in the legend of St Edmund', *PSIAH* 31 (1970), pp. 217–33.

Arthur B. Whittingham, 'Bury St. Edmunds Abbey and the churches of St Mary and St James', *Archaeological Journal* 108 (1952), pp. 168–89.

— *Bury St Edmunds Abbey* (London: HMSO, 1971).

Peter Wickins, *Victorian Protestantism and Bloody Mary: The Legacy of Religious Persecution in Tudor England* (Bury St Edmunds: Arena, 2012).

Margaret E. Wood, 'Moyse's Hall: a description of the building', *Archaeological Journal* 108 (1952), pp. 165–7.

Francis Woodman, 'Wastell, John (*d. c.*1518)', *ODNB*, vol. 57, pp. 542–3.

William Worcestre, *Itineraries of William Worcestre* ed. John H. Harvey (Oxford: Clarendon Press, 1969).

Richard Yates, *An Illustration of the Monastic Antiquities of the Town and Abbey of St Edmund's Bury* (London: J. B. Nichols & Son, 1843).

Francis Young, '"An horrid popish plot": the failure of Catholic Aspirations in Bury St. Edmunds, 1685–88', *PSIAH* 41 (2006), pp. 209–55.

— 'John Battely's *Antiquitates S. Edmundi Burgi* and its editors', *PSIAH* 41 (2008), pp. 467–79.

— *Where is St Edmund? The Search for East Anglia's Martyr King* (Ely: East Anglian Catholic History Centre, 2014).

— 'St Edmund, king and martyr in popular memory since the Reformation', *Folklore* 126 (2015) pp. 159–76.

— *The Gages of Hengrave and Suffolk Catholicism, 1640–1767* (Woodbridge: Catholic Record Society, 2015).

Index

Note: references to illustrations are indicated with **bold** print. References to footnotes are indicated with 'n'. Saints are indexed under their proper name.

A

Abbey Gate *see* gates, Abbey Gate
Abbot's Bridge 5, **89**, 172
Abbot's Palace 5, 8, 13, 83, **85**, 88, 91, 98, 105, 112, 113, 148, 155, 162, **163**
 see also London, Abbot's palace at
Adams, William, burgess 118
Adelham, Placid, monk 147
Adrian IV, pope 57
Ælfgar 25
Ælfgeth, pilgrim 33
Ælfric, bishop of Elmham 29, 31
Ælfwine, abbot of Ramsey 28
Ælfwine, bishop of Elmham 27, 28, 31, 146
Æthelberht II, king of the East Angles 30
Æthelflæd, queen 25
Æthelnoth, bishop of Elmham 29
Æthelstan, king of Wessex 20, 22, 23, 29, 132
Æthelwine, sacrist of Beodricsworth xv, 26, 33, 101, 112, 182, 187
Ailbold, priest 45
St Albans abbey 3, 52, 58, 74, 106, 146
aldermen 9, 79, 80, 83, 84, 87, 88, 90, 91–2, 97, 110, 115–16, 118, 140
Alebold, Abbot of Bury St Edmunds 47, 173
Alexander II, pope 39
Alexander III, pope 58
Alexander IV, pope 77, 79
Alexis Master, artist 52
Allen, William, cardinal 146–7, 168

almoner, office of 7
Almoner's Barns 91
Alnwick, William, bishop of Norwich 105, 107
Andrews, Thomas 155
Anna, king of the East Angles 32
Anselm, Abbot of Bury St Edmunds xiii, xv, 3, 14, 24, 44, 47–50, 51, 53, 54–5, 56, 59, 61, 69, 81, 104, 113, 173, 176n., 177, 180, 183, 187
Anselm, archbishop of Canterbury 47, 48, 53, 183
antisemitism 3, 53, 54, 59–60, 62
 see also Jews
Ap Rice, John, commissioner xvi, 127, 128, 129
aqueduct 70, 90
Aragon, Katherine of, queen 117–18, 121, 124n.
archaeology xiii, 3, 10, 11–12, 13, 15, 22, 23, 131, 151, 169–71
archdeacon
 of Bury St Edmunds 3, 7, 15, 83, 139–41
 of Sudbury 140–1
 see also sacrist, office of
archives, monastic xiii, 1, 8, 12, 83, 153
Arfast, bishop of Elmham
 see Herfast, bishop of Elmham
Arnold, Thomas, antiquary 10, 73, 168
Arthur, King 16
Arundel, Thomas, archbishop of Canterbury 103
Ashby, George, antiquary **160**, 162, 164
Assandun, battle of (1016) 27, 28
assizes 32, 138, 139
Astone, Andrew, monk 169
Attleborough, Humphrey, monk 136
Attleborough, Norfolk 154

Audley, Thomas 125
St Augustine of Canterbury 143, 146
Augustine, bishop of Nidaros 6
Avicenna 69
Avignon 95, 104
Avranches, Robert d', Abbot of Bury St Edmunds 47

B

Babington, William, Abbot of Bury St Edmunds 107–10, 175
Babwell, Suffolk 65, 80, 90, 92
Bacon, Nicholas 137–9, 142, 153
Badby, Thomas 155
Baker, Augustine, monk 145
Baldwin, Abbot of Bury St Edmunds xv, 3, 4, 9, 14, 27n., 29, 30, 32, 33, 35–47, 48, 50, 51, 55, 56, 67, 68, 77, 81, 83, 102, 113, 130, 73, 180, 181, 183, 187
Baldwin, prior 69, 173
Bale, John, reformer 154
Banham, Walter of, sacrist 70, 173
Banleuca xiii, xv, 5, 7, 9, 15, 25, 31, 44, 59, 62, 64, 69, 76, 77, 78, 80, 81, 84, 90, 105, 118, 134, 136–7, 139, 141, 159
Baret, John, burgess 110
Barnack, Lincs. 45
Barnes, John, monk 145
Barnes, Robert, reformer xiv, xvi, 120–1, 141
Barnwell, Cambs. 151
Barons' War 73, 75, 80, 81–2
Barrow, Suffolk 30, 125, 162
Barton, John, monk 136
Basel, council of 106
Basset, Philip 81
Battely, John, antiquary xiii, 10, **11**, 14, 151, **160**, 161–2, 164
Battely, Oliver, antiquary 10,

161
Bayfield, Richard, monk and Protestant martyr xiv, xvi, 120–1
Beaufort, Thomas, duke of Exeter xvi, 154, 162–4, 186
Beaumont, Robert de, earl of Leicester 60
Bec, abbey of 47, 48
Beccles, Suffolk 25
Becket, St Thomas 127
St Benedict, church of 28, 30, 56–7, 187
see also infirmary
St Benedict, Rule of 24, 28, 33, 42, 61, 76, 94, 103
Benedictine Congregation, English 97, 101, 143–4, 145, 147, 148
Bernham, William, Abbot of Bury St Edmunds 93, 94–5, 174, 186
Berton, John of, alderman 90, 91, 92
Berton, Richard of, alderman 90
Berwick, John of 82
Beodricesworth see Bury St Edmunds, town of
Bigod, Hugh, earl of Norfolk 60
Bigot, Roger le xv, 60
Bilney, Thomas, reformer 121
Black Death see plague
Blakeham, Benedict of, moneylender 58
Bloor, Aloysius, monk 149
Blythburgh, Suffolk 32
Bohun, John, Abbot of Bury St Edmunds 110, 113, 115, 175
Boniface, archbishop of Canterbury 77
Boniface IX, pope xvi, 101, 124
Boston, John, monk 96
St Botolph 32, 46, 87, 182, 183
Bradfield, John, monk 136
Bradfield St George, Suffolk 24
Bradshaw, Augustine, monk 144
Braganza, Catherine of, queen 147

Brainsford, John, suffragan bishop of Lincoln 121n.
Brakelond, Jocelin de, monk 3, 10, 54, 56, 60, 61, 62, 64n., 165
Brandon, Charles, duke of Suffolk 122
Brinkley, John, Abbot of Bury St Edmunds 95, 96–7, 101, 174, 186
Brinton, Suffolk 136
Bristol Abbey 3, 124n.
Bristol, marquess of see Hervey family
Brockley, Suffolk 125
Bromefield, Edmund, anti-Abbot xvi, 14, 96–8, 99, 174
Brooke, Norfolk 41
Brotherton, Thomas of, earl of Norfolk xvi, 154
Brundish, Edmund, prior 95, 96, 174, 181
Buckley, Sigebert, monk 143, 144
Bunting, William, Abbot of Bury St Edmunds xvi, 116, 175
Burgate, Suffolk 136
Burrough, James, antiquary 159, 161, 162, 164
Burton, Suffolk 34
Burton abbey 75
Bury Bible 3, 52–3, 54, 153
Bury bull 119–20
Bury St Edmunds, Liberty of 5, 137, 139, 141
see also banleuca
Bury St Edmunds Psalter 3, 28, 29, 68, 70n.
Bury St Edmunds, town of
Abbeygate Street 44, 92, 119, 149
Angel Hill **9**, 23, 35, 44, 119
Buttermarket 35
Churchgate Street 51, 119, **152**, 177
Cornhill 23, 35, 44, 59
Crown Street 132
gates 9, **43**, 44, 65, 80, 82, 90, 92, 99, 116, 118, 119, 122, 135, 136
government see aldermen
great axis 23, **152**

grid plan 3, 35, 44, 51
Guildhall Street 88, 99, 118, 119, 136
Hatter Street xiv, 60
limits of see banleuca
market 23, 32, 44, 84, 90, 92, 94, 99, 116, 135, 136, 138–9
Mustow Street 5, 23, 32n.
Northgate Street 30, 77
origins 22–4
St Mary's Square 23
Southgate Street 77, 119
Sparhawk Street 30
Bury Stirs 141

C
Cade, Jack, rebel 109
Caistor, Stephen of, monk 69
Cambridge 81, 116, 121, 127
Blackfriars 105
Corpus Christi College 3, 52, 153
Fitzwilliam Museum 169
Gonville and Caius College 161
St John's College 129
King's College 116, 169
Pembroke College 52, 128–9
University Library xiv, 153n., 167n.
Cambridge, John, prior 99, 174
Camden, William, antiquary 154–5
canon law 29, 47, 59, 66, 71, 89, 95, 103, 104, 107, 110, 147, 186
Canterbury cathedral 47–8, 53, 103, 116
Canute see Cnut, King
Carlyle, Thomas, essayist xi, 10, 166, 168
Caseneuve, Pierre de, hagiographer 73
Castle Acre, Norfolk 51, 61
Castone, Ralph, sacrist 90, 174
Cavendish, Suffolk 99
Cavendish, John, chief justice 99
Cecil, Robert 138
cellarer, office of 7, 62, 64, 91, 156, 159
cemetery see Churchyard, Great

INDEX

ceremonies *see* liturgy
chantries 86, 103, 110, 124, 136
chaplains, secular 8, 82, 86, 90–1, 99, 102, 128
Chapter 7, 71, 75, 77, 79, 82, 85, 87, 97, 101, 103, 105, 107, 109, 124, 125, 128
Chapter House 10, 61, 70, 71, 72, 74, 97, 102, 106, 169–70, 187
Charles I, king 144
Charnel, chapel of the xvi, 86–7, 136
charters 3, 7, 24–5, 27, 28–9, 31, 38, 40, 41, 47, 57, 71, 76, 81, 84–5, 86, 88, 90, 99, 101, 109, 116, 138, 139, 153, 159
see also forgery
Chartists 166
Chaucer, Geoffrey, poet 104, 107
Chelsworth, Suffolk 25
Chevington, Suffolk 92, 125
Christchurch, Canterbury *see* Canterbury cathedral
Church, Abbey (Church of Christ, St Mary and St Edmund)
  bells 52, 74, 102, 111, 112, 131, 186
  St Botolph, chapel of 87, 183
  Cross, chapel of the 32, 57, 183
  crypt 4, 5, 30, 45, 46, 50, 59, 102, 120, 130, 164, 170, **172**, 180, 183
  demolition xvi, 131, 141, 158
  St Denis, chapel of *see* St Denis, church of
  doors 52, 110, 177
  St Faith, chapel of 48, 180
  St Giles, chapel of 56, 180
  Lady Chapel xvi, 81–2, 164, 180, 183, 186, 187
  measurements 1
  nave altar 50, 102, 181
  St Nicasius, chapel of 183
  St Robert, chapel of 4, 59, 120, 183
  St Saba, chapel of 48, 103, 183

  sacristy 7, 32n., 34, 61, 88
  Samson's Tower 5, **68**, **135**
  shrine of St Edmund *see* St Edmund, shrine of
  spires xv, 67, 111, 112, 113, 177, 186
  St Stephen, chapel of
  towers xvi, 30, 50, 56, 61, 70, 74, 105, 110, 111–12, 177, 180, 181, 186, 187
  Trayle (door) 103
  west front 1n., 4, 5, 31, 44, 50, 51, 52, 55, **57**, 70, 155, 164, 167, 170, 177, **178–9**, 180
  see also Rotunda of St Mary and St Edmund
Churchyard, Great 1, 5, 45, 61, 62, 70, 81, 86, 95, 102, 136, 155, 157, 159, 187
Cistercians 53, 75, 124
Clare, Osbert of 48
Clare, Richard de, earl of Gloucester 76, 82
Clarke, Ernest, antiquary 10, 130, 169–70
Clement VI, pope 94–5
Clerk, Simon, master mason 116
Cloister 5, 8, 56, 70, 88, 102, 103, 106, 112, 113, 180, 186–7
Cloisters Cross 53–4, 59
Clopton, Peter of, prior 90, 174
Cluniacs 51, 145, 146
Cluny, abbey of 1
Cnut, king xi, 15, 27, 28–9, 32n., 40, 88, 146, 150
Cockfield, Suffolk 25, 34
Coddenham, William *see* Bunting, William, Abbot of Bury St Edmunds
Colchester, Abbot's palace at 7
Cole, William, antiquary 159
Cologne 110
Comnenus, Isaac, banner of 67, 182
Conception of the Blessed Virgin Mary, feast of the *see* Marian devotion
Coney Weston, Suffolk 31
confraternities 91, 103, 109, 163

Constance, council of 104
Convent (body of monks) 7, 15, 41, 62, 65, 71, 77, 82–3, 84, 90, 91, 95, 101, 104, 118, 127–8, 129, 159
Coote, Robert, Abbot of Bury St Edmunds 115–16, 175
Cope family 155
Corfe Castle 71
Cornwallis, John 137
Corporation of Bury St Edmunds 138–9
Cotton, Robert, antiquary 129
Cranmer, Thomas, archbishop of Canterbury 139
Cratfield, William, Abbot of Bury St Edmunds xvi, 94, 101–4, 124, 175
Cressy, Roger de 72
Cromwell, Thomas 122, 123, 127, 128, 129, 134
Culford, Suffolk 12, 34, 41, 85
Cullum, Thomas, physician 163
Curre, Nicholas, monk 144
Curteys, William, Abbot of Bury St Edmunds xvi, 14, 15, 94, 96, 104, 105–7, 110, 120, 153, 175
Curzun, Robert de 38, 40
St Cuthbert 20, 24, 130

D

D'Ewes, Simonds, antiquary 154
Danelaw 19, 27
Danes xv, 16, 18, 19, 20, 21, 24, 25, 27, 28, 146, 166, 182
Darcy, Thomas 137
Darkin, John, archaeologist 166
Davers, Charles 139
Deerhurst, Gloucs. 35, 37, 97
St Denis, abbey of 20, 30, 35, 37, 39, 40
St Denis, church of (Bury Edmunds) 44, 50, 180
Dennis, Thomas, prior 130, 175
Despenser, Henry, bishop of Norwich 99
Dewing, Edward, antiquary 168

Dienst, Brabant 92
Diss, Thomas, monk
Diss, William of, schoolmaster 61
dissolution xi, 13, 14, 1, 5, 8, 12, 13, 15, 31, 32, 35, 50, 53, 93, 114–15, 123–32
see also Church, Abbey, demolition
Dodsworth, Roger, antiquary 159
Domesday Book 8, 37, 41, 44
Dominicans 76, 105, 107, 124, 154
Douai, France 143, 144, 146, 149, 150, 168–9
Dover, Richard of, archbishop of Canterbury 58
Dovercourt, Essex 117
Draughton, Richard of, Abbot of Bury St Edmunds xvi, 87, 92, 93, 94, 174
Drury, Robert 119
Drury, William 125
Dugdale, William, antiquary 156, 159
Dunstable, Nicholas of, monk 71
Dunstan, archbishop of Canterbury 20, 22, 24
Dunwich, Peter, monk 136
Dunwich, Suffolk 60
Durham cathedral 24, 106, 130
Dykes-Bower, Stephen, architect 72

E

Eadmund, king of the East Angles *see* St Edmund
Eadwig 25
Eden family 140, 154
St Edmund
  body of xv, 16, 20–2, 23, 24, 26–7, 29, 30, 33, 34, 40, 64–5, 73–4, 102, 104, 117, 121, 130, 132, 147, 151, 154, 156, 159, 161, 182
  coinage of **16**, 18
  martyrdom of **17**, 18, 20–1, 40, **73**, 74, 102, 154, 161
  memorial coinage of 15, **19**
  miracles of 21, 22, 27, 52,
    65, 130, 181, 182
  relics of (secondary) 39
    (banner 60, 66, 182; cup 64; nail-parings 24, 127, 182; psalter 154; shirt (*camisia*) 64, 102, 182)
  shrine of xv, xvi, 8, 10, 15, 21, 24, 26, 27, 28, 30, 33, 34, 40, 41, 46, 55, 61, **63**, 64–5, 67, 70, 81, 90, 102, 105, 106, 111, 112, 113, 117, 119, 120, 124, 129–30, 154, 159, 161, 181, 182
  translations to:
    Beodericsworth 23–4, 154; London 26–7, 159, 182, 187; the Rotunda 30; Toulouse (alleged) 73–4
Edmund I, king xv, 3, 24–5, 159
Edmund II Ironside, king 27
St Edmund, Liberty of xv, 3, 5, 7, 31–2, 37, 38, 39, 46, 47, 76, 77, 80, 83, 84, 90, 98, 103, 121, 122, 134, 136–9, 140, 141, 142, 153
St Edmund, priory of (founded 1615) xiv, 134, 142–5, 147–50, 162, 168
St Edmund, Society of 148
St Edmundsbury cathedral *see* St James, Church of
St Edmundsbury and Ipswich, diocese of 50, 159
education 3, 42, 65–6, 83–4, 135, 136, 137, 155, 161
Edward the Confessor, king xv, 3, 7, 18, 31–2, 33, 35, 37, 38, 39, 42, 44, 62, 71, 76, 88, 130, 183
Edward the Elder, king 19
Edward I, king xvi, 62, 81, 82, 83, 84–6, 154
Edward II, king 88
Edward III, king 91, 92–3, 95, 99, 109, 159
Edward IV, king 110
Edward VI, king 65, 135, 136, 137
Eleanor of Aquitaine, queen 60, 79, 80, 83
elections, abbatial 7, 47, 50, 56, 58, 61, 71–2, 75, 76,
    77, 82, 87, 94, 95, 96–8, 101, 105, 107, 110, 116, 117, 118, 124, 132, 135, 173n.
Elias, sacrist 56–7, 173, 181, 187
Elizabeth I, queen 121, 137, 138, 139, 141, 153, 155
Ellingham, Peter of, alderman 84
Ellis, Phillip, monk 148
Elmswell, Suffolk 25, 34, 104, 105, 135
Ely, Cambs. xv, 20, 22, 27, 37, 38, 50, 70, 73–4, 75, 76, 81, 82, 86, 103, 129, 169
Emma, Queen 29, 31
Erasmus, Desiderius 120, 127
St Etheldreda 20, 32
Ethelred, king 25, 27
Eugenius IV, pope 107
Everisdun, John of, monk 169
Evesham Abbey 124, 142
Exeter, William, Abbot of Bury St Edmunds xvi, 104–5, 175
Eye, John, sacrist 118, 175
Eye, Suffolk 137
Eyre, John 155

F

Fair, Bury 3, 122, 149
Feckenham, John, abbot of Westminster 142, 143
fires 8
  of 1150 xv, 56
  of 1198 xv, 64–5, 181
  of 1465 xvi, 14, 15, 52, 94, 110–13, 130, 145, 177
  of 1608 144
St Firminus *see* St Jurmin
Fisher, John, bishop of Rochester 127
fisheries 28, 41
Flempton, Suffolk 125
Fleury, Abbo of, hagiographer xv, 18, 19, 28, 33, 40
Forgery 24, 25, 27, 29, 35, 37, 38–9, 40, 92
Fornham, battle of (1173) xv, 60
Fornham All Saints, Suffolk 25, 34, 108, 125
Fornham St Genevieve, Suffolk 60, 80

INDEX

Fountains abbey 3
Framlingham, Suffolk 140, 142
Francis I, king of France 122
Franciscans xv, xvi, 14, 75, 76, 77–80, 81, 82, 90–1, 92, 97, 98, 107, 124, 156, 157
fraternity, honorary members of 106, 109, 163
Fraunceys, John, rebel 88
St Fremund 106
Frenze, Norf. 129
Fressingfield, Suffolk 110
Friars *see* Dominicans, Franciscans
Frink, Elizabeth, sculptor 31

G

Gage, Edward, 1st baronet of Hengrave 145
Gage-Rokewode, John, antiquary 10, 164–6
Gaire, George, monk 144
Galen 3, 44
Gardiner, Robert, alderman 115
Gardiner, Stephen, bishop of Winchester 140, 154
Gascoigne, Placid, monk 144
Gately, Everard of, monk 82
gates 1, 90, 123
  Abbey Gate **xvii**, 4, 5, 32n., 83, 88, 91, 92, **93**, **97**, **100**, 155, 177
  St James' Gate (Norman Tower) xii, 4, 5, **49**, 51, 55, 102, 119, **152**, 177
  St Margaret's Gate 61, 105
Gaunt, John of, duke of Lancaster xvi, 103, 162
Gervase, George, monk and martyr 143–4
Gifford, William Gabriel, archbishop-duke of Rheims 144, 145
Gilbert, bishop of London 50
Gillingwater, Edmund, antiquary 164
Glastonbury Abbey 3, 16, 80, 110, 127, 146–7
Gloucester, Humphrey duke of xvi, 94, 104, 106, 108–9
Gloucester Abbey 3, 124n.
Gloucester Hall, Oxford 103, 104, 106, 107, 121, 144

Godfrey, sacrist 48, 50, 183
Grammar School *see* education
Graveley, Robert of, sacrist 71, 173, 182
Gravesend, Richard of, dean of Lincoln 77
Great Barton, Suffolk 139
Great Livermere, Suffolk 10, 169
Great Saxham, Suffolk 125
Greek, study of 48, 69
Greene, Margaretta Katherine 166–8
Greenstead, Essex 27
Gregory VII, pope 39
Gregory IX, pope 75, 76, 79
St Gregory, priory of (Douai) 143–4, 149, 150, 168
Grey, Frances, duchess of Suffolk 122
Grey, Jane, royal pretender 140
Grosseteste, Robert 48, 69
Gruffydd ap Nicholas 108
Grundisburgh, Suffolk 32
guestmaster, office of 7, 82
Guild of Youth, rebellion of (1264) xvi, 80
Guildhall 88, 99, 118
Guildhall feoffees 136, 137
guilds
  of the Assumption 136
  of St Botolph and St Nicholas 136
  Candlemas Guild 93, 136
  Guild Merchant 136
  of St Peter 136

H

Haberden, Suffolk 91, 119
Hadleigh, Suffolk 121, 140, 157
Hadley, John, monk 136
Hægelisdun 20, 22, 24, 40
Halesworth, Thomas, alderman 97
Halls, John 148
Hankinson, Bennet, monk 147
Harbridge, Roger of 77
Hardwick, Suffolk 125
Hargrave, Suffolk 125
Harleston, Suffolk 116, 164
Harlow, Essex 101, 103, 122, 128
Harthacnut, king 40, 88

Hastings, battle of (1066) 37, 38
Hastings, Henry of 80
Hatfield Regis, Essex xvi, 104
Hawkins, William, schoolmaster xiv, 157–8
Hawkyns, John, alderman 118
Hawstead, Suffolk 25, 125
Hawstead, Aylott, monk 136
Hearne, Thomas, antiquary 153
Hebrew, study of 69
Hengham, Richard *see* Ingham, Richard, Abbot of Bury St Edmunds
Hengrave, Suffolk 10, 125, **126**, 142, 145, 164, 165
Henry I, king xv, 47, 48, 50, 71
Henry II, king **58**, 60, 61, 67
Henry III, king 76, 79, 80–1, 84
Henry V, king 104–5, 163
Henry VI, king xvi, 94, 104–6, 108, 109, 110, 124, 163
Henry VII, king xvi, 116, 124, 154
Henry VIII, king xi, xvi, 1, 114, 117, 118, 119, 121–2, 123, 124, 126, 127, 131, 132, 137, 140, 141, 142, 147, 153, 154–5
Henry the Young King 60
Heptonstall, Thomas, titular Abbot of Bury St Edmunds 149
Herfast, bishop of Elmham xv, 39–41, 42, 45, 46
Hermann the Archdeacon, hagiographer 22, 24, 27, 33, 34, 40, 41, 44, 50, 76, 102, 120
Hervey, sacrist 52, 173, 177
Hervey family 125, 164, 166, 169, 170
Hessett, Robert, monk 136
Hills, Graham, antiquary 10, 166
Hinderclay, Suffolk 41
Hitchcock, William, monk 130
Holderness Barns 91
Holme, St Benedict's abbey at 27–8, 91, 123

Holt, Jeremiah 129
Hoo, William of, sacrist 12, 83, 174
Horningsheath (Horringer), Suffolk 25, 34, 70, 125, 136
hospitals
 of St John (*Domus Dei*) 76–7, 82, 103
 of St Nicholas 103, 136
 of St Peter xiii, 136
 of St Petronilla 136
 of St Saviour xv, xvi, 65, 86, **108**, 109, 145
Howard family 137, 138
Hoxne, Suffolk 40, 120, 154
Hubert, archbishop of Canterbury 66
Hugh I, Abbot of Bury St Edmunds 54, 56, 58, 59–61, 62, 173
Hugo, Master, artist xv, 3, 51–5, 56, 177, 181, 186
Hunstanton, Henry of, Abbot of Bury St Edmunds 95, 174

I
Icklingham, Suffolk 65, 76
Ickworth, Suffolk 125
Iconotypicon Buriense 156
Indulgences 41, 81, 105, 109, 110
infirmarian, office of 8, 69
Infirmary xv, 5, 28, 56, 61, 70, 91, 103, 112, 113, 170, 187
 see also medicine
Innocent III, pope 69, 71
Innocent IV, pope 76
interdict, papal 67, 71
Ipswich xvi, 23, 50, 84, 94, 116, 117, 118, 119, 121, 127, 128, 141–2
Isabella, queen xvi, 88
Isle, Richard of the (de Insula), Abbot of Bury St Edmunds 75, 81, 173, 174
Islip, John, abbot of Westminster 122
Ixworth, Robert *see* Coote, Robert, Abbot of Bury St Edmunds
Ixworth, Suffolk 41

J
Jacobitism 148
James I, king 138
James II, king 120n., 148, 161
James, Montague Rhodes, antiquary 10, 15, 96, 106, 110, 129, 145, 168–70, 177
St James, church of xvi, 3, 4, 13, 23, 48, 50, 51, 55, 72, 86, 90, 91, 102, 116, 136, 141–2, 154, 155, 166, 167, 170, 171, 177
Jermyn family 125, 138, 155
Jerusalem, kingdom of 52
Jesuits 120n., 148, 162
Jesus, college of 136
Jews xv, 53–4, 56, 58–60, 62, 69, 77, 120, 157, 186
 see also anti-semitism
Jocellus, monk 64
John, king xv, 14, 56, 66, 67, 71–2, 80
St Jurmin 32, 46, 182
Jurnet, moneylender 58

K
King, Edward, antiquary 164, 170
Kirby Cane, Norfolk 31
Kirby, John, Protestant martyr 141
Kirkstead, Henry of, prior xvi, 96, 174
Knights of St Edmund xv, 38, 60, 66, 80, 182
Kytson, Thomas 125, 142

L
Lackford, Suffolk 31, 34, 125
Lambarde, William, antiquary 154
Lambert, abbot of Angers 39
Lambspring, abbey of 144, 149, 150
Lancaster, duchy of 137, 140
Lancastrianism 103, 106, 116, 124
Lanfranc, archbishop of Canterbury 39
Langham, Simon, sacrist 95, 174
Langlifa, hermit 45
Langton, Stephen, archbishop of Canterbury 72
Laon cathedral 51
Lark, river 5, **23**, 30, 83, 105, Larkin, Laurence, abbot of St Edmund's, Douai 149
Larling plaque 30
Latham, Augustine, monk 147
St Laurence, priory of (Dieulouard) 144, 150
Lavenham, John, sacrist 92n., 174, 180, 182, 183
Lavenham, Suffolk 130
Legh, John xvi, 127, 128
Leland, John, antiquary 1, 4, 53, 129, 151–3, 159
Leofstan, Abbot of Bury St Edmunds 18, 31 – 4, 38, 41, 67, 156, 173, 182, 183, 187
library, monastic xvi, 1, 10, 12, 14, 44, 48, 67–9, 89, 96, 106, 113, 128–9, 151, 169
Lidgate, Suffolk 104n.
Lincoln cathedral 153
Linnet, river 70
Little Saxham, Suffolk 125
Little Whelnetham, Suffolk 136
Liturgy 28, 42, 48, 54, 102, 186
Loddon, Norfolk 31
Lollardy 98, 105, 107, 120, 121
London xv, 1, 26, 33, 38, 40, 50, 54, 66, 73, 75, 76, 80, 85, 88, 90, 91, 92, 98, 101, 105, 107, 119, 126, 134, 156, 158, 159, 169, 182, 187
 Abbot's palace at (Bevis Marks) 7, 57–8, 81
Long Melford, Suffolk 99, 116, 132, 175
Lorraine, Marie of, abbess of Chelles 144, 145
Losinga, Herbert de, bishop of Norwich 46, 47, 51
Louis VIII, king of France 73, 130
Louis XII, king of France 122
Lucca, Italy 32, 39, 183
Lutheranism 120, 121, 141
Luton, Simon of, Abbot of Bury St Edmunds xvi, 76,

INDEX

77–82, 83, 84, 161, 164, 174, 183, 186, 187
Lydgate, John, monk xvi, 15, 94, 104–7, 120, 164

M
Mackinlay, Joseph, monk 149
Magna Carta xv, 14, 56, 71–4, 78
Maldon, battle of (991) 25
Maldon, Reginald, monk 142
Malmesbury abbey 3
Maltby, H. J. M., archaeologist 170
Manhall, Essex 74
St Margaret, chapel of 5, 44–5, 102, 105, 157
Marian devotion 48, 82, 120
Markant family 125
Martin V, pope 104
Marwell, Hants. 62
Mary I, queen 131n., 135–6, 140–1, 142
St Mary, church of xv, xvi, 4, 5, 16, 22–3, 24, 29, 45, 46, 48, 55, 78, 86, 90, 91, 102, 104, 110, 117, 131–2, 136, 155, 159, 177
Mary Rose Tudor, queen of France *see* Tudor, Mary, queen of France
Maxwell, Lawrence, lollard 120
medicine 3, 8, 35, 42–4, 61, 68, 69, 98
 see also infirmarian; infirmary
Mendlesham, Suffolk 141
Middlington, Ralph of 84
Mildenhall, Suffolk 31, 62, 76, 99, 140
Mimara, Ante Topic, art dealer 53
Minster of St Edmund *see* Church, Abbey
mint xv, 13, 32, 38, **58**, 83, 92–3
Modercope, Ælfric 31
Monks Eleigh, Suffolk 103
Monte Cassino, abbey of 142
Montfort, Simon de 80
Morcere, moneyer 32
Moulton, Suffolk 142
Mowbray, John de, duke of Norfolk 109
Moyse's Hall 59, 170, 177n.

murders xv, 59–60, 87, 95, 101

N
Nedeham, Robert, monk 130
Newmarket, Suffolk 105
Newport, Richard of, sacrist 74, 174, 187
Newton, Suffolk 41
Nicholas V, pope 109
Nix, Richard, bishop of Norwich 118, 119, 122
Norman Conquest 12, 14, 27n., 35, 37, 38, 39, 59, 79
Norman French 41, 42, 82, 102–3
Norman Tower *see* gates, St James' Gate
Northwold, Hugh of, Abbot of Bury St Edmunds xv, 14, 56, 70–4, 75, 76, 82, 173
Northwold, John of, Abbot of Bury St Edmunds 14, 82–7, 181, 183
Norton, Suffolk 136
Norwich 46, 58, 59, 60, 91, 94, 121, 158
 cathedral 46, 47, 51, 59, 121
Norwich, diocese of 103, 158
Novices 61, 96, 102–3, 183
Nowton, Suffolk 125

O
obedientaries *see* cellarer, office of; sacrist, office of
Oldcoates, Philip 72
Ording of Stow, Abbot of Bury St Edmunds 50, 54, 55, 56–7, 66, 74, 173, 176n., 181, 187
Ortiger, Stephen, titular Abbot of Bury St Edmunds xi, 149
Oswald, king of Northumbria 21
Oswin, shrine-keeper 24, 182
Otho, papal legate 76
Otto, king of the Romans 67
Ottobuono, papal legate 81
outlaws 31, 92

P
pagans 21, 22, 27, 30, 32, 48
pageants 72

Pakenham, Suffolk 31
Palgrave, Suffolk 34, 82
Paris, Matthew, chronicler 76
Parker, Matthew, archbishop of Canterbury 52, 129, 142n., 153
Parker, William, monk 148–9
Parliaments
 of 1296 xvi, 85–6
 of 1447 xvi, 94, 107–9
Parys, Phillip, commissioner xvi, 129
Paston family 125
Peasants' Revolt (1381) xvi, 14, 98–101
Penda, king of Mercia 22
St Peter's basilica, Rome 1, 51
Peterborough Abbey 3, 45, 116, 124n.
Pettinger, Dunstan, monk 144
pilgrimage 8, 28, 35, 41, 45–6, 50, 51, 59, 64, 65, 71, 72, 81, 107, 120, 123, 135, 147, 182, 183, 187
pittancer, office of 7–8, 61
pittances 7–8, 42
Pius IV, pope 142, 147
plague xiii, xvi, 94–6, 98, 130, 162
Pole, Reginald, cardinal archbishop of Canterbury 140
Pole, William de la, duke of Suffolk 108
Pollard, Richard, commissioner xvi, 129
poor men, rising of the (1528) xvi, 119
Portmanmoot 7, 139
Preston, Gilbert of, judge 79–80
prior, office of 7, 15, 39, 62
Prior's House 5, 170, 187
Puritans 141, 155, 159

Q
Quo Warranto 81, 84

R
Rædwald, king of the East Angles 22
Ramsey abbey xv, 20, 25, 28, 37
Rattlesden, Thomas, Abbot of Bury St Edmunds 116, 175

rebellions
  of 1264 see Guild of Youth, rebellion of (1264)
  of 1290 xvi, 84–5
  of 1305 xvi, 87
  of 1327 xvi, 87–92
  of 1381 see Peasants' Revolt
Rede, Suffolk 125
Redgrave, Suffolk 34, 116, 137, 142
Reeve, John, Abbot of Bury St Edmunds xvi, 15, 115, 116–32, 134, 140, 149, 151, 159, 170, 175
Revolution, French 148–9
Rhys ap Rhys, prince 86
Richard I, king xv, 54, 62, 66, 67
Richard II, king 99, 101
Riche, Richard, commissioner 130
Rickinghall, Suffolk 34
Rievaulx abbey 3
Ringstead, Thomas see Dennis, Thomas, prior
Risby, Suffolk 25, 125, 170
Robert of Bury St Edmunds ('Little St Robert') xv, 4, 59–60, 62, 120, 183
Rochester, Solomon of, judge 84
Roe, Alban, monk and martyr 144, 145
Roger, abbot of St Augustine's, Canterbury 79
Rome 1, 32, 39, 46, 47, 51, 61, 66, 67, 75, 76, 77, 79, 82, 91, 96–7, 101, 104, 105, 107, 109–10, 123, 145, 183
Rotunda of St Mary and St Edmund xv, xvi, 29–30, 46, 50, 70, 81, 131, 180, 181, 187
Rougham, Edward, sacrist and archdeacon of Bury St Edmunds 120–1, 141, 175
Rougham, Suffolk 34, 141
Rufus, Alan, count of Brittany 41, 154
ruins, Abbey xi, xiii, xiv, **xviii**, 1, 3, **4**, 5, 10, 12, 13, 15, 30, 31, **45**, 46, 51, 68, 86, 111, 131, **133**, 134, 151,

155, 157–8, 162–4, 166–8, 170–1, **172**, **178–9**, **184–5**
Rushbrook, Henry of, Abbot of Bury St Edmunds 75–6, 174, 187
Rushbrooke, Suffolk 136, 155
Russel, Robert, prior 76, 77, 81, 174

S
sacrist, office of 7, 15, 62, 83–4, 88, 91, 110, 135, 139–40, 159, 173–5
Salisbury, John, bishop of Sodor and Man 121
Samson of Tottington, Abbot of Bury St Edmunds xi, xv, 3, 7, 8, 10, 14, 50, 54, 56, 59, 60, 61–71, 74, 77, 83, 84, 86, 87, 90, 135, 146, 148, 166, 168, 170, 173, 177, 180, 181, 182, 187
Sancroft, William, archbishop of Canterbury 161
Sayer, Robert Gregory, monk 142
schism, papal 104
Scotland 52, 85–6
Seymour, Edward, duke of Somerset 137
sheriff, Abbot of Bury St Edmunds as 7, 31, 137
sheriff of Norfolk and Suffolk 91, 137
Shipdam, John, lawyer 97
Shirehouse Heath 139
Shottisham, John of, monk 85
shrine-keepers 8, 64
Sigebert, king of the East Angles 21, 22–4, 32
sign-language, monastic 103
Smart, William, alderman of Ipswich 128
Smith, Jankyn, burgess 110
Smith, John, alderman 118
Smith, Thomas, clothier 116
Smyth, John, commissioner xvi, 129
Somerset House 147
Song School see education
Southwold, Suffolk 38
Southwood, Suffolk 125
Spearhafoc, abbot of Abingdon 32

Spelman, Henry, antiquary 156–7, 159
Speyer cathedral 1
Stacy, John, lollard 120
Stamford, Lincs. 59
Stanton, Hervey de, judge 88
Stapleford Abbotts, Essex 67
Star Chamber, court of 117–19
Stephen, king 54
steward of the Liberty of St Edmund see St Edmund, Liberty of
Stoke-by-Nayland, Suffolk 25, 121
Stonham Aspal, Suffolk 129
Stowe, John, antiquary 57–8, 107
Stratford Langthorn, Essex 80
Sturgeon family 125
sub-prior, office of 7, 15, 87
Submission of the Clergy and Restraint of Appeals, Act for the 123
Sudbury, Simon of, archbishop of Canterbury 99
Sudbury, Suffolk 99, 121, 154
Sudbury, archdeacon of 140, 141
Supremacy, oath of xvi, 123, 127, 147
Sutton Hoo ship burial 30
Swaffham, John, sacrist 154, 175
Sweyn Forkbeard, king of Denmark xv, 9, 25, 27, 84, 129, 182

T
Talbot, prior 52, 69, 173
Taloun, John, moneyer 92
Taxster, John de, monk 59, 80
Tay Fen 16, 84
Taylor, Rowland, archdeacon of Bury St Edmunds 139–40, 141
Taynton, Oxon. 35, 37
Tenison, Thomas, archbishop of Canterbury 161
Tewkesbury abbey 3
Theodred, bishop of London xv, 19–20, 25
Thetford, Norf. 40
  battle of (869) 16, 18
Thingoe, hundred of 31,

124–5, 139, 165
Thorkil, earl 28
Thornham Parva, Suffolk 136
Thurketel 41
Thwaite, Suffolk 136
Timworth, John, Abbot of Bury St Edmunds 97–8, 99, 101, 175
Tostock, Suffolk
Tottington, Samson of *see* Samson of Tottington
Tottington, Thomas of, Abbot of Bury St Edmunds 87, 180
Toulouse 73, 130
Tours cathedral 51
Tours, council of 58
Tudor, Mary, queen of France xvi, 122–3, 131, 135, 140
Tunstall, Cuthbert, bishop of London 121

U
Ufi, Abbot of Bury St Edmunds 18, 27, 28, 31, 161, 173
Urban IV, pope 79
Urban VI, pope 97
Urban VIII, pope 147, 149
Ussher, James, archbishop of Armagh 156

V
vacancies, abbatial 7, 47, 54, 59, 60, 61, 77, 79, 81, 82–3, 101
Valence, William de 80
Valognes, Peter de 38
Vertue, George, engraver xvii, 161
Vezano, Geoffrey of, papal legate 83
St Victor, Hugh of, theologian 54

Vikings
see Danes
visitations xvi, 58, 66, 75, 103, 118, 127–8

W
Walgrave, Francis, monk 145
Walkelin, bishop of Winchester 41, 46
Walpole, Edmund of, Abbot of Bury St Edmunds 76–7, 174, 187
Walsingham, Thomas of, monk 71
Walsingham, shrine of Our Lady of 118
Warenne, John de 80
Warkton, Northants. 7, 41, 42
Warkton, Ralph, monk 136
Warwick, Nicholas of, sacrist 67, 174
Wastell, John, master mason 116, 117, 135
Webling, Archibald 170
Weever, John, antiquary 158–9
Weldon, Ralph Bene't, monk 130, 148
Wendover, Roger of, chronicler 71, 73
Wentworth, Jane, demoniac 117
West Stow, Suffolk 125
West Suffolk, county of 3, 31, 141
see also St Edmund, Liberty of
Westbrom, Robert, rebel 99
Westley, Suffolk 25, 91, 125
Westminster 47, 61, 71, 108, 123
abbey 48, 121, 122, 124, 130, 141, 142–3, 145, 146
Westhorpe, Suffolk 122

Whepstead, Suffolk 34, 125
Whittingham, Arthur, archaeologist 4, 11–12, 15, 45, 83, 170, 177
Whyting, Richard, abbot of Glastonbury 147
Wiardel, William, sacrist 54, 62, 173
William of Norwich 59
William I, king xv, 37, 38, 39–40, 41, 42, 45
William II Rufus, king 42, 46, 47
William and Mary, king and queen 161
Williams, John, commissioner xvi, 129
Winchester 33, 40
cathedral 1, 48, 51, 70
Windsor castle xv, 66
Wisbech, Cambs. 129
Wolsey, Thomas, cardinal xvi, 116, 118–19, 121–2
Wodecroft, John, painter 87, 181
Woodditton, Cambs. 136
Woolhampton, Berks. 149–50
Woolpit 61
shrine of Our Lady at 120
Worcestre, William 162
Wordwell, Suffolk 41
Worlingworth, Suffolk 34
Wrawe, John, rebel 99
Wyclif, John, theologian 98

Y
Yates, Richard, junior, antiquary 10, 14, 164, **165**
Yates, Richard, senior 164
Yates, William 1n., 164
York 59, 60, 90
York, Richard duke of xvi, 109, 118

The Norwich Historic Churches Trust, entrusted with the care of 18 of Norwich's redundant medieval churches, works not only to maintain them but to increase awareness of architectural, historical and other related aspects of our medieval ecclesiastical heritage. These two volumes draw on papers from its 2014 and 2015 conferences, supplemented with a series of contributions about the Trust itself. *Of Churches, Toothache and Sheep* focuses on historical issues; *Redundancy and Renewal* on the problems of the buildings today. Both take a readable and wide-ranging view, stretching well beyond Norwich itself. All profits from the sale of both books go to support the work of the NHCT.

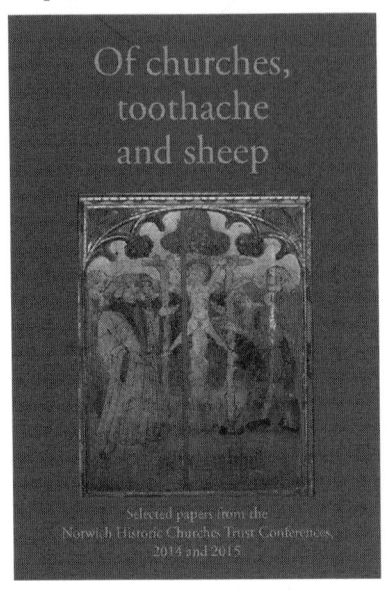

Contents:

Foreword *Brian Ayers;* Preface *Nicholas Groves;* Toothache, saints, and churches in medieval Norfolk, with particular reference to the City of Norwich *John Beal;* Theology to liturgy: the material culture of change in Norwich and Beyond, c.1450–1600 *Victor Morgan;* Norwich's Catholic chapels *Francis Young;* The sheep hath paid for all: church building and self-expression in the Late Middle Ages *Allan Barton;* Valuations of churches in medieval Norfolk *Elizabeth Gemmill;* The funeral of John Paston *Susan Curran*

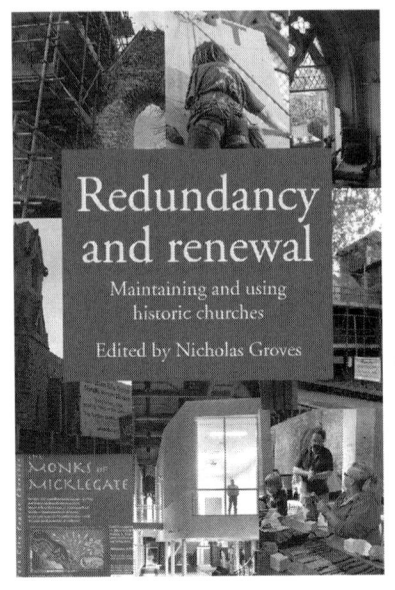

Contents:

Foreword *Nick Williams;* Preface *Nicholas Groves;* Historic churches: heritage and voluntary action *Robert Piggott;* A historical perspective on the reappropriation of urban closed churches for other purposes *Steven Saxby;* Working co-operatively with closed churches: the Holland Coastal Group *Stella Jackson;* 'With concern, but not without hope': an overview of the Norwich Historic Churches Trust *Nicholas Groves;* The Norwich Historic Churches Trust, returning churches to the community *Rory Quinn;* Heavenly Gardens *George Ishmael;* Confessions of a former tenant *Susan Curran;* New uses for religious heritage at the Churches Conservation Trust *Peter Aiers, Matthew McKeague and Edward Walkington*

For full details of these and other Lasse Press titles, visit

www.lassepress.com